Chest Pain

Guest Editors

GUY D. ESLICK, PhD
MICHAEL YELLAND, MBBS, PhD

MEDICAL CLINICS
OF NORTH AMERICA

www.medical.theclinics.com

March 2010 • Volume 94 • Number 2

SAUNDERS an imprint of ELSEVIER, Inc.

W.B. SAUNDERS COMPANY
A Division of Elsevier Inc.

1600 John F. Kennedy Boulevard ● Suite 1800 ● Philadelphia, Pennsylvania 19103-2899

http://www.theclinics.com

MEDICAL CLINICS OF NORTH AMERICA Volume 94, Number 2
March 2010 ISSN 0025-7125, ISBN-13: 978-1-4377-1835-5

Editor: Rachel Glover
Developmental Editor: Donald Mumford

Medical Clinics of North America (ISSN 0025-7125) is published bimonthly by Elsevier Inc., 360 Park Avenue South, New York, NY 10010-1710. Months of issue are January, March, May, July, September, and November. Periodicals postage paid at New York, NY, and additional mailing offices. Subscription prices are USD 204 per year for US individuals, USD 361 per year for US institutions, USD 105 per year for US students, USD 259 per year for Canadian individuals, USD 469 per year for Canadian institutions, USD 165 per year for Canadian students, USD 314 per year for international individuals, USD 469 per year for international institutions and USD 165 per year for international students. To receive student/resident rate, orders must be accompanied by name of affiliated institution, date of term, and the *signature* of program/residency coordinator on institution letterhead. Orders will be billed at individual rate until proof of status is received. Foreign air speed delivery is included in all *Clinics* subscription prices. All prices are subject to change without notice. **POSTMASTER:** Send address changes to *Medical Clinics of North America*, Elsevier Health Sciences Division, Subscription Customer Service, 3251 Riverport Lane, Maryland Heights, MO 63043. **Customer Service: Telephone: 1-800-654-2452** (U.S. and Canada); **1-314-447-8871** (outside U.S. and Canada). **Fax: 1-314-447-8029. E-mail: journalscustomerservice-usa@elsevier.com** (for print support); **journalsonlinesupport-usa@elsevier.com** (for online support).

Reprints. For copies of 100 or more of articles in this publication, please contact the Commercial Reprints Department, Elsevier Inc., 360 Park Avenue South, New York, NY 10010-1710. Tel.: 212-633-3812; Fax: 212-462-1935; E-mail: reprints@elsevier.com.

Medical Clinics of North America is also published in Spanish by McGraw-Hill Interamericana Editores S. A., P.O. Box 5-237, 06500 Mexico, D.F., Mexico.

Medical Clinics of North America is covered in *MEDLINE/PubMed (Index Medicus), Current Contents, ASCA, Excerpta Medica, Science Citation Index,* and *ISI/BIOMED.*

Printed in the United States of America.

GOAL STATEMENT

The goal of *Medical Clinics of North America* is to keep practicing physicians up to date with current clinical practice by providing timely articles reviewing the state of the art in patient care.

ACCREDITATION

The *Medical Clinics of North America* is planned and implemented in accordance with the Essential Areas and Policies of the Accreditation Council for Continuing Medical Education (ACCME) through the joint sponsorship of the University of Virginia School of Medicine and Elsevier. The University of Virginia School of Medicine is accredited by the ACCME to provide continuing medical education for physicians.

The University of Virginia School of Medicine designates this educational activity for a maximum of 15 *AMA PRA Category 1 Credits*™ for each issue, 90 credits per year. Physicians should only claim credit commensurate with the extent of their participation in the activity.

The American Medical Association has determined that physicians not licensed in the US who participate in this CME activity are eligible for a maximum of 15 *AMA PRA Category 1 Credits*™ for each issue, 90 credits per year.

Credit can be earned by reading the text material, taking the CME examination online at http://www.theclinics.com/home/cme, and completing the evaluation. After taking the test, you will be required to review any and all incorrect answers. Following completion of the test and evaluation, your credit will be awarded and you may print your certificate.

FACULTY DISCLOSURE/CONFLICT OF INTEREST

The University of Virginia School of Medicine, as an ACCME accredited provider, endorses and strives to comply with the Accreditation Council for Continuing Medical Education (ACCME) Standards of Commercial Support, Commonwealth of Virginia statutes, University of Virginia policies and procedures, and associated federal and private regulations and guidelines on the need for disclosure and monitoring of proprietary and financial interests that may affect the scientific integrity and balance of content delivered in continuing medical education activities under our auspices.

The University of Virginia School of Medicine requires that all CME activities accredited through this institution be developed independently and be scientifically rigorous, balanced and objective in the presentation/discussion of its content, theories and practices.

All authors/editors participating in an accredited CME activity are expected to disclose to the readers relevant financial relationships with commercial entities occurring within the past 12 months (such as grants or research support, employee, consultant, stock holder, member of speakers bureau, etc.). The University of Virginia School of Medicine will employ appropriate mechanisms to resolve potential conflicts of interest to maintain the standards of fair and balanced education to the reader. Questions about specific strategies can be directed to the Office of Continuing Medical Education, University of Virginia School of Medicine, Charlottesville, Virginia.

The faculty and staff of the University of Virginia Office of Continuing Medical Education have no financial affiliations to disclose.

The authors/editors listed below have identified no professional or financial affiliations for themselves or their spouse/partner:
Sami R. Achem, MD; Megha Agarwal, MD; Cristina Almansa, MD, PhD; Fraser J.H. Brims, MRCP, MD; William E. Cayley Jr, MD, MDiv; Henrik Wulff Christensen, DC, MD, PhD; Helen E. Davies, MRCP; Guy D. Eslick, PhD, MMedSc (Clin Epi), MMedStat (Guest Editor); Rachel Glover (Acquisitions Editor); Puja K. Mehta, MD; Jim Muir, MBBS, FACD, FACRRM (Hon); Amanke C. Oranu, MD; Simon F. Preuss, MD, PhD; Mette Jensen Stochkendahl, MSc; Jennifer Thull-Freedman, MD, MSc; Werner Vach, Dip Stats, PhD; Julia Vent, MD, PhD; Benjamin Wang, MD, FRCPC; Kamila S. White, PhD; Andrew Wolf, MD (Test Author); and Michael Yelland, MBBS, PhD, FRACGP, FAFMM, Grad Dip Musculoskeletal Med (Guest Editor).

The authors/editors listed below identified the following professional or financial affiliations for themselves or their spouse/partner:
Anthony F.T. Brown, MB, ChB, FRCP, FRCSEd, FACEM, FCEM received an once-off Honorarium from Elixir Health Care, Australia.
Louise Cullen, MBBS (Hons), FACEM is an industry funded research/investigator for Inverness Medical and Radiometer Pacific, and is on the Speakers' Bureau for Inverness Medical.
Y.C. Gary Lee, MBChB, FRACP, FCCP, PhD is a research/investigator for Rocket UK Ltd and is an industry funded research/investigator for Roche UK Ltd.
C. Noel Bairey Merz, MD is a consultant for Bristol-Myers Squibb, Curtis Green LLP, Cook Inc, Gilead Sciences and Axis Healthcare Comm LLC (Gilead), Navvis Healthcare (VHA), NHLBI, Pollock Communications, Practice Point Communications Inc, Society for Women's Health Research, Itamar Medical Inc, and Virginia Commonwealth University (McCue Prize); receives lecture honorarium from Brentwood Country Club, Mayo foundation for Medical Education, Medical Education Speakers Net, Rush-Copley Medical Center, SCS Healthcare (CV Therapeutics), St. John's Regional Medical Center, Oxnard, Tarzana Medical Center, University of Oklahoma Health, Washington University of St. Louis, West Hills Hospital, and Pri-Med-Scienta Healthcare Education; and owns stock in Medtronic and Johnson & Johnson.
Marc A. Rozner, PhD, MD is on the Speakers' Bureau for Baxter Anesthesia Pharmaceuticals.
Sunil K. Sahai, MD was on the Speakers' Bureau for Sanofi Aventis 2005-12/31/2009.
Martin Than, MBBS, FRCSEd(A&E), FACEM, FCEM is an industry funded research/investigator for Inverness Medical and Abbott, and is on the Speakers' Bureau for Inverness Medical.
Michael F. Vaezi, MD, PhD, MSc (Epi) has a research grant with Takeda.
Ali Zalpour, PharmD, BCPS is on the Speakers' Bureau for Easi Pharmaceuticals.

Disclosure of Discussion of Non-FDA Approved Uses for Pharmaceutical Products and/or Medical Devices.

The University of Virginia School of Medicine, as an ACCME provider, requires that all faculty presenters identify and disclose any off-label uses for pharmaceutical and medical device products. The University of Virginia School of Medicine recommends that each physician fully review all the available data on new products or procedures prior to clinical use.

TO ENROLL

To enroll in the Medical Clinics of North America Continuing Medical Education program, call customer service at 1-800-654-2452 or visit us online at http://www.theclinics.com/home/cme. The CME program is available to subscribers for an additional fee of USD 205.

RELATED INTEREST

Clinics in Chest Medicine, March 2010 (Volume 31, Issue 1)
Interventional Pulmonology
Atul C. Mehta, MD, *Guest Editor*

THE CLINICS ARE NOW AVAILABLE ONLINE!

Access your subscription at:
www.theclinics.com

Contributors

GUEST EDITORS

GUY D. ESLICK, PhD, MMedSc (Clin Epi), MMedStat
Program in Molecular and Genetic Epidemiology, Harvard School of Public Health, Boston, Massachusetts; School of Public Health; Department of Gastroenterology, Nepean Clinical School, The University of Sydney, Sydney, New South Wales, Australia

MICHAEL YELLAND, MBBS, PhD, FRACGP, FAFMM, Grad Dip Musculoskeletal Med
Associate Professor in Primary Health Care, School of Medicine, Logan Campus, Griffith University, Meadowbrook, Queensland, Australia

AUTHORS

SAMI R. ACHEM, MD, FACP, FACG, AGAF
Professor of Medicine, Division of Gastroenterology and Hepatology, Mayo Clinic Florida, Jacksonville, Florida

MEGHA AGARWAL, MD
Women's Heart Center, Heart Institute, Cedars-Sinai Medical Center, Los Angeles, California

CRISTINA ALMANSA, MD, PhD
Visiting Scientist, Division of Gastroenterology and Hepatology, Mayo Clinic Florida, Jacksonville, Florida

FRASER J.H. BRIMS, MRCP, MD
Respiratory Department, Portsmouth Hospitals NHS Trust, Portsmouth, United Kingdom; Respiratory Department, Sir Charles Gairdner Hospital, Perth, Australia

ANTHONY F.T. BROWN, MB, ChB, FRCP, FRCSEd, FACEM, FCEM
Professor of Emergency Medicine, School of Medicine, University of Queensland, Mayne Medical School; Senior Staff Specialist, Department of Emergency Medicine, Royal Brisbane and Women's Hospital, Herston, Brisbane, Queensland, Australia

WILLIAM E. CAYLEY Jr, MD, MDiv
Associate Professor, Department of Family Medicine, University of Wisconsin School of Medicine and Public Health, UW Health Eau Claire Family Medicine Residency, Eau Claire, Wisconsin

HENRIK WULFF CHRISTENSEN, DC, MD, PhD
Director, Research Department, Nordic Institute of Chiropractic and Clinical Biomechanics, Forskerparken, Odense, Denmark

LOUISE CULLEN, MBBS (Hons), FACEM
Senior Lecturer, School of Medicine, University of Queensland, Mayne Medical School; Staff Specialist, Department of Emergency Medicine, Royal Brisbane and Women's Hospital, Herston, Brisbane; PhD candidate, School of Public Health, Queensland University of Technology, Brisbane, Queensland, Australia

HELEN E. DAVIES, MRCP
Oxford Centre for Respiratory Medicine, Churchill Hospital, Oxford, United Kingdom

GUY D. ESLICK, PhD, MMedSc (Clin Epi), MMedStat
Program in Molecular and Genetic Epidemiology, Harvard School of Public Health, Boston, Massachusetts; School of Public Health; Department of Gastroenterology, Nepean Clinical School, The University of Sydney, Sydney, New South Wales, Australia

Y.C. GARY LEE, MBChB, FRACP, FCCP, PhD
Professor, Respiratory Department, Sir Charles Gairdner Hospital; School of Medicine & Pharmacology and Lung Institute of Western Australia, University of Western Australia, Perth, Australia

PUJA K. MEHTA, MD
Women's Heart Center, Heart Institute, Cedars-Sinai Medical Center, Los Angeles, California

C. NOEL BAIREY MERZ, MD, FACC
Women's Heart Center, Heart Institute, Cedars-Sinai Medical Center, Los Angeles, California

JIM MUIR, MBBS, FACD, FACRRM(Hon)
Director, Department of Dermatology, Mater Misericordiae Hospital, South Brisbane, Queensland, Australia

AMANKE C. ORANU, MD
Division of Gastroenterology, Hepatology and Nutrition, Center for Swallowing and Esophageal Disorders, Vanderbilt University Medical Center, Nashville, Tennessee

SIMON F. PREUSS, MD, PhD
Department of Otorhinolaryngology, Head and Neck Surgery, University of Hospital Cologne, Cologne, Germany

MARC A. ROZNER, MD, PhD
Professor of Anesthesiology and Perioperative Medicine, Professor of Cardiology, The University of Texas M.D. Anderson Cancer Center; Adjunct Professor of Integrative Biology and Pharmacology, The University of Texas Health Science Center at Houston, Houston, Texas

SUNIL K. SAHAI, MD
Associate Professor of Medicine, Department of General Internal Medicine, Ambulatory Treatment, and Emergency Care; Medical Director, Internal Medicine Perioperative Assessment Center, The University of Texas M.D. Anderson Cancer Center, Houston, Texas

METTE JENSEN STOCHKENDAHL, MSc
Researcher, Institute of Sports Science and Clinical Biomechanics, University of Southern Denmark; Research Department, Nordic Institute of Chiropractic and Clinical Biomechanics, Forskerparken, Odense, Denmark

MARTIN THAN, MBBS, FRCSEd(A&E), FACEM, FCEM
Senior Clinical Lecturer, Christchurch School of Medicine, University of Otago; Consultant in Emergency Medicine, Department of Emergency Medicine, Christchurch Hospital, Christchurch, New Zealand

JENNIFER THULL-FREEDMAN, MD, MSc
Assistant Professor, Department of Paediatrics, Division of Paediatric Emergency Medicine, University of Toronto; Staff Physician, The Hospital for Sick Children, Toronto, Ontario, Canada

WERNER VACH, DIP STATS, PhD
Professor of Clinical Epidemiology, Institute of Medical Biometry and Medical Informatics, University Medical Center Freiburg, Freiburg, Germany

MICHAEL F. VAEZI, MD, PhD, MSc (Epi)
Division of Gastroenterology, Hepatology and Nutrition, Center for Swallowing and Esophageal Disorders, Vanderbilt University Medical Center, Nashville, Tennessee

JULIA VENT, MD, PhD
Department of Otorhinolaryngology, Head and Neck Surgery, University of Hospital Cologne, Cologne, Germany

BENJAMIN WANG, MD, FRCPC
Division of Rheumatology, Mayo Clinic Florida, Jacksonville, Florida

KAMILA S. WHITE, PhD
Assistant Professor of Psychology, Department of Psychology, University of Missouri-St. Louis, St. Louis, Missouri

MICHAEL YELLAND, MBBS, PhD, FRACGP, FAFMM, Grad Dip Musculoskeletal Med
Associate Professor in Primary Health Care, School of Medicine, Logan Campus, Griffith University, Meadowbrook, Queensland, Australia

ALI ZALPOUR, PharmD, BCPS
Clinical Pharmacist, Department of General Internal Medicine, Ambulatory Treatment, and Emergency Care, The University of Texas M.D. Anderson Cancer Center, Houston, Texas

Contents

Anginal chest pain is one of the most common complaints in the outpatient setting. While much of the focus has been on identifying obstructive atherosclerotic coronary artery disease (CAD) as the cause of anginal chest pain, it is clear that microvascular coronary dysfunction (MCD) can also cause anginal chest pain as a manifestation of ischemic heart disease, and carries an increased cardiovascular risk. Epicardial coronary vasospasm, aortic stenosis, left ventricular hypertrophy, congenital coronary anomalies, mitral valve prolapse, and abnormal cardiac nociception can also present as angina of cardiac origin. For nonacute coronary syndrome (ACS) stable chest pain, exercise treadmill testing (ETT) remains the primary tool for diagnosis of ischemia and cardiac risk stratification; however, in certain subsets of patients, such as women, ETT has a lower sensitivity and specificity for identifying obstructive CAD. When combined with an imaging modality, such as nuclear perfusion or echocardiography testing, the sensitivity and specificity of stress testing for detection of obstructive CAD improves significantly. Advancements in stress cardiac magnetic resonance imaging enables detection of perfusion abnormalities in a specific coronary artery territory, as well as subendocardial ischemia associated with MCD. Coronary computed tomography angiography enables visual assessment of obstructive CAD, albeit with a higher radiation dose. Invasive coronary angiography remains the gold standard for diagnosis and treatment of obstructive lesions that cause medically refractory stable angina. Furthermore, in patients with normal coronary angiograms, the addition of coronary reactivity testing can help diagnose endothelial-dependent and -independent microvascular dysfunction. Lifestyle modification and pharmacologic intervention remains the cornerstone of therapy to reduce morbidity and mortality in patients with stable angina. This review focuses on the pathophysiology, diagnosis, and treatment of stable, non-ACS anginal chest pain.

Chest pain from respiratory causes is a common complaint and may indicate the presence of a serious or even life-threatening pathologic condition. Most chest pains are the result of irritation or inflammation of the parietal pleura, as the visceral pleura is insensate, although pain may arise from direct malignant invasion or trauma to the chest wall. Rapid recognition with appropriate understanding of the anatomy and physiology of chest pain from respiratory causes is vital to ensure timely and appropriate therapy.

Noncardiac chest pain (NCCP) is not only a difficult disorder to define but is also complex in characterization and treatment. Patients with NCCP are a challenge to primary care and subspecialty services such as cardiology and gastroenterology. NCCP is often a heterogeneous disorder with many potential causes including gastroenterologic diagnoses. This article presents the current evidence for gastroesophageal reflux disease as a cause of NCCP and highlights the best currently available tests for this group of patients.

Dysphagia is an important alarm symptom, commonly associated with chest pain; it is often associated with reflux disease, xerostomia, or tumors of the head and neck. However, simple diagnoses such as aspiration of a foreign body can be overseen and may result in major complications, such as perforation and mediastinitis. It is thus of crucial importance that a thorough gastrointestinal, cardiac, and radiologic examination precede a rigid esophagoscopy by an otolaryngologist. In this article the differential diagnoses of dysphagia are discussed, and the otolaryngologist's approach to diagnosis and therapy are explained.

The musculoskeletal system is a recognized source of chest pain. However, despite the apparently benign origin, patients with musculoskeletal chest pain remain under-diagnosed, untreated, and potentially continuously disabled in terms of anxiety, depression, and activities of daily living. Several overlapping conditions and syndromes of focal disorders, including Tietze syndrome, costochondritis, chest wall syndrome, muscle tenderness, slipping rib, cervical angina, and segmental dysfunction of the cervical and thoracic spine, have been reported to cause pain. For most of these syndromes, evidence arises mainly from case stories and empiric knowledge. For segmental dysfunction, clinical features of musculoskeletal chest pain have been characterized in a few clinical trials. This article summarizes the most commonly encountered syndromes of focal musculoskeletal disorders in clinical practice.

Fibromyalgia (FM) remains an enigmatic and challenging clinical entity to manage, given its far-reaching spectrum of symptoms, chronicity, associated psychopathology, and lack of clinically available diagnostic tests. However, recent insights into the pathophysiology of FM offer hope that this condition, as with all members of the central sensitization syndromes, can be more readily diagnosed, measured, and treated. This paper presents the epidemiology features and pathogenesis of FM in the context of evaluating NCCP as a prototype among central pain sensitization syndromes. Evidence for the multimodality approach to treatment of this condition is also presented.

Chest pain prompts an estimated 4.6 million people in the United States to seek emergency medical care each year. Chest pain is common in patients with coronary artery disease (CAD). Chest pain is also common in patients without CAD or other cardiac causes for their chest pain, sometimes called non-cardiac chest pain. Psychological assessment and treatment may clinically aid patients with chest pain in ways that may influence disease onset, maintenance, and progression and may improve quality of life. This article highlights factors important for psychological assessment and treatment of patients with chest pain.

There are several skin and breast lesions that can cause pain or tenderness. In most cases the presence of a skin lesion, if not its definitive diagnosis, will be clinically evident. In most instances treatment of these painful skin lesions is by simple excision, which will also provide histologic confirmation of the diagnosis. It would be rare for a cutaneous cause of skin pain to be mistaken for another cause. The prodromal pain of herpes zoster is most likely to cause diagnostic confusion. The painful skin lesions are usually identified by the patient as being the source of their discomfort. The specific diagnosis may not be apparent without submission of lesional tissue for histology. Chest pain is an uncommon presenting symptom of benign and malignant breast lesions. Breast examination and investigation may be appropriate when other causes of chest pain are not evident.

Chest pain is common in children seen in emergency departments, ambulatory clinics, and cardiology clinics. Although most children have a benign cause of their pain, some have serious and life-threatening conditions. The symptom must be carefully evaluated before reassurance and supportive care are offered. Because serious causes of chest pain are uncommon and not many prospective studies are available, it is difficult to develop evidence-based guidelines for evaluation. The clinician evaluating a child with chest pain should keep in mind the broad differential diagnosis and pursue further investigation when the history and physical examination suggest the possibility of serious causes.

Preface

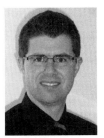
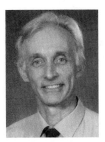

Guy D. Eslick, PhD, MMedSc (Clin Epi), MMedStat

Michael Yelland, MBBS, PhD, FRACGP, FAFMM, Grad Dip Musculoskeletal Med

Guest Editors

It is with great excitement that we welcome you to this issue of *Medical Clinics of North America*, which is devoted to chest pain, one of the most common reasons for individuals presenting to an Emergency Department. Chest pain is a most challenging and complex symptom. Most individuals who present with chest pain are given no diagnosis or prognosis, which makes many individuals concerned that they may have a potentially fatal form of chest pain. The number of chest pain presentations is increasing not only in Western countries but also in Asia and other developing countries. Chest pain can be chronic and debilitating, and other forms of chest pain can be acutely fatal. For physicians, the most challenging aspect of chest pain is differentiating between cardiac and noncardiac chest pain in a timely and efficient manner. Providing a diagnosis for all patients will lead to a reduced level of anxiety and improved quality of life; a greater impetus on patient education and understanding will result in a decrease in repeat presentations and reduced work load for hospital physicians. In this issue of *Medical Clinics of North America* we have selected cutting-edge topics that we hope will be an asset to physicians working in emergency departments, internal medicine, primary care, and others. The topics selected are as broad as the potential number of chest pain conditions encountered by physicians in everyday practice.

In preparing this issue we selected the leading authorities in different areas of medicine, including cardiology, gastroenterology, otolaryngology, respiratory medicine, rheumatology, chiropractic, psychological medicine, dermatology, pediatrics, emergency medicine, and primary care. The authors have provided us with a unique collection of articles dedicated to understanding and improving the diagnosis and treatment of chest pain, and it was truly a pleasure reading and editing this outstanding collection of articles.

We would like to thank all of the authors who contributed their valuable time and expertise to this issue. We would also like to thank the editor of *Medical Clinics of North America*, Rachel Glover, for her patience and understanding when things were slow and valuable assistance in getting this important issue published. Guy Eslick would

Med Clin N Am 94 (2010) xiii–xiv
doi:10.1016/j.mcna.2010.01.013
0025-7125/10/$ – see front matter © 2010 Elsevier Inc. All rights reserved.

medical.theclinics.com

like to thank Enid, Marielle, and the littlest one, Guillaume, for their support and love, and would like to dedicate this work to Leslie Vincent Stapleton, his Grandfather, who died of a heart attack after sheep shearing on March 17, 1965, aged 59 years. Michael Yelland would like to thank his wife, Carmel Simpson, for her love and support during the production of this issue, and to dedicate this work to his father, John Yelland, who died suddenly of a heart attack in 2000.

We hope this timely collection of outstanding articles devoted to chest pain will provide physicians with useful and practical information that will assist them in diagnosing and treating patients with chest pain with care and reassurance.

Guy D. Eslick, PhD, MMedSc (Clin Epi), MMedStat
Program in Molecular and Genetic Epidemiology
Harvard School of Public Health
677 Huntington Avenue
Building 2, 2nd Floor, Room 209
Boston, MA 02115, USA

Michael Yelland, MBBS, PhD, FRACGP, FAFMM, Grad Dip Musculoskeletal Med
School of Medicine, Logan Campus
Griffith University
Meadowbrook, Logan, Queensland, Australia

E-mail addresses:
geslick@hsph.harvard.edu (G.D. Eslick)
m.yelland@griffith.edu.au (M. Yelland)

Nonacute Coronary Syndrome Anginal Chest Pain

Megha Agarwal, MD, Puja K. Mehta, MD,
C. Noel Bairey Merz, MD*

KEYWORDS

- Chronic stable angina • Chest pain • Stress testing
- Atherosclerosis • Microvascular angina

Anginal chest pain is one of the most common complaint encountered by family physicians, internists, and emergency room physicians. Patients with escalating chest pain symptoms, electrocardiographic (ECG) abnormalities consistent with acute myocardial ischemia or infarction, or hemodynamic instability suggestive of an acute coronary syndrome (ACS), which includes unstable angina (UA), ST-elevation myocardial infarction (STEMI), and non–ST-elevation myocardial infarction (NSTEMI), should be triaged to the emergency department. Non-ACS anginal chest pain, termed chronic stable angina (CSA), can also have devastating consequences; therefore, a considerable amount of time and resources is appropriately spent in risk stratifying the patient who complains of chest pain in an office-based setting. The challenge for the clinician is to determine cardiac from noncardiac chest pain, and use a systematic approach for testing and therapy based on patient risk factors and characteristics. This review focuses on our current understanding of non-ACS anginal chest pain, its pathophysiology, diagnostic modalities, and treatment.

PATHOPHYSIOLOGY

The acute reduction in coronary blood flow (CBF) leads to a decline in oxygen supply, resulting in development of an ACS. Similarly, a chronic limited ability to increase

There are no relevant conflicts of interest of any of the authors to be disclosed.

This work was supported by contracts from the National Heart, Lung and Blood Institutes, nos. N01-HV-68161, N01-HV-68162, N01-HV-68163, N01-HV-68164, a GCRC grant MO1-RR00425 from the National Center for Research Resources, and grants from the Gustavus and Louis Pfeiffer Research Foundation, Denville, NJ, the Women's Guild of Cedars-Sinai Medical Center, Los Angeles, CA, the Edythe L. Broad Women's Heart Research Fellowship, Cedars-Sinai Medical Center, Los Angeles, CA, and the Barbra Streisand Women's Cardiovascular Research and Education Program, Cedars-Sinai Medical Center, Los Angeles, CA, USA.

Women's Heart Center, Heart Institute, Cedars-Sinai Medical Center, 444 South San Vicente Boulevard, Suite 600, Los Angeles, CA 90048, USA

* Corresponding author.

E-mail address: merz@cshs.org

oxygen supply to the myocardium in the setting of increased oxygen demand results in CSA.[1] Because myocytes already extract about 75% of the oxygen in coronary blood at rest, a higher demand is primarily met by increasing CBF.[2,3] Myocardial ischemia results from hypoxia, which disrupts oxidative metabolic pathways; cellular anaerobic pathways are activated and mediators such as lactate are produced, which results in the sensation of pain.[4]

Coronary Atherosclerosis and Obstructive Coronary Artery Disease

In the largest diameter epicardial coronary vessels, CBF is primarily limited due to obstructive atherosclerotic coronary artery disease (CAD). Originally thought to be dominantly a lipid storage disease, our current understanding of the pathogenesis of atherosclerosis implicates endothelial injury and inflammation.[5–9] Inflammation-induced atherosclerosis does not occur linearly.[10] Instead, bursts of atherosclerotic plaque progression occur and are accompanied by physical disruption to endothelial cells, hemorrhage into the plaque, clot formation, and vascular remodeling. Studies of vessels at autopsy show that as the number of atheromatous plaques increases, deposition occurs principally within the vascular wall, with compensatory enlargement of the external vessel.[11] This process permits maintenance of the lumen size. Once this compensatory mechanism is exhausted, the plaque begins to bulge into the lumen, causing obstruction to CBF during periods of increased oxygen demand.[1,6,11] As a result, atherosclerosis produces symptomatic chest pain relatively later in its course of development.

While elevated low-density lipoprotein (LDL) cholesterol still remains a major contributor to atherosclerosis and adverse ischemic heart disease (IHD) events, effective therapies that target LDL reduce coronary events by only 33% over a 5-year treatment period.[6] This observation has led to the conclusion that additional chemical and mechanical insults also trigger endothelial injury, including altered sheer stress, high oxidative stress, smoking, and insulin resistance.[8,9]

Microvascular Coronary Dysfunction

Myocardial ischemia can produce anginal chest pain without angiographically obstructive CAD, often due to microvascular coronary dysfunction (MCD). A relatively common occurrence of MCD appears to be in women who present with evidence of myocardial ischemia, identified by a myocardial infarction (MI) or abnormal stress testing in the absence of obstructive CAD. Autopsy reports in patients with normal angiograms and angina have revealed myointimal proliferation, endothelial degeneration, and lipid deposits in the microvasculature.[12] Multiple angiographic studies have demonstrated abnormal endothelium-dependent function in subjects with angina, evidence of ischemia, and no obstructive CAD.[13–15] Patients with angina and MCD have elevated levels of serum inflammatory markers, such as C-reactive protein (CRP), suggesting an underlying inflammatory process as well.[16] There is a significant peri- and postmenopausal female predominance in this condition, leading to a suspected pathogenic role of estrogen deficiency[17]; however, this remains controversial.

Coronary Artery Spasm

Additional causes of anginal chest pain to consider include coronary artery vasospasm (CAS),[18] also known as Prinzmetal angina,[19–21] which involves epicardial coronary vasoconstriction secondary to smooth muscle dysregulation, and may lead to transient reduction in myocardial oxygen supply. Again, inflammation is thought to initiate damage as patients with CAS tend to have higher levels of circulating leukocytes, CRP, and interleukin-6 (IL-6) compared with control populations.[22,23]

Inflammatory mediators promote smooth muscle cell (SMC) migration into the intima. Endothelial damage exposes SMC to agents that cause vasoconstriction.[24] Of note, intimal thickening in CAS patients is not a localized phenomenon, as intravascular ultrasound images and angiography have shown diffuse intimal thickening in patients with spasm.[25]

Aortic Stenosis and Left Ventricular Hypertrophy

Aortic stenosis (AS) can indirectly affect CBF in normal arteries and can produce CSA in 30% to 40% of patients.[25,26] Physiologic hypertrophy of cardiac myocytes occurs to generate enough force to maintain cardiac output against the restricted valvular diameter.[26,27] Because patients may develop severe AS and not manifest symptoms, it is difficult to associate a degree of hypertrophy to development of anginal chest pain. Pressure overload resulting in compensatory left ventricular hypertrophy (LVH) results in impaired diastolic relaxation, increased end-diastolic pressure, and reduced gradient driven CBF, especially to the subendocardium.[28] CBF is further compromised due to tachycardia-induced decreased diastolic filling times and decreased capillary density in hypertrophied myocardium.[29,30] Impaired flow leads to ischemia, necrosis, and fibrosis, primarily in the subendocardial layer.[27] Weidemann and colleagues[31] reported severe myocardial fibrosis in this layer and observed an association with reduced stroke volume in these patients, which further exacerbates reductions in CBF.

Congenital Coronary Anomalies

Congenital coronary anomalies such as precapillary fistulas, myocardial bridging, whereby coronary arteries are embedded in contractile myocardial tissue, and most commonly, aberrant origins of coronary vessels (eg, ectopic origin of the right coronary artery, or the left coronary artery originating from the right coronary ostia and vice versa) can lead to angina.[32] Often not discovered well into adulthood, it has been speculated that coronary anomalies produce symptoms by local compression and cessation of distal flow or even CAS.[33,34] Chest pain may occur due to left-to-right shunting or a coronary steal phenomenon, which supplies the myocardium with poorly oxygenated blood at low perfusion pressures.[34] Presentation can range from reproducible typical angina, sudden death, cardiomyopathy, or lethal arrhthymias.[32]

Mitral Valve Prolapse

Mitral valve prolapse (MVP) has a population incidence of 1%, with 11% to 15% of those patients exhibiting symptoms of chest pain and dyspnea.[35] The pathophysiologic mechanisms behind chest pain in MVP have proven to be elusive. Vavuranakis and colleagues[36] conducted left ventricular hemodynamic studies in patients with MVP and control subjects, and found few differences between the 2 groups. One study compared panic disorders to MVP and found many similarities in the nature and frequency of the pain, which suggests that a component of the pain may be related to panic disorders.[37] MVP is currently not considered a diagnostic etiology for anginal chest pain.

Abnormal Cardiac Nociception

Patients can have a heightened perception of cardiac pain due to abnormalities in cardiac neural nociception pathways. This situation has been documented when anginal chest pain was reproduced during right heart stimulation with intracardiac infusion of saline.[38–40] In one study, the perception of pain occurred in the absence of ECG changes or evidence of left ventricular dysfunction, suggesting a nonischemic origin of pain.[40] Other studies even suggest altered central nervous system processing in these patients.[41,42] Because the atria and ventricles have dense sensory innervations, heightened sensitivity of chemical and mechanical receptors may be leading to the false sensation of ischemia.[40] This abnormality in cardiac nociception may require medications to treat neuropathic pain (such as imipramine).

DIAGNOSIS

Diagnosis of cardiac chest pain relies on history and physical, patient characteristics, and identification of coronary heart disease (CHD) risk factors.[43] Using age, sex, and characteristics of pain, the pretest probability of having obstructive CAD can be determined (**Table 1**).[43] If there is a low pretest probability of having CAD (<10%), further workup should focus on noncoronary causes of pain. The intermediate-risk group benefits the most from noninvasive testing, while further workup in high-probability patients should place more focus on prognostication instead of diagnosis, because CAD is likely based on history and risk factors (**Fig. 1**).[43,44] High-risk patients benefit more from coronary angiography rather than noninvasive testing first.[43,45–49] However, it should be noted that regardless of the patient's pretest probability of CAD, further testing is not recommended if life expectancy is limited.[48]

Electrocardiogram

The electrocardiogram (ECG) remains the most convenient, albeit a relatively insensitive method of diagnosing myocardial ischemia. An ECG is most useful when compared with a prior ECG when the patient was asymptomatic. A resting ECG may be normal in 50% of patients with CSA[50]; however, certain ECG patterns are suggestive of ischemia or an increased likelihood of morbidity and mortality from IHD. In both men and women, LVH as determined by ECG is associated with the development of CHD,[51,52] and serves as a strong, independent prognostic marker in patients with angina.[52] In a 30-year follow-up of the Framingham study, Kannel and colleagues[53] also found that nonspecific ST-T wave abnormalities were associated with a twofold increase in the risk for IHD morbidity and mortality in both men and women.

DeBacquer and colleagues[54] further separated ECG findings into major and minor ECG criteria. These investigators found that severe or moderate ST depression,

Table 1						
Pretest likelihood of obstructive CAD in symptomatic patients according to age and sex						
	Nonanginal Chest Pain		Atypical Angina		Typical Angina	
Age	Men	Women	Men	Women	Men	Women
y			%			
30–39	4	2	34	12	76	26
40–49	13	3	51	22	87	53
50–59	20	7	65	31	93	73
60–69	27	14	72	51	94	86

Each value represents the percentage of patients with obstructive coronary artery disease on catheterization.

Data from Snow V, Barry P, Fihn SD, et al. Evaluation of primary care patients with chronic stable angina: guidelines from the American College of Physicians. Ann Intern Med 2004;141(1):57–64.

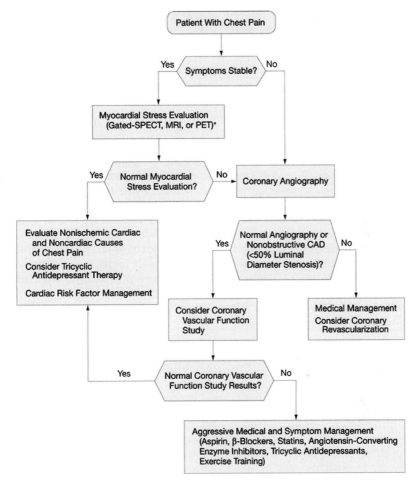

Fig. 1. Practical algorithm for management of patients with anginal chest pain symptoms and no obstructive coronary artery disease. MRI, magnetic resonance imaging; PET, positron emission tomography; CAD, coronary artery disease. Vascular function studies include coronary flow reserve and coronary acetylcholine testing. (*From* Bugiardini R, Bairey Merz CN. Angina with "normal" coronary arteries: a changing philosophy. JAMA 2005;293(4): 477–84; with permission.)

deep or moderate T-wave inversions, complete or second-degree atrioventricular (AV) block, complete right and left bundle branch block (RBBB and LBBB), frequent premature beats, and atrial fibrillation and flutter on ECG were highly predictive of all-cause mortality. ST-T wave changes are nonspecific, but in the setting of anginal chest pain may indicate ischemia. In addition, if ST-T wave changes occur at rest, this suggests the presence of significant obstructive CAD or an ACS.[48] Similarly, conduction defects are nonspecific, but may indicate multivessel disease.

Stress Testing

Stress testing is most often used to diagnose ischemia and to detect the amount of myocardium at risk. The main contraindications to stress testing include acute MI within 2 days of stress testing, symptomatic cardiac arrhythmia, severe AS, and decompensated heart failure.[47] Without contraindications the choice of stress test is dictated by prior cardiac history, baseline ECG, ability to exercise, as well as local expertise and availability.

Exercise Treadmill Testing

Exercise treadmill testing (ETT) is the recommended initial noninvasive test for risk stratification and diagnosis of CAD in intermediate probability patients who are able to exercise and have no abnormalities on resting ECG.[47] ETT is widely available at a relatively low cost,[55] and is useful because of its convenience and relative accuracy. The presence of LBBB, LVH, paced rhythm, intraventricular conduction delay, digoxin use, and Wolf-Parkinson-White syndrome on ECG[47,49] render an ETT nondiagnostic for ischemia detection. A cardiac imaging study typically is added to the ETT in these patients to enhance diagnostic sensitivity and specificity for detection of obstructive CAD.

ETT alone has a moderate sensitivity and specificity for obstructive CAD. A normal test may not exclude ischemia,[48,56] particularly in low-risk populations such as women.[47] Sex-related hormonal and anatomic differences between men and women may contribute to this difference, as well as the presence of MCD, which can cause ischemia in the absence of obstructive CAD.[55,57] Even after using a modified ETT protocol to account for some of the gender differences, the test remains of moderate diagnostic value in this subgroup.[57] Therefore, intermediate-risk female patients may be better suited to receive an imaging study.[55,56]

Stress Imaging

When imaging is added to ETT, via myocardial perfusion studies (MPS) or stress echocardiogram (SE), sensitivity is improved.[49] Imaging is preferred in patients with a history of prior revascularization as this allows localization of the myocardial ischemia.[47] Both imaging studies are superior to ETT because of their ability to quantify and localize ischemia, and to offer diagnostic data in patients with resting ECG abnormalities and in patients who cannot exercise. The 2 imaging modalities are comparable, and usage is primarily dependent on availability and local expertise; however, imaging studies are more expensive than ETT and less readily available.[49]

Stress echocardiography

SE remains a widely used method to determine left ventricular wall motion and valvular abnormalities. The addition of advanced echocardiographic techniques such as tissue Doppler and strain imaging allows for assessment of diastolic function, but is limited by patient characteristics (obesity, emphysema) that limit image quality. This limitation occurs in 5% to 10% of patients,[49] and is often technician dependent. SE has a higher specificity but is less sensitive than MPS for detecting ischemia.[49]

Stress myocardial perfusion study

A stress MPS with nuclear imaging identifies focal regions of hypoperfusion in the myocardium. MPS is especially preferred in women, obese patients, and patients with LBBB. However, MPS does expose patients to a moderate amount of ionizing radiation.[47,49,56]

Modalities of Stress

Both SE and MPS can be used with exercise or pharmacologic agents as a cardiac stressor, and both methods are equally accurate and safe in the diagnosis of ischemia.[58] If a patient is able to reach 85% to 90% of his or her predicted maximal heart rate with exercise, this form of stress is preferred as it provides information regarding the patient's functional capacity. If the patient is unable to exercise, a pharmacologic agent is preferred. Two main categories of pharmacologic stress are used: coronary vasodilators (adenosine and dipyridamole) and positive inotropic agents (dobutamine). Vasodilators dilate coronary arteries directly to increase flow. Inotropic agents indirectly increase coronary flow by increasing myocardial work load and oxygen requirements, mimicking the effects of physical exercise.

Coronary vasodilators

Pharmacologic vasodilators provide the largest increase in CBF.[59] With adenosine, this effect is short lived. Dipyridamole inhibits adenosine metabolism, therefore the vasodilatory effect lasts longer. Adenosine can cause AV block, which is rare with dipyridamole because inhibition of adenosine metabolism does not produce a sufficient enough concentration to induce AV block. Moreover, adenosine is known to induce bronchospasm in asthmatics. Dipyridamole, instead, is safe in patients with reactive airways producing no evidence of wheezing.[47,49,58]

Positive inotropic agents

Dobutamine is the preferred positive inotropic agent for patients who have had recent respiratory failure or bronchospasm.[47,49,58] This agent accelerates conduction through the sinoatrial (SA) and AV nodes[58] and is, therefore, contraindicated in patients with supraventricular and ventricular tachycardias.[47] Further, dobutamine promotes myocardial ectopy and is unsafe in acute post-MI patients.[60,61]

Advanced Cardiac Imaging

Advanced cardiac imaging allows assessment not only of obstructive and nonobstructive CAD but also of plaque composition, subendocardial myocardial perfusion, coronary flow reserve, myocardial metabolism, and left ventricular function. Cardiac magnetic resonance imaging (CMRI), positron emission tomography (PET), and coronary computed tomography angiography (CCTA), have transformed clinical cardiology. Even single photon emission computed tomography (SPECT) has evolved with improved resolution cameras and more sensitive tracers. The clinician's challenge is determining which test is appropriate for an individual patient and whether advanced imaging adds further to risk stratify the patient.

Cardiac magnetic resonance imaging

Stress CMRI is done with a vasodilatory pharmacologic agent (usually adenosine), and provides comprehensive assessment of myocardial function, perfusion, and structural details. In addition to very high spatial and temporal resolution images, CMRI can detect and quantify areas of necrosis and scar tissue, quantify perfusion deficits at the level of the subendocardium (**Fig. 2**), define structural abnormalities, and evaluate ventricular function.[62] Patterns of enhancement can identify myocarditis, significant epicardial coronary disease, or subendocardial ischemia secondary to MCD, which may be missed by other stress tests. The test does not expose the patient to ionizing radiation.[63] CMRI use is limited in patients with metallic hardware such as pacemakers, and has long acquisition times that can lead to patient discomfort and claustrophobia.[47,49,56,62,63]

Positron emission tomography

PET imaging uses glucose metabolism to assess myocardial viability. PET's high sensitivity and contrast resolution provide accurate ischemia detection and confers a high predictive value for future cardiac events.[64] PET scans also have improved

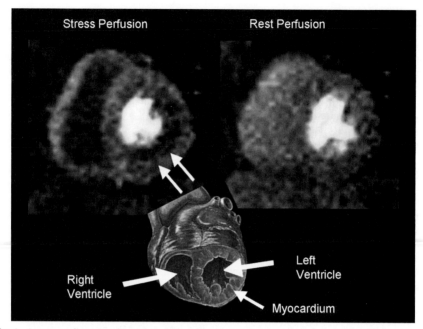

Fig. 2. Stress cardiac MRI. (*Right*) Cardiac MRI depicting normal myocardial perfusion at rest. (*Left*) Under stress, arrows identify radiolucent region of subendocardial hypoperfusion of the left ventricle, suggestive of microvascular coronary disease.

sensitivity in detecting multivessel CAD,[65] preventing balanced ischemia from going undetected. New radiotracers are being developed that target inflammation, identifying sites of active atherosclerotic plaques,[65] which are more likely to rupture or progress. In theory, a high accuracy can eliminate unnecessary and costly interventions, and balance the high cost of the imaging test itself.[64] Unfortunately, no randomized controlled trials have been performed for PET imaging in comparison with traditional diagnostic techniques and therefore no formal recommendation can be made.

Computed tomography

Coronary artery calcification can be determined by computed tomography (CT). Newer multidetector CT scans can often visualize the coronary artery lumen and characterize plaque in many subjects. Meta-analysis has shown that patients with an increased coronary calcium score (CCS) are at a higher risk for CAD.[66] Calcium deposition increases with age and with progression of atherosclerotic lesions; however, the two are not directly correlated. Lesions with significant calcifications may not show signs of critical stenosis and vice versa[67] It has not been established whether treating an asymptomatic patient with a positive CCS confers any benefit, therefore more research is needed before further recommendations are made.[47,49] CCTA can also be used to assess patency of coronary artery bypass grafts (CABG), coronary artery anomalies, and coronary fistulas.[68] CCTA may have a role in evaluating chest pain in patients with an atypical presentation or equivocal ETT, and in premenopausal women.[69]

Coronary angiography

Whereas noninvasive imaging and stress testing aid in the diagnosis and assessment of IHD, the gold standard for definitive diagnosis of CAD remains invasive coronary angiography (CA).[47] CA allows visualization of the site and severity of a coronary lesion. Routine use of CA without prior noninvasive testing is not recommended unless a patient has a high pretest probability of CAD, absolute contraindications to stress testing, or medically refractory angina. High cost, associated morbidity and mortality due to the procedure, as well as the inability to identify which plaques are liable to future rupture make CA a poor initial test in the diagnosis of CSA.[56]

Coronary Reactivity Testing

Coronary reactivity testing (CRT) can be used to diagnose MCD in patients with persistent chest symptoms, evidence of myocardial ischemia, and nonobstructive coronaries.[70] The test involves passing a Doppler flow wire into the coronary artery and injecting vasoactive agents (adenosine, acetylcholine, and nitroglycerin), and measuring the resultant change in the velocity of blood flow.[71] The test helps to differentiate between endothelial-dependent and -independent and coronary artery diameter MCD, as well as coronary artery spasm.

TREATMENT

Management of CSA is geared toward symptom reduction and prevention of adverse events such as acute MI, cardiac death, and revascularization procedures. Data from the Clinical Outcomes Utilizing Revascularization and Aggressive Drug Evaluation (COURAGE) trial show that an approach of optimizing medical therapy (OMT) and aggressive risk factor management in patients with CSA is as beneficial as percutaneous coronary intervention (PCI) and OMT,[72,73] and is recommended by the American College of Cardiology (ACC) and the American Heart Association (AHA).[47,49]

Medical Therapies to Reduce Adverse Cardiovascular Events

Antiplatelet medications act to prevent coronary thrombosis. Low-dose aspirin (81–162 mg/d) has a favorable risk to benefit ratio and is cost effective, making it an ideal agent.[49] Higher doses of aspirin do not appear to confer any additional antithrombotic benefits and increase the risk of gastrointestinal (GI) side effects.[74] For patients who are intolerant to aspirin, clopidogrel is an equally to slightly more efficacious anti-thrombotic medication.[5] Combination of aspirin and clopidogrel is a mainstay of therapy in patients after PCI; however, combination therapy is not typically warranted in CSA.[49]

Statin medications lower cholesterol and have anti-inflammatory effects that help reduce the risk of adverse cardiovascular events. Therapeutic goals are determined by assessing a patient's risk factors and the presence of CHD, or a CHD equivalent.[75] CSA is a CHD subtype; therefore, current recommendations are to maintain LDL levels less than 100 mg/dL. If a patient is considered to be very high risk or if a patient has a baseline LDL of less than 100 mg/dL and is high risk, an LDL goal of less than 70 mg/dL can be considered.[75]

Angiotensin-converting enzyme (ACE) inhibitors improve prognosis in the treatment of hypertension, heart failure, or left ventricular dysfunction, and in diabetic patients. Based on these findings, ACE inhibitors are recommended for treatment of CSA only if these comorbidities exist.[49]

Antianginal and Anti-Ischemic Therapies

β-Blockers decrease oxygen demand and increase diastolic filling time. This process results in increased myocardial perfusion and decreased oxygen needs, which reduces angina symptoms and ischemia.[47] At present, studies confirm the antianginal benefit of β blockade[76]; however, clinical trials have not evaluated the effect on mortality in patients with CSA.[49] Instead, studies have confirmed an improvement in mortality of post-MI and heart failure patients after receiving β-blockers.[77] Therefore, the ACC/AHA recommend β blockade for antianginal symptom control in post-MI and heart failure patients to improve prognosis.[47] If a patient is unable to tolerate a β-blocker, a nondihydropyridine calcium channel blocker (CCB), such as diltiazem, may be used.[49]

In contrast to nondihydropyridine CCBs, clinical trials show that dihydropyridine CCBs (amlodipine) decrease adverse cardiovascular events at 2 years,[78] although this was not statistically significant. These agents did, however, effectively reduce angina symptoms, resulting primarily from systemic vasodilation that decreases cardiac work. In addition, dihydropyridine CCBs also dilate coronary vessels and counteract vasospasm, making them ideal antianginals in vasospastic coronary angina.[47] To enhance the antianginal effect, dihydropyridine CCBs may be combined with β blockade. This union counteracts reflex sympathetic activation of the heart by dihydropyridine CCBs.

β-Blockers also improve mortality in patients post MI. Based on these findings, the ACC/AHA recommends that selection of either agent as an antianginal be based on individual tolerance and coexistent disease; unless the patient has a history of MI, β blockade is preferred. If all disease factors are equally weighted then β blockade is recommended as first line over a CCB.[47,49]

When β-blockers and CCBs are ineffective in controlling angina, long-acting nitrates may be used. These agents reduce the frequency and severity of anginal attacks; however, they have not been tested regarding their impact on mortality.[49] Nitrates cause venodilation, which reduces end-diastolic volume and pressure, leading to increased subendocardial perfusion. Patients may become tolerant to the effects of nitrates; therefore, appropriate dosing should consider a daily nitrate-free interval of 12 hours.[49]

Rapidly acting, short-acting nitrates provide "situational prophylaxis" and can abort an acute angina attack.[49] Because of this immediate relief, short-acting nitrates can be prescribed for a wide variety of patients with angina.[49] Excessive usage may result in dose-dependent headache, flushing, and postural hypotension. Most important, excessive usage should warn patients to seek further medical attention.

Ranolazine

In 2006, the Food and Drug Administration approved the first sodium ion channel (I_{Na}) inhibitor, ranolazine, for the symptomatic control of CSA. Ranolazine exerts its antianginal effect without affecting heart rate and blood pressure,[79] making it an ideal drug of choice in bradycardic and hypotensive patients. Both the Combination Assessment of Ranolazine in Stable Angina (CARISA) and the Monotherapy Assessment of Ranolazine in Stable Angina (MARISA) trials showed that ranolazine increased symptom-related exercise duration.[80,81] The Efficacy of Ranolazine in Chronic Angina (ERICA) and CARISA trials showed a decreased frequency of anginal symptoms and decreased use of short-acting nitrates.[80,82] Unlike nitrates, ranolazine shows no evidence of tolerance at 12 weeks of therapy.[80] The recently published Metabolic Efficiency with Ranolazine for Less Ischemia in Non-ST Elevation Acute Coronary Syndromes (MERLIN)-TIMI 36 trial confirms the aforementioned findings, but concludes that ranolazine did not affect the incidence of cardiovascular mortality or MI.[83–85] Subgroup analyses did demonstrate a significant beneficial effect in women, possibly due to a higher prevalence of MCD.[84] Hence, for symptom control and improved prognosis, the medication should be used in conjunction with β-blockers and CCBs.[49]

Revascularization Therapies

If a patient continues to have persistent angina after using multiple medications, or if imaging shows a large area of myocardium at risk, revascularization should be considered.[49] In addition, if the benefit of revascularization outweighs the risk, or the patient prefers an interventional approach after a discussion of risks and benefits, revascularization may also be considered. PCI and CABG are 2 well-established treatment options. The goal of these interventions once again is to decrease occurrence of symptoms and to improve survival.

PCI may be considered an alternative to CABG in improving quality of life; however, clinical trial summaries demonstrate that there is no benefit in mortality.[49] Balloon angioplasty is now infrequently used as a stand-alone therapy due to high rates of restenosis; it is usually combined with either a bare metal stent or a drug-eluting stent, depending on lesion and patient characteristics. For stable angina, PCI should be mainly reserved for single-vessel disease in moderate to severely symptomatic patients who have failed medical therapy. Due to advanced equipment and increasing physician experience, multivessel disease can also be treated with PCI, given that coronary anatomy is not high risk and therefore more suitable for CABG.[49] Once again, risk of the procedure must be weighed against benefit of angina relief.

CABG can reduce mortality in medium- to high-risk patients and in the presence of specific multivessel disease anatomy including greater than 50% left main artery stenosis, greater than 70% proximal stenosis of 3 major coronary arteries, or greater than 70% proximal left anterior descending artery stenosis and any 2 other major coronary arteries.[49,86] CABG is beneficial in reducing symptoms; however, the incidence of MI is not affected.[87] These considerations are important because of the operative morbidity and mortality associated with this intervention.

SUMMARY

Cardiac risk factors and inflammation lead to the development of obstructive CAD and MCD, which are common causes of CSA chest pain. AS, LVH, CAS, congenital coronary anomalies, and abnormal cardiac nociception are also causes of CSA. ETT is typically the first step in the diagnosis of CAD in intermediate-risk patients who are able to exercise and have a normal baseline ECG. However, ETT has a modest sensitivity and specificity in women, who are more likely to have angina caused by MCD in the absence of obstructive CAD. There are many other stress imaging modalities available for detection of ischemia, including SPECT, PET, SE, MPS, and stress CMRI. The test of choice depends on the patient characteristics and local testing center expertise. CCS and CCTA may allow for noninvasive visualization of obstructive CAD, but invasive CA remains the gold standard for detection and treatment of obstructive CAD. CRT should be considered in patients with CSA, if there is objective evidence of myocardial ischemia and nonobstructive coronary arteries, to evaluate for MCD. Management for CSA includes aggressive lifestyle and risk factor modification to control cardiac risk factors; pharmacologic interventions such as β-blockers, nitrates, CCBs, antiplatelet agents, and statins remain the standard of care. Ranolazine is the most recent antianginal medication available and is effective, especially women. If, however, maximal medication therapy fails to resolve symptoms, interventional therapy in the form of PCI or CABG can reduce frequency of symptoms. Although there are many therapies available, the optimal management of CSA, especially in patients with no obstructive CAD, remains to be delineated. Further mechanistic understanding studies that lead to new interventions are needed to reduce the burden of angina in our society.

REFERENCES

1. Pepine Carl J, Nichols Wilmer W. The pathophysiology of chronic ischemic heart disease. Clin Cardiol 2007;30(S1):I4–9.
2. Rubio R, Berne RM. Regulation of coronary blood flow. Prog Cardiovasc Dis 1975;18(2):105–22.
3. Tune JD, Gorman MW, Feigl EO. Matching coronary blood flow to myocardial oxygen consumption. J Appl Physiol 2004;97(1):404–15.
4. Foreman RD. Mechanisms of visceral pain: from nociception to targets. Drug Discov Today Dis Mech 2004;1(4):457–63.
5. A randomised, blinded, trial of clopidogrel versus aspirin in patients at risk of ischaemic events (CAPRIE). Lancet 1996;348(9038):1329–39.
6. Libby P. Inflammation in atherosclerosis. Nature 2002;420(6917):868–74.
7. Libby P, Theroux P. Pathophysiology of coronary artery disease. Circulation 2005; 111(25):3481–8.
8. Ross R. The pathogenesis of atherosclerosis: a perspective for the 1990s. Nature 1993;362(6423):801–9.
9. Traub O, Berk BC. Laminar shear stress: mechanisms by which endothelial cells transduce an atheroprotective force. Arterioscler Thromb Vasc Biol 1998;18(5): 677–85.
10. Bruschke AV, Kramer JR Jr, Bal ET, et al. The dynamics of progression of coronary atherosclerosis studied in 168 medically treated patients who underwent coronary arteriography three times. Am Heart J 1989;117(2):296–305.
11. Glagov S, Weisenberg E, Zarins CK, et al. Compensatory enlargement of human atherosclerotic coronary arteries. N Engl J Med 1987;316(22):1371–5.
12. Mosseri M, Yarom R, Gotsman MS, et al. Histologic evidence for small-vessel coronary artery disease in patients with angina pectoris and patent large coronary arteries. Circulation 1986;74(5):964–72.
13. Cannon RO 3rd, Watson RM, Rosing DR, et al. Angina caused by reduced vasodilator reserve of the small coronary arteries. J Am Coll Cardiol 1983;1(6): 1359–73.
14. Egashira K, Inou T, Hirooka Y, et al. Evidence of impaired endothelium-dependent coronary vasodilatation in patients with angina pectoris and normal coronary angiograms. N Engl J Med 1993;328(23):1659–64.
15. Opherk D, Zebe H, Weihe E, et al. Reduced coronary dilatory capacity and ultrastructural changes of the myocardium in patients with angina pectoris but normal coronary arteriograms. Circulation 1981;63(4):817–25.
16. Sakr SA, Abbas TM, Amer MZ, et al. Microvascular angina. The possible role of inflammation, uric acid, and endothelial dysfunction. Int Heart J 2009;50(4): 407–19.
17. Kaski JC. Cardiac syndrome X in women: the role of oestrogen deficiency. Heart 2006;92(Suppl 3):iii5–9.
18. Mohri M, Koyanagi M, Egashira K, et al. Angina pectoris caused by coronary microvascular spasm. Lancet 1998;351(9110):1165–9.
19. Hodgson JM, Marshall JJ. Direct vasoconstriction and endothelium-dependent vasodilation. Mechanisms of acetylcholine effects on coronary flow and arterial

diameter in patients with nonstenotic coronary arteries. Circulation 1989;79(5): 1043–51.

20. Okumura K, Yasue H, Horio Y, et al. Multivessel coronary spasm in patients with variant angina: a study with intracoronary injection of acetylcholine. Circulation 1988;77(3):535–42.

21. Prinzmetal M, Kennamer R, Merliss R, et al. Angina pectoris I. A variant form of angina pectoris; preliminary report. Am J Med 1959;27:375–88.

22. Hung MJ, Cherng WJ, Yang NI, et al. Relation of high-sensitivity C-reactive protein level with coronary vasospastic angina pectoris in patients without hemodynamically significant coronary artery disease. Am J Cardiol 2005;96(11): 1484–90.

23. Li JJ, Zhang YP, Yang P, et al. Increased peripheral circulating inflammatory cells and plasma inflammatory markers in patients with variant angina. Coron Artery Dis 2008;19(5):293–7.

24. Kawano H, Ogawa H. Endothelial function and coronary spastic angina. Intern Med 2005;44(2):91–9.

25. Miyao Y, Kugiyama K, Kawano H, et al. Diffuse intimal thickening of coronary arteries in patients with coronary spastic angina. J Am Coll Cardiol 2000;36(2): 432–7.

26. Julius BK, Spillmann M, Vassalli G, et al. Angina pectoris in patients with aortic stenosis and normal coronary arteries. Mechanisms and pathophysiological concepts. Circulation 1997;95(4):892–8.

27. Gould KL. Why angina pectoris in aortic stenosis. Circulation 1997;95(4):790–2.

28. Hittinger L, Mirsky I, Shen Y-T, et al. Hemodynamic mechanisms responsible for reduced subendocardial coronary reserve in dogs with severe left ventricular hypertrophy. Circulation 1995;92(4):978–86.

29. Masuyama T, Uematsu M, Doi Y, et al. Abnormal coronary flow dynamics at rest and during tachycardia associated with impaired left ventricular relaxation in humans: implication for tachycardia-induced myocardial ischemia. J Am Coll Cardiol 1994;24(7):1625–32.

30. Gould KL, Carabello BA. Why angina in aortic stenosis with normal coronary arteriograms? Circulation 2003;107(25):3121–3.

31. Weidemann F, Herrmann S, Stork S, et al. Impact of myocardial fibrosis in patients with symptomatic severe aortic stenosis. Circulation 2009;120(7):577–84.

32. Angelini P, Velasco JA, Flamm S. Coronary anomalies: incidence, pathophysiology, and clinical relevance. Circulation 2002;105(20):2449–54.

33. Angelini P. Functionally significant versus intriguingly different coronary artery anatomy: anatomo-clinical correlations in coronary anomalies. G Ital Cardiol 1999;29(6):607–15.

34. Levin DC, Fellows KE, Abrams HL. Hemodynamically significant primary anomalies of the coronary arteries. Angiographic aspects. Circulation 1978;58(1):25–34.

35. Freed LA, Levy D, Levine RA, et al. Prevalence and clinical outcome of mitral-valve prolapse. N Engl J Med 1999;341(1):1–7.

36. Vavuranakis M, Kolibash AJ, Wooley CF, et al. Mitral valve prolapse: left ventricular hemodynamics in patients with chest pain, dyspnea or both. J Heart Valve Dis 1993;2(5):544–9.

37. Alpert MA, Mukerji V, Sabeti M, et al. Mitral valve prolapse, panic disorder, and chest pain. Med Clin North Am 1991;75(5):1119–33.

38. Cannon R 3rd, Quyyumi A, Schenke W, et al. Abnormal cardiac sensitivity in patients with chest pain and normal coronary arteries. J Am Coll Cardiol 1990; 16(6):1359–66.

39. Chauhan A, Mullins P, Thuraisingham S, et al. Abnormal cardiac pain perception in syndrome X. J Am Coll Cardiol 1994;24(2):329–35.

40. Shapiro LM, Crake T, Poole-Wilson PA. Is altered cardiac sensation responsible for chest pain in patients with normal coronary arteries? Clinical observation during cardiac catheterisation. Br Med J (Clin Res Ed) 1988;296(6616):170–1.

41. Rosen SD, Paulesu E, Wise RJ, et al. Central neural contribution to the perception of chest pain in cardiac syndrome X. Heart 2002;87(6):513–9.

42. Valeriani M, Sestito A, Pera DL, et al. Abnormal cortical pain processing in patients with cardiac syndrome X. Eur Heart J 2005;26(10):975–82.

43. Snow V, Barry P, Fihn SD, et al. Evaluation of primary care patients with chronic stable angina: guidelines from the American College of Physicians. Ann Intern Med 2004;141(1):57–64.

44. Bugiardini R, Bairey Merz CN. Angina with "normal" coronary arteries: a changing philosophy. JAMA 2005;293(4):477–84.

45. Fraker TD Jr, Fihn SD, Gibbons RJ, et al. 2007 chronic angina focused update of the ACC/AHA 2002 guidelines for the management of patients with chronic stable angina: a report of the American College of Cardiology/American Heart Association Task Force on Practice Guidelines Writing Group to develop the focused update of the 2002 guidelines for the management of patients with chronic stable angina. J Am Coll Cardiol 2007;50(23):2264–74.

46. Fraker TD Jr, Fihn SD, Gibbons RJ, et al. 2007 chronic angina focused update of the ACC/AHA 2002 Guidelines for the management of patients with chronic stable angina: a report of the American College of Cardiology/American Heart Association Task Force on Practice Guidelines Writing Group to develop the focused update of the 2002 Guidelines for the management of patients with chronic stable angina. Circulation 2007;116(23):2762–72.

47. Gibbons RJ, Balady GJ, Bricker JT, et al. ACC/AHA 2002 guideline update for exercise testing: summary article: a report of the American College of Cardiology/American Heart Association Task Force on Practice Guidelines (Committee to Update the 1997 Exercise Testing Guidelines). Circulation 2002;106(14):1883–92.

48. Williams SV, Fihn SD, Gibbons RJ. Guidelines for the management of patients with chronic stable angina: diagnosis and risk stratification. Ann Intern Med 2001;135(7):530–47.

49. Fox K, Garcia MA, Ardissino D, et al. Guidelines on the management of stable angina pectoris: executive summary: the Task Force on the Management of Stable Angina Pectoris of the European Society of Cardiology. Eur Heart J 2006;27(11):1341–81.

50. Connolly DC, Elveback LR, Oxman HA. Coronary heart disease in residents of Rochester, Minnesota IV. Prognostic value of the resting electrocardiogram at the time of initial diagnosis of angina pectoris. Mayo Clin Proc 1984;59(4):247–50.

51. Kannel WB, Dawber TR, Kagan A, et al. Factors of risk in the development of coronary heart disease—six year follow-up experience. The Framingham Study. Ann Intern Med 1961;55:33–50.

52. Daly C, Norrie J, Murdoch DL, et al. The value of routine non-invasive tests to predict clinical outcome in stable angina. Eur Heart J 2003;24(6):532–40.

53. Kannel WB, Anderson K, McGee DL, et al. Nonspecific electrocardiographic abnormality as a predictor of coronary heart disease: the Framingham study. Am Heart J 1987;113(2 Pt 1):370–6.

54. De Bacquer D, De Backer G, Kornitzer M, et al. Prognostic value of ECG findings for total, cardiovascular disease, and coronary heart disease death in men and women. Heart 1998;80(6):570–7.

55. Nasir K, Redberg RF, Budoff MJ, et al. Utility of stress testing and coronary calcification measurement for detection of coronary artery disease in women. Arch Intern Med 2004;164(15):1610–20.

56. Sharples L, Hughes V, Crean A, et al. Cost-effectiveness of functional cardiac testing in the diagnosis and management of coronary artery disease: a randomised controlled trial. The CECaT trial. Health Technol Assess 2007;11(49):iii–iv, ix-115.

57. Lewis JF, McGorray S, Lin L, et al. Exercise treadmill testing using a modified exercise protocol in women with suspected myocardial ischemia: findings from the National Heart, Lung and Blood Institute-sponsored women's ischemia syndrome evaluation (WISE). Am Heart J 2005;149(3):527–33.

58. Travain MI, Wexler JP. Pharmacological stress testing. Semin Nucl Med 1999; 29(4):298–318.

59. Leppo JA. Comparison of pharmacologic stress agents. J Nucl Cardiol 1996;3(6 Pt 2):S22–6.

60. Leppo JA, O'Brien J, Rothendler JA, et al. Dipyridamole-thallium-201 scintigraphy in the prediction of future cardiac events after acute myocardial infarction. N Engl J Med 1984;310(16):1014–8.

61. Mahmarian JJ, Mahmarian AC, Marks GF, et al. Role of adenosine thallium-201 tomography for defining long-term risk in patients after acute myocardial infarction. J Am Coll Cardiol 1995;25(6):1333–40.

62. Schwitter J, Nanz D, Kneifel S, et al. Assessment of myocardial perfusion in coronary artery disease by magnetic resonance: a comparison with positron emission tomography and coronary angiography. Circulation 2001;103(18):2230–5.

63. Gershlick AH, de Belder M, Chambers J, et al. Role of non-invasive imaging in the management of coronary artery disease: an assessment of likely change over the next 10 years. A report from the British Cardiovascular Society Working Group. Heart 2007;93(4):423–31.

64. Bengel FM, Higuchi T, Javadi MS, et al. Cardiac positron emission tomography. J Am Coll Cardiol 2009;54(1):1–15.

65. Knuuti J, Bengel FM. Positron emission tomography and molecular imaging. Heart 2008;94(3):360–7.

66. Dendukuri N, Chiu K, Brophy J. Validity of electron beam computed tomography for coronary artery disease: a systematic review and meta-analysis. BMC Med 2007;5(1):35.

67. Redberg RF, Shaw LJ. A review of electron beam computed tomography: implications for coronary artery disease screening. Prev Cardiol 2002;5(2):71–8.

68. Achenbach S, Hoffmann U, Ferencik M, et al. Tomographic coronary angiography by EBCT and MDCT. Prog Cardiovasc Dis 2003;46(2):185–95.

69. Garcia MJ. Non-invasive tests in coronary artery disease: are we facing a fork in the road? Heart 2007;93(4):413–4.

70. Lerman A, Sopko G. Women and cardiovascular heart disease: clinical implications from the women's ischemia syndrome evaluation (WISE) study: are we smarter? J Am Coll Cardiol 2006;47(3 Suppl 1):S59–62.

71. Phan A, Shufelt C, Merz CN. Persistent chest pain and no obstructive coronary artery disease. JAMA 2009;301(14):1468–74.

72. Boden WE, O'Rourke RA, Teo KK, et al. Optimal medical therapy with or without PCI for stable coronary disease. N Engl J Med 2007;356(15):1503–16.

73. Katritsis DG, Ioannidis JP. Percutaneous coronary intervention versus conservative therapy in nonacute coronary artery disease: a meta-analysis. Circulation 2005;111(22):2906–12.

74. Baigent C, Sudlow C, Collins R, et al. Collaborative meta-analysis of randomised trials of antiplatelet therapy for prevention of death, myocardial infarction, and stroke in high risk patients. BMJ 2002;324(7329):71–86.

75. Grundy SM, Cleeman JI, Bairey Merz CN, et al. Implications of recent clinical trials for the National Cholesterol Education Program Adult Treatment Panel III Guidelines. J Am Coll Cardiol 2004;44(3):720–32.

76. Pepine C, Cohn P, Deedwania P, et al. Effects of treatment on outcome in mildly symptomatic patients with ischemia during daily life. The Atenolol silent ischemia study (ASIST). Circulation 1994;90(2):762–8.

77. Yusuf S, Wittes J, Friedman L. Overview of results of randomized clinical trials in heart disease I. Treatments following myocardial infarction. JAMA 1988;260(14): 2088–93.

78. Nissen SE, Tuzcu EM, Libby P, et al. Effect of antihypertensive agents on cardiovascular events in patients with coronary disease and normal blood pressure: The CAMELOT study: a randomized controlled trial. JAMA 2004;292(18): 2217–25.

79. Chaitman BR. Ranolazine for the treatment of chronic angina and potential use in other cardiovascular conditions. Circulation 2006;113(20):2462–72.

80. Chaitman BR, Pepine CJ, Parker JO, et al. Effects of ranolazine with atenolol, amlodipine, or diltiazem on exercise tolerance and angina frequency in patients with severe chronic angina: a randomized controlled trial. JAMA 2004;291(3):309–16.

81. Chaitman BR, Skettino SL, Parker JO, et al. Anti-ischemic effects and long-term survival during ranolazine monotherapy in patients with chronic severe angina. J Am Coll Cardiol 2004;43(8):1375–82.

82. Stone PH, Gratsiansky NA, Blokhin A, et al. Antianginal efficacy of ranolazine when added to treatment with amlodipine: the ERICA (efficacy of ranolazine in chronic angina) trial. J Am Coll Cardiol 2006;48(3):566–75.

83. Melloni C, Newby LK. Metabolic Efficiency with Ranolazine for Less Ischemia in Non-ST elevation acute coronary syndromes (MERLIN TIMI-36) study. Expert Rev Cardiovasc Ther 2008;6(1):9–16.

84. Morrow DA, Scirica BM, Karwatowska-Prokopczuk E, et al. Effects of ranolazine on recurrent cardiovascular events in patients with non-ST-elevation acute coronary syndromes: the MERLIN-TIMI 36 randomized trial. JAMA 2007;297(16): 1775–83.

85. Wilson SR, Scirica BM, Braunwald E, et al. Efficacy of ranolazine in patients with chronic angina: observations from the randomized, double-blind, placebo-controlled MERLIN-TIMI (metabolic efficiency with ranolazine for less ischemia in non-ST-segment elevation acute coronary syndromes) 36 trial. J Am Coll Cardiol 2009;53(17):1510–6.

86. Jones RH, Kesler K, Phillips HR 3rd, et al. Long-term survival benefits of coronary artery bypass grafting and percutaneous transluminal angioplasty in patients with coronary artery disease. J Thorac Cardiovasc Surg 1996;111(5):1013–25.

87. Rihal CS, Raco DL, Gersh BJ, et al. Indications for coronary artery bypass surgery and percutaneous coronary intervention in chronic stable angina: review of the evidence and methodological considerations. Circulation 2003;108(20): 2439–45.

Respiratory Chest Pain: Diagnosis and Treatment

Fraser J. H. Brims, MRCP, MD[a,b], Helen E. Davies, MRCP[c],
Y.C. Gary Lee, MBChB, FRACP, PhD[b,c,d],*

KEYWORDS

- Respiratory • Chest pain • Pneumothorax • Pneumonia
- Pleural infection • Pulmonary embolism

Chest pain from respiratory disease is common. In the United States in 2006, 10% of all admissions to emergency departments were a result of diseases of the respiratory system, and chest pain was the most frequent presenting complaint.[1] The nature and underlying pathophysiology of respiratory chest pain are poorly understood and studies of its quantification, clinical course, and management are limited.

Respiratory chest pain most commonly arises from parietal pleura (including the diaphragmatic pleura), chest wall, and the mediastinal structures.[2] The lung parenchyma and the visceral pleura are insensitive to most painful stimuli. This review summarizes the available literature and the authors' clinical experiences in the diagnoses of common respiratory conditions associated with chest pain, and provides an overview of therapeutic options.

ORIGINS OF RESPIRATORY CHEST PAINS

The main site of respiratory chest pain is the parietal pleura. The pleura costalis, or parietal pleura, lines the inner thoracic cavity, including the diaphragm and mediastinum, whereas the pleura pulmonalis, or visceral pleura, covers the entire surface of the lung, including the interlobar fissures.[3] Although the two surfaces

Conflict of interests: None of the authors has a conflict of interests to declare.
Professor Lee receives a project grant from the State Health Advisory Council of Western Australia, the NH&MRC (Australia), the Raine Foundation of Western Australia, and the MRC (UK).
[a] Respiratory Department, Portsmouth Hospitals NHS Trust, Portsmouth, UK
[b] Respiratory Department, Sir Charles Gairdner Hospital, Perth, Australia
[c] Oxford Centre for Respiratory Medicine, Churchill Hospital, Oxford, OX3 7LJ, UK
[d] School of Medicine and Pharmacology and Lung Institute of Western Australia, University of Western Australia, Perth, Australia
* Corresponding author.
E-mail address: gary.lee@uwa.edu.au

Med Clin N Am 94 (2010) 217–232
doi:10.1016/j.mcna.2010.01.003

medical.theclinics.com

embryologically originate from the same coelomic membrane, their microscopic anatomy differs, with clinically important distinctions. The peripheral part of the diaphragm and costal portion of the parietal pleura are innervated by somatic intercostal nerves, thus pain felt in these areas is often localized to the cutaneous distribution of the involved neurons over the adjacent chest wall. The central portion of the diaphragm is innervated by the phrenic nerve, and central diaphragm irritation is referred to the ipsilateral shoulder tip or even the neck. The visceral pleura is extensively innervated by pulmonary branches of the vagus nerve and sympathetic trunk, with no specific nociceptors.[2] Therefore, the presence of a localized pleuritic chest pain indicates involvement of the parietal pleura. Recent animal studies suggested that pleural adhesions bridging the visceral and parietal pleurae may become innervated, although this has not been documented in humans.[4] The remainder of this review focuses on clinical conditions involving the parietal pleura.

Pains arising from the parietal pleura or chest wall are often exaggerated during deep respiration, coughing/sneezing, or body trunk movement involving the chest wall. The intensity may vary amongst patients with the same pathology, from asymptomatic to agonizing, and is not an indicator of the underlying cause. The description of the pain may also vary significantly amongst patients, for example, from sharp to dull, from burning to catching. The temporal evolution of the pain can be useful. Sudden onset of pain may accompany spontaneous pneumothorax or a rib fracture, whereas pain arising from malignant involvement of the pleura is often of insidious onset. Intercostal neuritis has been listed as a differential diagnosis of respiratory chest pain, but is rare.[5]

Parietal pleural inflammation is commonly termed pleurisy, a localized inflammation of the parietal pleura, which clinically produces a sharp localized pain, made worse on deep inspiration or coughing, and occasionally twisting or bending movements. A pleural rub may be heard over the site of localized pleuritic pain. Although dry pleurisy occurs, pleural inflammation is generally associated with an exudative pleural effusion.

Direct infiltration of the chest wall by a malignancy involving the parietal pleura frequently produces a chronic dull ache localized to the relevant anatomic region, although referred neuropathic pain from intercostal nerve involvement is possible. Less frequently, trauma to the chest wall, ribs, or vertebrae may present in a similar way. Selected specific disease processes that give rise to pain from the parietal pleura or chest wall are discussed later.

CLINICAL ASPECTS

Exudative pleural effusion affects as many as 1800 patients per million population every year.[6] Most of these patients have evidence of parietal pleural inflammation, which may arise from more than 40 different diseases, many of which can present with chest pain. The most common causes of pleuritis and exudative effusions are lung infections (parapneumonic effusions), pleural malignancies (primary pleural mesothelioma or metastatic cancers to the pleura), and systemic disorders (eg, autoimmune diseases).[7]

Pleural inflammation is characterized by neutrophil influx to the pleural cavity, a complicated process mediated by cytokines, especially interleukin eight.[8] Inflammation is often accompanied by increased vascular permeability and resultant plasma extravasation, leading to the accumulation of pleural effusions. These can be detected clinically by percussion (stony) dullness, and by imaging. Thoracic ultrasound and computed tomography (CT) are more sensitive in detecting the presence of pleural fluid than plain radiographs.[9]

Patients with chest pain from pleural inflammation usually have an exudative pleural fluid, characterized by elevated pleural fluid protein and lactate dehydrogenase concentrations, and leukocytosis. Markers of high metabolic activities (eg, low pH and glucose levels) are commonly seen with intense pleuritis (eg, empyema) and in pleural malignancies.

Inflamed pleura may appear thickened on CT scans, especially when performed with a pleural phase contrast protocol. Fluorodeoxyglucose positron emission tomography (PET) can reveal increased uptake of tracer material along the pleural surface, although it may not define the underlying cause. Ultrasound and CT may also reveal features that indicate other conditions, such as malignant invasion of the pleura or periosteum, which may explain the presence of chest pain. CT with pulmonary angiography (CTPA) is useful for detecting pulmonary emboli and any associated lung infarct as a cause of pain.

Tissue biopsies are often required to determine the pleural pathology and can be obtained by closed (blind) biopsies if generalized pleuritis is expected (eg, granulomatous inflammation such as tuberculosis), or under direct vision during thoracoscopy or thoracotomy.[10]

Pleural inflammation often resolves, either spontaneously or following treatment of the underlying diseases, without consequences. Chronic pleuritis and ongoing pain can occur. This chronic inflammation may result in pleural fibrosis and thickening, with restrictive changes in lung functions.[11] Examples include the development of diffuse pleural thickening following resolution of benign asbestos pleural effusions or tuberculous pleuritis. Common conditions leading to pleuritis and chest pain are discussed later.

MANAGEMENT PRINCIPLES

The general principle for the control of all pain is to initiate prompt, appropriate treatment, at the correct dosage, ensuring a favorable benefit to adverse effect profile. The World Health Organization introduced the conceptual framework of the pain ladder, guiding physicians to adopt a stepwise approach to the treatment of patients with pain.[12] Although originally described for patients with cancer-related pain, the concept is now widely used for the management of all types of pain. In the absence of high-quality clinical data, the use of such a systematic approach for respiratory, especially pleural, chest pain seems logical. Simple analgesics (eg, acetaminophen, acetylsalicylic acid) and nonsteroidal antiinflammatory drugs (NSAIDs) can be used regularly and in combination if necessary, for mild pain. Meta-analyses of clinical trials[13–17] suggest NSAIDs (eg, ketoprofen or ibuprofen) are more effective than opiates in controlling general postoperative pain. Conventional teaching often suggests NSAIDs are particularly effective against pleuritic pain, although this has not been formally tested.

Opioids (eg, codeine, oxycodone, dihydrocodeine) can be added, if simple analgesia is insufficient. Doses should be adjusted individually according to the degree of analgesia and side effects (eg, nausea and constipation). Stronger opioids (eg, morphine, fentanyl, or buprenorphine) may be indicated, especially for patients with underlying malignant disease. Parenteral administration may be necessary if oral analgesic drugs are not tolerated.

Adjuvant analgesic medications may be added in combination with the agents listed earlier. Their use for patients with acute pleuritic chest pain is limited but may have a role in those with neuropathic pain (eg, using tricyclic antidepressants or anticonvulsants)[18] and persistent pain syndromes.

The use of intrapleural local anesthetic agents for postoperative (eg, thoracotomy[19–28] and sympathectomy[29]) and posttrauma pain[30,31] has been studied with varying results. One randomized trial showed decreased pain with the use of intrapleural local anesthetic in patients with spontaneous pneumothorax.[32]

Radiotherapy

Radiotherapy has a role in palliating localized pain from malignancies, especially from tumor infiltration of parietal pleura or ribs (**Fig. 1**). For example, radiotherapy can relieve chest wall pain in more than 60% of patients with mesothelioma, although a sustained effect may not be achieved.[33,34] Side effects include tiredness, esophagitis at higher doses, local skin soreness, loss of hair in the irradiated area, and nausea, vomiting, or diarrhea (particularly if the lower chest is being treated). Pain relief from rib metastases can be achieved in approximately 80% of patients, with most of those achieving complete control within 4 weeks.[35] The effect is independent of underlying histologic tumor type and radiotherapy fractionation regimen.[36] Recurrence of metastatic bone pain at a previously irradiated site may be amenable to repeated treatment.[37]

Nerve Blocks

Intercostal nerve blocks using local anesthetic injection (eg, 0.25–0.5% bupivacaine or 1%–2% lidocaine) provide reversible regional analgesia and are effective in controlling acute pain (eg, with rib fractures, or postthoracotomy) and chronic thoracic pain. In patients with pain of neuropathic origin, repeated blocks may afford permanent relief. Pneumothorax is a known but uncommon complication (1%). Paravertebral nerve blocks may be a useful adjunct in the treatment of postthoracotomy/thoracoscopy pain, multiple rib fractures, and chronic pain syndromes.[38,39]

Thoracic epidural with local anesthetic plus opioid, and intrathecal opioid analgesic techniques can provide effective pain control in postthoracotomy patients.[40]

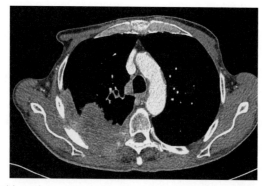

Fig. 1. A 67-year-old smoker presented with an 18-month history of progressively severe gnawing pain in his right shoulder and posterior chest wall. On examination he had marked wasting and paresthesia of his right upper limb and hand. Regular acetaminophen and nonsteroidal antiinflammatory agents had been of limited benefit. This axial CT image shows a right-sided soft-tissue mass invading his adjoining rib and destroying the transverse process and pedicle of the vertebra. A histologic diagnosis of non–small cell lung cancer was made (Pancoast tumor) with his pain secondary to tumor extension into the adjacent brachial plexus, parietal pleura, vertebral bodies, and ribs. Successful palliation of pain was achieved following radiotherapy treatment.

Neurosurgical Measures

Various surgical interventions have been used successfully in selected patients to provide pain relief.

Percutaneous cervical cordotomy interrupts the spinothalamic tract at the C1/C2 levels to abolish pain sensation on the contralateral side. It is used in selected patients with malignancies, especially mesothelioma,[41] and severe chest pain refractory to other approaches. Cervical cordotomy is performed under local anesthesia using fluoroscopic or CT control. Potential complications include permanent ipsilateral limb weakness (0%–3%), bladder, bowel, or sexual dysfunction, and respiratory failure.[42] The latter may occur as a result of destruction of the reticulospinal fibers responsible for spontaneous respiration. A greater degree of functional impairment is seen following a bilateral procedure and with higher levels of analgesia.[43] The analgesic effect of cordotomy diminishes with time and there is a risk of development of delayed dysaesthesic pain. Hence, it is usually offered only to those with limited life expectancy from advanced malignancies.

Neurosurgical techniques for pain control may be considered for selected patients when conservative strategies for pain control have been exhausted. Neuromodulation procedures aim to preferentially stimulate nonnociceptive fibers to alleviate pain.

Deep brain stimulation is effective in well-selected patients with refractory neuropathic or nociceptive thoracic pain.[44] The exact underlying neural mechanism of action is unknown. Central neuroablative procedures such as cingulotomy are occasionally used as a last resort to relieve intractable pain. Modulation of the sensory component of pain is believed to play a key role. It is best considered in patients with a limited life expectancy (eg, mesothelioma or metastatic malignant disease), as recurrence of pain can be troublesome.[45] Dorsal root entry zone lesioning modulates pain pathways by using thermocoagulation, laser, or ultrasound to selectively cut nociceptive afferent fibers within the dorsal nerve root as they enter the spinal cord. Its main indication is in the control of deafferentation pain; however, it may be considered for neuropathic pain syndromes.

Other Considerations

Psychological factors may exacerbate patients' perception, and fear, of their pain and measures to minimize emotional distress can be as important as medication in optimizing pain control.[46] Physiotherapy input may be valuable in patients with pneumonia in whom pleuritic chest pain limits effective sputum clearance. Patients often seek complementary medical therapies, although no data from randomized clinical trials exist to support their routine use in acute pleuritic chest pain.

COMMON CONDITIONS CAUSING RESPIRATORY CHEST PAIN
Malignant Pleural Diseases

Dyspnea and chest pain are the most common presenting symptoms of cancer involvement of the pleura and chest wall. Pleural malignancies can originate from the pleura (the most common of which is pleural mesothelioma) or present as metastases from extrapleural cancers, especially lung and breast carcinomas.

In the United States, lung cancer is the second most common solid organ malignancy and in 2008 was responsible for an estimated 181,840 deaths.[47] Chest pain associated with lung cancer is frequently a dull ache on the affected side, which may signify the presence of malignant pleural or chest wall infiltration. The classic Pancoast tumor in the lung apex may present with pain from brachial plexus invasion and localized shoulder and chest pain. Patients with lung cancer and chest pain often have additional symptoms (eg, dyspnea, cough, hemoptysis, and weight loss).

Malignant pleural mesothelioma is an incurable cancer, and its incidence is rising exponentially in western Europe.[48] In the United Kingdom, 1 patient dies from mesothelioma every 4 hours. Mesothelioma affects 2500 to 3000 patients each year in the United States.[49] Patients often present with breathlessness and chest pain, both of which can be debilitating. The median survival is less than 12 months.[50,51] In 1 study 44% of the patients developed chest pain during the course of disease,[52] although this is likely an underestimation compared with our experience. The tumor arises from the parietal pleura and the visceral pleura is secondarily affected. Mesothelioma has a high propensity to spread along the serosal surfaces, to the contralateral pleura, the peritoneum, and to pleural puncture sites, producing needle-track metastases. Especially in the advanced stages, pain can be diffuse and involve distant sites, and its management can be challenging.[53]

Malignant pleural disease affects about 660 patients per million population each year. Up to 25% of those with lung carcinoma, 95% of patients with mesothelioma, and about 30% of patients with breast cancer develop a pleural effusion during their disease course.[54] Positive histocytologic confirmation is required for diagnosis, usually by pleural fluid cytology or via thoracoscopic or CT-guided pleural biopsy. In patients with chemotherapy-sensitive tumors (eg, lymphoma), pain may resolve/improve when tumors regress after treatment. However, cure is usually not possible in most cases of pleural malignancy. Management is thus directed toward improving symptom control (especially pain and dyspnea) and quality of life. Localized pain can respond to radiotherapy, especially when pharmacologic approaches fail (see **Fig. 1**). In refractory cases, intercostal nerve block can be tried. Limited surgical resection has been used in occasional cases (eg, for ulcerated needle-track metastases). In selected mesothelioma patients with protracted and diffuse chest pain, cervical cordotomy can provide dramatic clinical benefit.

Pleurodesis or other fluid drainage strategies (eg, indwelling pleural catheters) can help control effusion-related breathlessness. The pleural fluid per se does not cause pain.

Clinicians should also bear in mind that patients with any underlying malignancy are also at higher risk of developing pleuritic chest pain from nonmalignant causes (eg, pulmonary embolism [PE] and pneumonia). A community-based study in the United States has shown an increased risk of venous thromboembolism and a 4.1- to 6.5-fold increased risk of developing PE in these patients.[55]

PE

The annual incidence of PE is up to 200 cases per million people.[55,56] Patients may classically present with sudden onset of chest pain, dyspnea, and possibly collapse.[57] In 1 study, two-thirds of patients experienced pleuritic chest pain, which, together with dyspnea, were the 2 most common symptoms (**Fig. 2**).[58] Concurrent illnesses, such as pneumonia or underlying cancers, are frequent and can also give rise to pain. A recent meta-analysis of 550 hospitalized patients with acute chronic obstructive pulmonary disease (COPD) from the United States and Europe concluded that the prevalence of PE is up to 24.7% in this population.[59]

The pleuritic chest pain characteristic of PE may develop after the initial symptoms and is caused by irritation to the parietal pleura following local inflammation and infarction of the underlying visceral pleura overlying the lung segment affected by the embolus. Some patients may experience a central pain believed to be a result of distension of mechanoreceptors in the pulmonary artery.[60]

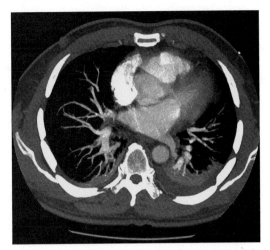

Fig. 2. A 58-year-old patient presented with pleuritic chest pain and dyspnea following hip surgery. CTPA showed bilateral pulmonary emboli, peripheral atelectasis, and a small pleural effusion.

Two recent studies described the characteristics of pleural effusions in patients diagnosed with PE.[61,62] Detailed discussion of the diagnosis and management of PE can be found in recent clinical guidelines,[63] and is outside the scope of this review.

Pneumonia and Pleural Infection

Pneumonia classically presents with fever, cough productive of purulent sputum, leukocytosis, and often pleuritic chest pain localized to the area overlying the infection. In the United States and Europe, community-acquired pneumonia (CAP) has an incidence of 500 to 1100 per million adults,[64–66] and is markedly higher in elderly people. Hospitalization rates for CAP are consistently high (between 110 and 400 cases per million population) in several North American and European series.[65–67]

Nearly half of all patients with pneumonia may have pleuritic chest pain[68] and 13% still complained of pain after 30 days.[69] The pain is believed to arise from parietal pleural inflammation secondary to infective involvement of the peripheral lung parenchyma. The lack of peripheral parenchymal involvement may explain why pleuritis is uncommon in patients with chronic airway (but not distal lung parenchymal) inflammation, such as bronchiectasis and cystic fibrosis. Chest pain was not listed as a presenting complaint in a recent report from Mexico on severe pneumonia associated with H1N1 viral infection.[70] Details on diagnosis and management of pneumonia can be found elsewhere (eg, British Thoracic Society guidelines).[71]

The frequent involvement of the pleura is supported by the finding that 40% of patients with pneumonia develop exudative parapneumonic effusions during their disease course.[72] Pleural infection develops as a result of secondary infection of these simple parapneumonic effusions. Such patients may continue to complain of pleuritic chest pain and are likely to have clinical features consistent with infection (fever and raised inflammatory markers) and a pleural effusion. The size of the effusion varies, and cannot be used to predict infective cause. Treatment is based on drainage of the infected material and antimicrobial therapy as guided by national communicable disease surveillance reports and international guidelines.[73]

Pneumothorax

A pneumothorax refers to the presence of air within the pleural space and may occur spontaneously, after trauma, post-surgery, or via iatrogenic means. Spontaneous pneumothorax may develop in patients with no known underlying lung disease (primary pneumothorax) and in those with known underlying lung disease (secondary pneumothorax), especially COPD. A spontaneous pneumothorax of either cause is likely to present with a sudden onset of ipsilateral pleuritic chest pain, with variable degrees of breathlessness, depending on the severity of the underlying lung disease. In one study of 155 patients, 90% had pain[74] and all patients had pain in a smaller study of 17 children with spontaneous pneumothoraces.[75] The precise cause of the pain is not known, although recent experimental evidence suggests pleural inflammation (often eosinophilic) does occur with pneumothorax.[76,77] Ongoing chest pain in patients with pneumothorax should alert the clinicians to either a persistent airleak or concomitant pleuropulmonary diseases.

Spontaneous pneumomediastinum is a rare condition defined by the presence of free air in the mediastinum that is not preceded by trauma or interventional procedures. A recent report from the Mayo Clinic identified that two-thirds of patients present with pleuritic chest pain, with an additional pneumothorax evident in one-third of cases.[78] In most cases the pneumomediastinum resolved with conservative management.

Connective Tissue Disease

Pleuritis and pleural effusions are common in connective tissue diseases, affecting up to 50% of patients with systemic lupus erythematosus (SLE) and 5% of patients with rheumatoid arthritis. Pleuritis and pleural effusions in SLE are often bilateral and typically exudative (occasionally hemorrhagic) with a lymphocytosis (if chronic).[79] NSAIDs may relieve pleuritic chest pain, and corticosteroid treatment may produce a swift clinical response if the patient remains symptomatic. Pleural effusions as a consequence of drug-induced lupus erythematosus are rare.

Wegener's granulomatosis is associated with pleural effusion in approximately 30% of patients and responds to treatment of the underlying condition with immunosuppressant therapy. Pleural effusion may occur in up to 30% of those with Churg-Strauss syndrome; typically the fluid is rich in eosinophils. The effusions are not usually of any clinical consequence and most resolve with corticosteroids.

Tracheobronchitis

Patients with tracheobronchitis may complain of a central burning sensation localized to the sternal region. This symptom may occur in otherwise normal subjects or those with underlying lung disease, such as COPD, who may more frequently suffer bronchitis. A similar sensation is occasionally reported during heavy exercise or hyperventilation, particularly in cold environments.[2]

Rare Conditions

Pulmonary arterial hypertension (PAH) can be idiopathic, or occur in association with underlying pulmonary and systemic conditions.[80] PAH of any cause can present with various symptoms, including fatigue, lethargy, worsening dyspnea, and, rarely, chest pain. The exact mechanism by which the chest pain occurs is unclear, with more typical anginal pain sometimes described, even in the presence of normal coronary arteries[81]; pulmonary artery dilatation and stretching or right ventricular ischemia may contribute. Patients with secondary PAH often have symptoms that reflect the underlying cause, for example recurrent pulmonary thromboembolic disease, or collagen vascular disease.

Rarely, asbestos-related pleural plaques have been associated with an angina-like chest pain[82]; there is no treatment possible or required for asbestos-related pleural plaques.

Epidemic myalgia (Bornholm disease) is caused by viral infection from the Coxsackie B virus. It most commonly affects young adults in late summer and autumn in the northern hemisphere and is characterized by upper respiratory tract illness followed by pleuritic chest pain with a normal chest radiograph. Treatment is supportive and the illness usually clears within a week, although relapses are characteristic, particularly during the weeks following the acute illness.

IATROGENIC CAUSES OF CHEST PAIN

Pleural interventions, frequently needed for diagnostic and management of pleural effusions, are another important, but often neglected, cause of chest pain. Careful attention to provision of local and systemic anesthesia can help minimize iatrogenic chest pain from pleural procedures.

Thoracentesis

Pleural aspiration (thoracentesis) is performed daily around the world, most commonly for the diagnosis of pleural effusions. Pain mainly arises as a consequence of puncture of the skin and parietal pleural surface. Inadvertent contact with the rib surface can result in severe pain, caused by stimulation of numerous nociceptors present on the periosteal surface. Diligent and generous use of local anesthesia (eg, up to 3 mg/kg of 1% lidocaine) to the skin, intercostal tissues, and parietal pleura is recommended before aspiration. Anaesthetizing the periosteum of the rib for simple thoracentesis is often unnecessary if good technique is ensured, but can be useful before closed needle pleural biopsy.

Chest pain may also be related to the evacuation of pleural fluid, especially with rapid or large volume (usually several liters) drainage. Its nature may vary from a vague aching discomfort to severe pleuritic pain. Slowing the rate of drainage can ease this discomfort; negative pressure suction is best avoided as it frequently aggravates pain. Reexpansion pulmonary edema, although rare, is a potentially life-threatening complication, especially after evacuation of a large effusion in patients with a chronically collapsed lung.[83,84]

Chest Tube Insertion

Chest pain is common during and following intercostal chest drain insertion (thoracostomy). Adequate use of local anesthesia (see section on pain management), often together with conscious sedation, is recommended. The pain is presumed to result from direct irritation of the (often inflamed) pleura or periosteum by the chest tube, together with trauma to the skin and underlying tissue during the insertion process.

Larger bore chest tubes have been associated with a higher level of discomfort, and 2 studies reported that all patients experienced moderate or intense pain at some point during chest drainage.[85,86] Severe pain and anxiety of 9 or 10 (on a scale of 1 to 10) was reported in 50% of patients during chest tube drainage in 1 study.[87] Large-bore (28–32 F) chest tubes were favored by many clinicians in the management of pleurodesis for malignant pleural effusions in a survey of 859 pulmonologists from 5 English-speaking countries.[88] Guidelines (eg, the British Thoracic Society Pleural Guidelines 2010) presume that small-bore catheters result in less pain but robust, validated study data supporting this are scant.[89] A randomized clinical trial comparing the optimal chest tube size for pleurodesis is currently under way in the United Kingdom.

Indwelling tunneled ambulatory pleural catheters are increasingly used for the management of recurrent pleural effusion.[79] Chest pain is common in the first week following insertion, with patients often reporting a bruised sensation related to dissection of the subcutaneous tract. This pain is usually mild and can be controlled with regular analgesia (eg, acetaminophen or NSAIDs). Pain experienced with indwelling catheters is significantly less than those associated with intercostal chest drain insertion and pleurodesis in treating malignant pleural effusions.[90]

Thoracoscopy/Thoracotomy

Thoracoscopy is often required for diagnosis of pleural effusions, and video-assisted thoracoscopy can further be used for lung biopsy or lobectomy. Thoracotomy is the conventional method employed for lung resection, amongst other indications. Rib displacement and, occasionally, resection is required during the procedure.

Persistent pain (chronic intercostal neuralgia) is common following these procedures. Furrer and colleagues[91] reported that one-third of 30 patients reported persistent pain or discomfort 3 to 18 months following video-assisted thoracic surgery (VATS) and thoracotomy. Dajczman and colleagues[92] found that in 56 postthoracotomy patients, 9% suffered from severe chronic pain requiring daily analgesia, nerve blocks, acupuncture, or referral to pain specialist clinics. A retrospective survey[93] reported persistent postthoracotomy pain for more than 6 months in 44% of patients; and a further study of 60 patients noted chronic pain in 19 of 60 patients following thoracotomy, especially if pleurectomy was performed.[94] A systematic review favored VATS over thoracotomy, reporting lower analgesia requirements and a shorter length of hospital stay.[95]

Pleurodesis

Iatrogenic induction of pleural fibrosis to obliterate the pleural cavity (pleurodesis) is performed therapeutically for recurrent pleural effusions or pneumothoraces. Whether performed by chemical (injection of a sclerosing agent) or surgical means (eg, mechanical pleural abrasion, pleurectomy), the principle is to damage the pleural mesothelial surface.[96] The resultant inflammation, if sufficiently intense, heals with pleural fibrosis. This intense pleuritis is known to cause severe pain. More than 60% of patients in 1 observational study reported moderate to severe pain with pleurodesis.[97] In the International Survey of Pleurodesis Practice, pain was the most commonly reported complication by pulmonologists, irrespective of sclerosing agents used.[88]

No quality data exist on the best analgesic regimes for pleurodesis. Most physicians use opiate for pleurodesis pain.[88] Respiratory society guidelines recommend instillation of lidocaine before the pleurodesing agent[10] and up to 90% of physicians routinely used intrapleural lidocaine in the International Survey of Pleurodesis Practice.[88] Readers should be aware that this practice is based on conventional wisdom, and has not been tested in clinical studies. Premedication with opioids or conscious sedation should be used, provided no contraindications exist. Patients undergoing pleurodesis are often at risk of respiratory compromise; lower doses or alternative agents may need to be considered.[98,99] Antiinflammatory effects from NSAIDs and corticosteroids can theoretically reduce efficacy of pleurodesis by dampening pleural inflammation. This result has been shown in animal studies[100,101] and is the subject of a multicenter, randomized controlled trial.

SUMMARY

Chest pain is a common clinical presentation in patients with respiratory diseases. Respiratory pain has been poorly studied. Better knowledge of the pain, its character, origin, regulation, and quantification will help guide clinicians to appropriate differential diagnoses and improve management. Clinical examination and radiological imaging are important in directing clinicians to appropriate further investigations. Optimal treatment of pain associated with common respiratory diseases remains uncertain in most cases, and focused studies are urgently needed.

ACKNOWLEDGMENTS

The authors thank Dr Naj Rahman and Dr Deepak Ravindran for their help in the preparation of this manuscript.

REFERENCES

1. Pitts SR, Niska RW, Xu J, et al. National Hospital Ambulatory Medical Care Survey: 2006 emergency department summary. Hyattsville (MD): National Center for Health Statistics; 2008. Contract No.: Document Number.
2. Albert R. Chest pain. In: Albert RK, Spiro SG, Jett JR, editors. Clinical pulmonary medicine. 3rd edition. Philadelphia: Elsevier; 2008. p. 317–24.
3. Gray H. Gray's anatomy. In: Pick TP, Howden R, editors. 15th edition. New York: Crown Publishers Inc; 1988. p. 969–70.
4. Montes JF, Garcia-Valero J, Ferrer J. Evidence of innervation in talc-induced pleural adhesions. Chest 2006;130(3):702–9.
5. Murray J, Gebhart G. Chest pain. In: Murray J, Nadel J, Mason R, et al, editors. Textbook of respiratory diseases. 4th edition. Philadelphia: WB Saunders & Co; 2005. p. 848–65.
6. Marel M, Zrustova M, Stasny B, et al. The incidence of pleural effusion in a well-defined region. Epidemiologic study in central Bohemia. Chest 1993;104(5): 1486–9.
7. Lee YCG, Light R. Pleural effusion: overview. In: Laurent G, Shapiro S, editors. Encyclopedia of respiratory diseases. Oxford (UK): Elservier; 2006. p. 353–8.
8. Wilson NA, Mutsaers S, Lee YCG. Immunology in pleural diseases. In: Light R, Lee YCG, editors. Textbook of pleural diseases. 2nd edition. London: Arnold; 2008. p. 71–100.
9. Gleeson FV, Lee YCG. Practical imaging in pleural sepsis. In: Desai S, Franquet T, Hartman T, Wells A, editors. Pulmonary imaging. London: Taylor & Francis Book Ltd; 2008. p. 99–105.
10. Antunes G, Neville E, Duffy J, et al. BTS guidelines for the management of malignant pleural effusions. Thorax 2003;58(Suppl 2):ii29–38.
11. Light RW, Lee YCG. Pneumothorax, chylothorax, hemothorax and fibrothorax. In: Murray J, Nadel J, Mason R, et al, editors. Textbook of respiratory diseases. 5th edition. Philadelphia: WB Saunders & Co, in press.
12. World Health Organization. WHO's pain ladder. 2009. [updated 2009; cited December 2009]; Available at: http://www.who.int/cancer/palliative/painladder/en/index.html. Accessed December 1, 2009.
13. Oxford league table of analgesic efficacy. Oxford: Bandolier Evidence Based Healthcare. 2007 [updated 2007; cited December 2009]; Available at: http://

www.medicine.ox.ac.uk/bandolier/booth/painpag/Acutrev/Analgesics/Leagtab. html. Accessed December 1, 2009.

14. Barden J, Derry S, McQuay HJ, et al. Single dose oral ketoprofen and dexketoprofen for acute postoperative pain in adults. Cochrane Database Syst Rev 2009;(4):CD007355.

15. Collins SL, Moore RA, McQuay HJ, et al. Single dose oral ibuprofen and diclofenac for postoperative pain. Cochrane Database Syst Rev 2000;(2):CD001548.

16. Collins SL, Moore RA, McQuay HJ, et al. Oral ibuprofen and diclofenac in postoperative pain: a quantitative systematic review. Eur J Pain 1998;2(4):285–91.

17. McQuay HJ, Carroll D, Moore RA. Injected morphine in postoperative pain: a quantitative systematic review. J Pain Symptom Manage 1999;17(3):164–74.

18. Dworkin RH, Backonja M, Rowbotham MC, et al. Advances in neuropathic pain: diagnosis, mechanisms, and treatment recommendations. Arch Neurol 2003; 60(11):1524–34.

19. Tetik O, Islamoglu F, Ayan E, et al. Intermittent infusion of 0.25% bupivacaine through an intrapleural catheter for post-thoracotomy pain relief. Ann Thorac Surg 2004;77(1):284–8.

20. Aykac B, Erolcay H, Dikmen Y, et al. Comparison of intrapleural versus intravenous morphine for postthoracotomy pain management. J Cardiothorac Vasc Anesth 1995;9(5):538–40.

21. Raffin L, Fletcher D, Sperandio M, et al. Interpleural infusion of 2% lidocaine with 1:200,000 epinephrine for postthoracotomy analgesia. Anesth Analg 1994; 79(2):328–34.

22. Miguel R, Hubbell D. Pain management and spirometry following thoracotomy: a prospective, randomized study of four techniques. J Cardiothorac Vasc Anesth 1993;7(5):529–34.

23. Elman A, Debaene B, Magny-Metrot C, et al. Interpleural analgesia with bupivacaine following thoracotomy: ineffective results of a controlled study and pharmacokinetics. J Clin Anesth 1993;5(2):118–21.

24. Schneider RF, Villamena PC, Harvey J, et al. Lack of efficacy of intrapleural bupivacaine for postoperative analgesia following thoracotomy. Chest 1993; 103(2):414–6.

25. Inderbitzi R, Flueckiger K, Ris HB. Pain relief and respiratory mechanics during continuous intrapleural bupivacaine administration after thoracotomy. Thorac Cardiovasc Surg 1992;40(2):87–9.

26. Symreng T, Gomez MN, Rossi N. Intrapleural bupivacaine v saline after thoracotomy–effects on pain and lung function–a double-blind study. J Cardiothorac Anesth 1989;3(2):144–9.

27. Mann LJ, Young GR, Williams JK, et al. Intrapleural bupivacaine in the control of postthoracotomy pain. Ann Thorac Surg 1992;53(3):449–53 [discussion: 53–4].

28. Gaeta RR, Macario A, Brodsky JB, et al. Pain outcomes after thoracotomy: lumbar epidural hydromorphone versus intrapleural bupivacaine. J Cardiothorac Vasc Anesth 1995;9(5):534–7.

29. Assalia A, Kopelman D, Markovits R, et al. Intrapleural analgesia following thoracoscopic sympathectomy for palmar hyperhidrosis: a prospective, randomized trial. Surg Endosc 2003;17(6):921–2.

30. Knottenbelt JD, James MF, Bloomfield M. Intrapleural bupivacaine analgesia in chest trauma: a randomized double-blind controlled trial. Injury 1991;22(2): 114–6.

31. Short K, Scheeres D, Mlakar J, et al. Evaluation of intrapleural analgesia in the management of blunt traumatic chest wall pain: a clinical trial. Am Surg 1996; 62(6):488–93.
32. Engdahl O, Boe J, Sandstedt S. Interpleural bupivacaine for analgesia during chest drainage treatment for pneumothorax. A randomized double-blind study. Acta Anaesthesiol Scand 1993;37(2):149–53.
33. Waite K, Gilligan D. The role of radiotherapy in the treatment of malignant pleural mesothelioma. Clin Oncol (R Coll Radiol) 2007;19(3):182–7.
34. Bissett D, Macbeth FR, Cram I. The role of palliative radiotherapy in malignant mesothelioma. Clin Oncol (R Coll Radiol) 1991;3(6):315–7.
35. McQuay HJ, Carroll D, Moore RA. Radiotherapy for painful bone metastases: a systematic review. Clin Oncol 1997;9(3):150–4.
36. Price P, Hoskin PJ, Easton D, et al. Prospective randomised trial of single and multifraction radiotherapy schedules in the treatment of painful bony metastases. Radiother Oncol 1986;6(4):247–55.
37. Mithal NP, Needham PR, Hoskin PJ. Retreatment with radiotherapy for painful bone metastases. Int J Radiat Oncol Biol Phys 1994;29(5):1011–4.
38. Eason MJ, Wyatt R. Paravertebral thoracic block–a reappraisal. Anaesthesia 1979;34(7):638–42.
39. Karmakar MK. Thoracic paravertebral block. Anesthesiology 2001;95(3): 771–80.
40. Joshi GP, Bonnet F, Shah R, et al. A systematic review of randomized trials evaluating regional techniques for postthoracotomy analgesia. Anesth Analg 2008; 107(3):1026–40.
41. Jackson MB, Pounder D, Price C, et al. Percutaneous cervical cordotomy for the control of pain in patients with pleural mesothelioma. Thorax 1999;54(3): 238–41.
42. Lipton S. Percutaneous cervical cordotomy. Proc R Soc Med 1973;66(7):607–9.
43. Kuperman AS, Krieger AJ, Rosomoff HL. Respiratory function after cervical cordotomy. Chest 1971;59(2):128–32.
44. Bittar RG, Kar-Purkayastha I, Owen SL, et al. Deep brain stimulation for pain relief: a meta-analysis. J Clin Neurosci 2005;12(5):515–9.
45. Yen CP, Kung SS, Su YF, et al. Stereotactic bilateral anterior cingulotomy for intractable pain. J Clin Neurosci 2005;12(8):886–90.
46. Fallon M, Hanks G, Cherny N. Principles of control of cancer pain. BMJ 2006; 332(7548):1022–4.
47. Jemal A, Siegel R, Ward E, et al. Cancer statistics, 2008. CA Cancer J Clin 2008; 58(2):71–96.
48. Peto J, Decarli A, La Vecchia C, et al. The European mesothelioma epidemic. Br J Cancer 1999;79(3–4):666–72.
49. Yang H, Testa JR, Carbone M. Mesothelioma epidemiology, carcinogenesis, and pathogenesis. Curr Treat Options Oncol 2008;9(2–3):147–57.
50. Robinson BW, Lake RA. Advances in malignant mesothelioma. N Engl J Med 2005;353(15):1591–603.
51. Curran D, Sahmoud T, Therasse P, et al. Prognostic factors in patients with pleural mesothelioma: the European Organization for Research and Treatment of Cancer experience. J Clin Oncol 1998;16(1):145–52.
52. Ribak J, Lilis R, Suzuki Y, et al. Malignant mesothelioma in a cohort of asbestos insulation workers: clinical presentation, diagnosis, and causes of death. Br J Ind Med 1988;45(3):182–7.

53. West SD, Lee YC. Management of malignant pleural mesothelioma. Clin Chest Med 2006;27(2):335–54.
54. Mishra E, Davies HE, Lee YC. Malignant pleural disease in primary lung cancer. In: Spiro S, Janes S, Huber R, editors. Thoracic malignancies. European respiratory monograph. 3rd edition. Sheffield (UK): European Respiratory Society Journals Ltd; 2009. p. 318–55.
55. Heit JA, Silverstein MD, Mohr DN, et al. Risk factors for deep vein thrombosis and pulmonary embolism: a population-based case-control study. Arch Intern Med 2000;160(6):809–15.
56. Anderson FA Jr, Spencer FA. Risk factors for venous thromboembolism. Circulation 2003;107(23 Suppl 1):I9–16.
57. Stein PD, Terrin ML, Hales CA, et al. Clinical, laboratory, roentgenographic, and electrocardiographic findings in patients with acute pulmonary embolism and no pre-existing cardiac or pulmonary disease. Chest 1991;100(3):598–603.
58. Worsley DF, Alavi A. Comprehensive analysis of the results of the PIOPED Study. Prospective Investigation of Pulmonary Embolism Diagnosis Study. J Nucl Med 1995;36(12):2380–7.
59. Rizkallah J, Man SF, Sin DD. Prevalence of pulmonary embolism in acute exacerbations of COPD: a systematic review and metaanalysis. Chest 2009;135(3):786–93.
60. Rubin LJ. Pathology and pathophysiology of primary pulmonary hypertension. Am J Cardiol 1995;75(3):51A–4A.
61. Yap E, Anderson G, Donald J, et al. Pleural effusion in patients with pulmonary embolism. Respirology 2008;13(6):832–6.
62. Porcel JM, Madronero AB, Pardina M, et al. Analysis of pleural effusions in acute pulmonary embolism: radiological and pleural fluid data from 230 patients. Respirology 2007;12(2):234–9.
63. Kearon C, Kahn SR, Agnelli G, et al. Antithrombotic therapy for venous thromboembolic disease: American College of Chest Physicians evidence-based clinical practice guidelines. (8th edition). Chest 2008;133(Suppl 6):454S–545S.
64. Jokinen C, Heiskanen L, Juvonen H, et al. Incidence of community-acquired pneumonia in the population of four municipalities in eastern Finland. Am J Epidemiol 1993;137(9):977–88.
65. Foy HM, Cooney MK, Allan I, et al. Rates of pneumonia during influenza epidemics in Seattle, 1964 to 1975. JAMA 1979;241(3):253–8.
66. Lave JR, Fine MJ, Sankey SS, et al. Hospitalized pneumonia. Outcomes, treatment patterns, and costs in urban and rural areas. J Gen Intern Med 1996;11(7):415–21.
67. Community-acquired pneumonia in adults in British hospitals in 1982–1983: a survey of aetiology, mortality, prognostic factors and outcome. The British Thoracic Society and the Public Health Laboratory Service. Q J Med 1987;62(239):195–220.
68. Fine MJ, Stone RA, Singer DE, et al. Processes and outcomes of care for patients with community-acquired pneumonia: results from the Pneumonia Patient Outcomes Research Team (PORT) cohort study. Arch Intern Med 1999;159(9):970–80.
69. Brandenburg JA, Marrie TJ, Coley CM, et al. Clinical presentation, processes and outcomes of care for patients with pneumococcal pneumonia. J Gen Intern Med 2000;15(9):638–46.

70. Perez-Padilla R, de la Rosa-Zamboni D, Ponce de Leon S, et al. Pneumonia and respiratory failure from swine-origin influenza A (H1N1) in Mexico. N Engl J Med 2009;361(7):680–9.

71. Lim WS, Baudouin SV, George RC, et al. British Thoracic Society guidelines for the management of community acquired pneumonia in adults: update 2009. Thorax 2009;64(Suppl III):iii1–iii55.

72. Koegelenberg CF, Diaconi AH, Bolligeri CT. Parapneumonic pleural effusion and empyema. Respiration 2008;75(3):241–50.

73. American Thoracic Society. Available at: www.thoracic.org/sections/publications/statements/index.html. Accessed December 1, 2009.

74. Seremetis MG. The management of spontaneous pneumothorax. Chest 1970; 57(1):65–8.

75. Wilcox DT, Glick PL, Karamanoukian HL, et al. Spontaneous pneumothorax: a single-institution, 12-year experience in patients under 16 years of age. J Pediatr Surg 1995;30(10):1452–4.

76. Kalomenidis I, Moschos C, Kollintza A, et al. Pneumothorax-associated pleural eosinophilia is tumour necrosis factor-alpha-dependent and attenuated by steroids. Respirology 2008;13(1):73–8.

77. Kalomenidis I, Guo Y, Peebles RS, et al. Pneumothorax-associated pleural eosinophilia in mice is interleukin-5 but not interleukin-13 dependent. Chest 2005;128(4):2978–83.

78. Iyer VN, Joshi AY, Ryu JH. Spontaneous pneumomediastinum: analysis of 62 consecutive adult patients. Mayo Clin Proc 2009;84(5):417–21.

79. Davies HE, Lee YCG. Pleural effusion, empyema and pneumothorax. In: Albert RK, Spiro S, Jett J, editors. Clinical pulmonary medicine. 3rd edition. Philadelphia: Elsevier; 2008. p. 853–67.

80. Farber HW, Loscalzo J. Pulmonary arterial hypertension. N Engl J Med 2004; 351(16):1655–65.

81. Stuckey D. Cardiac pain in association with mitral stenosis and congenital heart disease. Br Heart J 1955;17(3):397–408.

82. Mukherjee S, de Klerk N, Palmer LJ, et al. Chest pain in asbestos-exposed individuals with benign pleural and parenchymal disease. Am J Respir Crit Care Med 2000;162(5):1807–11.

83. Mahajan VK, Simon M, Huber GL. Reexpansion pulmonary edema. Chest 1979; 75(2):192–4.

84. Trapnell DH, Thurston JG. Unilateral pulmonary oedema after pleural aspiration. Lancet 1970;1(7661):1367–9.

85. Fox V, Gould D, Davies N, et al. Patients' experiences of having an underwater seal chest drain: a replication study. J Clin Nurs 1999;8(6):684–92.

86. Owen S, Gould D. Underwater seal chest drains: the patient's experience. J Clin Nurs 1997;6(3):215–25.

87. Luketich JD, Kiss M, Hershey J, et al. Chest tube insertion: a prospective evaluation of pain management. Clin J Pain 1998;14(2):152–4.

88. Lee YC, Baumann MH, Maskell NA, et al. Pleurodesis practice for malignant pleural effusions in five English-speaking countries: survey of pulmonologists. Chest 2003;124(6):2229–38.

89. Clementsen P, Evald T, Grode G, et al. Treatment of malignant pleural effusion: pleurodesis using a small percutaneous catheter. A prospective randomized study. Respir Med 1998;92(3):593–6.

90. Musani AI, Haas AR, Seijo L, et al. Outpatient management of malignant pleural effusions with small-bore, tunneled pleural catheters. Respiration 2004;71(6): 559–66.

91. Furrer M, Rechsteiner R, Eigenmann V, et al. Thoracotomy and thoracoscopy: postoperative pulmonary function, pain and chest wall complaints. Eur J Cardiothorac Surg 1997;12(1):82–7.

92. Dajczman E, Gordon A, Kreisman H, et al. Long-term postthoracotomy pain. Chest 1991;99(2):270–4.

93. Kalso E, Perttunen K, Kaasinen S. Pain after thoracic surgery. Acta Anaesthesiol Scand 1992;36(1):96–100.

94. Passlick B, Born C, Sienel W, et al. Incidence of chronic pain after minimal-invasive surgery for spontaneous pneumothorax. Eur J Cardiothorac Surg 2001; 19(3):355–8 [discussion: 8–9].

95. Sedrakyan A, van der Meulen J, Lewsey J, et al. Video assisted thoracic surgery for treatment of pneumothorax and lung resections: systematic review of randomised clinical trials. BMJ 2004;329(7473):1008.

96. Davies HE, Lee YCG. Pleurodesis. In: Light R, Lee YCG, editors. Textbook of pleural diseases. London: Arnold Press; 2008. p. 569–82.

97. Pulsiripunya C, Youngchaiyud P, Pushpakom R, et al. The efficacy of doxycycline as a pleural sclerosing agent in malignant pleural effusion: a prospective study. Respirology 1996;1(1):69–72.

98. McNicol E, Horowicz-Mehler N, Fisk RA, et al. Management of opioid side effects in cancer-related and chronic noncancer pain: a systematic review. J Pain 2003;4(5):231–56.

99. Wilder-Smith CH. Pain treatment in multimorbid patients, the older population and other high-risk groups. The clinical challenge of reducing toxicity. Drug Saf 1998;18(6):457–72.

100. Teixeira LR, Vargas FS, Acencio MM, et al. Influence of antiinflammatory drugs (methylprednisolone and diclofenac sodium) on experimental pleurodesis induced by silver nitrate or talc. Chest 2005;128(6):4041–5.

101. Lardinois D, Vogt P, Yang L, et al. Non-steroidal anti-inflammatory drugs decrease the quality of pleurodesis after mechanical pleural abrasion. Eur J Cardiothorac Surg 2004;25(5):865–71.

Noncardiac Chest Pain: Gastroesophageal Reflux Disease

Amanke C. Oranu, MD, Michael F. Vaezi, MD, PhD, MSc (Epi)*

KEYWORDS

- Noncardiac chest pain • Gastroesophageal reflux disease
- Clinical presentation • Diagnosis

Noncardiac chest pain (NCCP) is not only a difficult disorder to define but is also complex in characterization and treatment.[1–3] It represents a symptom of chest pain not of cardiac etiology characterized as burning or squeezing in nature with or without radiation. A cardiac cause must be ruled out in every patient in whom a work-up of potential NCCP is being considered. Approximately 20% to 30% of patients with chest pain have normal cardiac catheterization and may be classified as NCCP, representing more than 200,000 new cases annually in the United States.[4] Patients with NCCP are a challenge to primary care and subspecialty services such as cardiology and gastroenterology. These patients are likely to have a high level of health care use and undergo many tests and empiric therapies, and they are usually poorly satisfied with the care provided.[5] NCCP is often a heterogeneous disorder with many potential causes including gastroenterologic diagnoses (**Box 1**).

Gastroesophageal reflux disease (GERD) represents 1 of the most common gastroenterologic causes of NCCP.[1–3] Nearly 25% to 60% of patients with NCCP have abnormal prolonged ambulatory pH findings.[6] In this group of patients, the presence of baseline heartburn may be helpful but not definitive for the association of GERD with patients' chest pain episodes. The current dilemma in this disorder is identifying when GERD may be responsible for the patient's presentation and what to do if empiric therapy fails to resolve the patient's symptoms. This article presents the current evidence for GERD as a cause of NCCP and highlights the best currently available tests for this group of patients.

Division of Gastroenterology, Hepatology and Nutrition, Center for Swallowing and Esophageal Disorders, Vanderbilt University Medical Center, TVC 1660, Nashville, TN 37232-5280, USA
* Corresponding author.
E-mail address: Michael.vaezi@vanderbilt.edu

Med Clin N Am 94 (2010) 233–242
doi:10.1016/j.mcna.2010.01.001
0025-7125/10/$ – see front matter © 2010 Elsevier Inc. All rights reserved.

Box 1
Potential gastroenterologic causes of NCCP

- Gastroesophageal reflux disease (GERD)
- Esophageal motility disorder
- Esophageal hypersensitivity
- Biliary colic
- Pancreatitis
- Hepatitis
- Pneumoperitoneum
- Peptic ulcer disease
- Splenomegaly

CLINICAL PRESENTATION

GERD-related NCCP may resemble angina. The pain may be described as squeezing or burning in the substernal location with possible radiation to the neck, arms or back. It may be worse postprandially and in the supine position and occasionally post exercise or during emotional stress. Heavy exercise may induce the typical symptoms of GERD, such as heartburn and regurgitation, and may cause NCCP. The pain may last minutes or hours and may be intermittent for days. Symptoms usually resolve with antacids, proton pump inhibitors (PPIs), or rest. The presence of typical GERD symptoms such as heartburn and regurgitation are independently associated with NCCP[7] although they do not predict response to PPI therapy. In a population study by Eslick[1] 53% and 58% of patients with NCCP had concomitant heartburn and regurgitation. Therefore, both conditions may coexist but the causal link may be more difficult to establish. In a recent study[8] the presence of classic reflux symptoms and response to antacid therapy were important in establishing GERD-related NCCP.

PATHOPHYSIOLOGY

An esophageal origin for recurring NCCP was considered likely by William Osler in 1892 who first suggested that esophageal spasm might play a role in patients' symptoms. However, later studies using ambulatory pH monitoring tests and pressure monitoring suggested that reflux of gastric content, mainly acid, may be the most common cause of patients' symptoms of chest pain.[1–3] Chemostimulation and mechanostimulation are the 2 broad concepts put forward as the main pathogenesis of reflux-induced symptoms.[9,10] Esophageal pain may be a manifestation of nociceptor activation by chemoreceptors responding to chemical or thermal stimulation or mechanostimulation responding to esophageal wall stretch.[11] Once activated, the receptors transmit their signal through small unmyelinated C-fibers; the pain is usually perceived as dull, burning, gradual, and poorly localized. In contrast, when the signals are transmitted with myelinated fibers, the perception is of sharp, sudden, and well-localized pain. The activated esophageal wall nociceptors transmit their signal peripherally and centrally. The latter is required for pain perception. It is suggested that, because the esophagus and heart share a common innervation, esophageal nociceptor activation may influence coronary circulation.[12] In this study, the investigators found a significant reduction in coronary blood flow with esophageal acid perfusion, which was also associated with typical angina pain. This finding was attributed to an esophagocardiac inhibitory reflex. Similar reduction in coronary blood flow was identified by Rosztoczy and colleagues[13] in 45% of patients with NCCP.

GERD may also cause a hypersensitivity response manifested as NCCP. Peripheral sensitization of esophageal sensory afferents may lead to heightened response to even normal physiologic acid reflux. Infusion of 0.1 N hydrochloric acid in normal subjects was found to reduce the perception threshold for pain.[14,15] The reduction in the pain threshold is most likely caused by increased central excitability by activation of the nociceptive C-fibers. Some also suggest autonomic dysfunction in patients with NCCP.[16] In a study of NCCP and healthy volunteers, Tougas and colleagues[16] showed that patients with acid sensitivity had a higher baseline heart rate and lower baseline vagal activity than acid-insensitive patients. Acid perfusion cardiac outflow increased in patients with acid sensitivity and not in those with insensitive esophagus.

Distention of the esophagus may also play a role in spatial summation, as a result of input from multiple neuronal cells that are more in the upper striated muscle part of the esophagus. Esophageal distention with or without priming of esophageal mucosa by exposure to gastric content has some effect on the mechanostimulator pathway of GERD. The biomechanical and sensory characteristics of the upper, middle, and distal esophagus of 11 healthy volunteers were evaluated by Patel and Rao.[17] This group reported a lower threshold of pain sensation in the proximal esophagus compared with the other esophageal segments and postulated that the proximal esophagus might have a larger number of mechanoreceptors than the distal esophagus with distention in the proximal esophagus contributing to the generation of symptoms during a reflux.[17] The priming of the esophagus after exposure to gastric content was evaluated by Fass and colleagues[18] and DeVault[19] who unlike Mehta and colleagues[20] and Peghini and colleagues[21] found no accentuation of mechanical stimulation after acid exposure. Sarkar and colleagues[22] demonstrated induction of hypersensitivity in the proximal esophagus after exposure of distal esophagus to hydrochloric acid suggesting that the latency of esophageal evoked potential is reduced thus leading to visceral hypersensitivity. Sustained contraction of the esophageal longitudinal muscle is also suggested as a potential causative factor in patients with NCCP.[23] In this study, the investigators suggested that heartburn was associated with short duration of contraction and chest pain was associated with longer contraction duration.

In addition to reflux of acid, nonacid causes may be important in NCCP. Siddiqui and colleagues[24] assessed the causative role of bile acids in esophageal symptoms with a modified Bernstein acid-infusion test and esophageal barostat balloon distensions, in healthy individuals and patients with nonerosive disease. 0.1 M hydrochloric acid; 2 mM and 5 mM chenodexycholic acid and ursodeoxycholic acid infusions were used at least 7 days apart. Significantly higher pain thresholds (with regard to volume and time) were found for ursodeoxycholic acid than for chenodexycholic acid, than for acid infusion, suggesting a possible role for bile acids in the generation of esophageal symptoms and pain.[24]

DIAGNOSTIC TESTING

Given the lack of sensitivity of the current diagnostic testing in NCCP, no test can be considered as the gold standard. The most commonly used tests include barium swallow, upper endoscopy, ambulatory pH (with or without impedance monitoring), and PPI trial. Barium esophagram has a low sensitivity (20%–30%) in diagnosing GERD,[25,26] and should be considered when there is an associated complication such as dysphagia in patients with GERD or NCCP. In addition, reflux of barium during an esophagram is of questionable significance and can seen in up to 20% of healthy people.[27] Upper endoscopy is valuable for diagnosing esophageal mucosal injury related to GERD such as erosive esophagitis, ulceration, peptic stricture, and Barrett esophagus. However, patients with NCCP have lower incidence of esophageal findings at endoscopy. Thus, the clinical yield of this test is low in this group of patients.[28]

Ambulatory 24-hour pH monitoring is regarded as an important physiologic test in diagnosing GERD. It has a sensitivity ranging from 79% to 96% and specificity from 85% to 100%.[29–31] Normal pH findings on 24-hour esophageal pH monitoring are present in up to 25% of patients with erosive esophagitis and 50% of patients with nonerosive reflux disease.[32–34] This is most commonly caused by diet and lifestyle modification during the study period as a result of the nasopharyngeal location of the traditional pH catheter. The introduction of a wireless ambulatory pH capsule and longer duration (48 hours) of recording has somewhat improved the sensitivity of pH testing.[35] In patients with NCCP, pH monitoring is abnormal in 50% to 60% of patients. Hewson and colleagues[36] reported prevalence of abnormal pH in 48% of 100 patients with NCCP; 60% had a positive symptom index (SI). The overzealous conclusion from this study was that pH monitoring and SI measurement is the single best test in patients with NCCP. However, a subsequent study did not confirm these conclusions[37] reporting that SI positivity was not a common occurrence in NCCP. Multichannel intraluminal impedance with a pH sensor allows the detection of acidic and weakly acidic reflux.[38] This recent technique dramatically improved the detection of reflux, regardless of its pH. Well-controlled studies in NCCP patients using impedance monitoring are needed to assess the role of weakly or nonacid reflux.

The PPI trial is currently the most attractive alternative to the modalities discussed earlier because it combines knowledge of symptomatic response with a therapeutic trial of acid suppression. The test uses a short course of high dose PPI to diagnose GERD in those with NCCP. The main requirement of the PPI trial is to achieve a significant symptomatic improvement from as many patients as possible within a short time period. Diagnostic accuracy of a PPI trial is summarized in **Table 1**.[32,39–44] In most studies the test was considered to be positive if symptom assessment scores improved by 50% to 75% compared with baseline. Overall these trials suggest a sensitivity ranging from 69% to 92% and a specificity ranging from 67% to 86% for a PPI trial in NCCP. A recent meta-analysis[45] of randomized controlled studies in NCCP suggested that PPI therapy reduces symptoms in NCCP and may be useful as a diagnostic test in identifying abnormal esophageal acid reflux. The study reported a pooled risk ratio for continued chest pain after PPI therapy of 0.54 (95% confidence interval [CI] 0.41–0.71). The overall number to treat to achieve benefit was 3 (95% CI 2–4). The pooled sensitivity, specificity, and diagnostic odds ratio for the PPI test versus pH monitoring and esophagogastroduodenoscopy (EGD) were 80%, 73%, and 14% (95% CI 5.5–34.9). However, the studies were heterogeneous and small in sample size with evidence of publication bias. In a different meta-analysis,[46] the investigators used 6 of the published controlled trials and found that the use of a PPI trial as a diagnostic test for GERD in NCCP has an acceptable sensitivity and specificity and may be used as an initial test. The investigators reported an overall sensitivity and specificity of 80% and 74%. The PPI trial showed significant higher discriminative power with a summary diagnostic odds ratio of 19.4 (95% CI 8.5–43.8) compared with 0.61 (95% CI 0.2–1.9) in the placebo group. Thus, there seems to be adequate evidence in support of a PPI trial as the initial test of choice in patients with NCCP to assess if symptoms may be from GERD and this may be cost effective.[32,47] The PPI test saved US$575 per patient with NCCP and the test was associated with 79% and 81% reduction in the use of pH monitoring and EGD, respectively.

Table 1
PPI trial studies in NCCP

References	Dosing	No. of Patients	Symptom Improvement (%)	Sensitivity (%)	Specificity (%)
Young et al[39]	Omeprazole 80 mg/d 1 day	30	75	90	80
Squillace et al[40]	Omeprazole 80 mg/d 1 day	17	50	69	75
Xia et al[41]	Lansoprazole 30 mg/d 4 weeks	68	50	92	67
Pandak et al[42]	Omeprazole 40 mg twice a day 2 weeks	37	50	90	67
Fass et al[32]	Omeprazole 40 mg every morning and 20 mg every evening 7 days	37	50	78	86
Fass et al[43]	Lansoprazole 60 mg every morning and 30 mg every evening 7 days	40	50	78	82
Fass et al[44]	Rabaprazole 20 mg every morning and 20 mg every evening 7 days	20	50	83	75

Provocative tests such as the edrophonium test (Tensilon test) or the Bernstein test are no longer recommended or commonly used in the evaluation of patients with NCCP. Edrophonium, a short-acting acetylcholinesterase inhibitor, increases esophageal motility by increasing the amplitude and duration of esophageal contractions.[1] This test initially showed clinical presentation of chest pain in 50% of patients; however, a response to this test does not indicate a motility disorder as the cause of the patients' symptoms. The Bernstein test requires perfusion of 0.1 N hydrochloric acid into the esophagus in an attempt to reproduce the patients' symptoms of NCCP if GERD related. It has low sensitivity and with the emergence of PPIs it has become less valuable in NCCP.

MANAGEMENT

In patients with NCCP in whom a PPI trial is successful in improving symptoms, tapering of the dose of PPI to once daily and subsequently to the minimal dose of acid suppression is recommended. The role of lifestyle modification in GERD and even in NCCP is questionable.[48] The recent American Gastroenterological Association guidelines for treating GERD question the role of lifestyle changes such as raising the head of the bed, avoiding fat, chocolate, alcohol, caffeine, mints, or garlic.[48] There is no concrete evidence for their effectiveness. However, weight loss in those who may be overweight or obese is recommended and may result in improvement of GERD and subsequently NCCP. Similarly, given the lower efficacy of H2-receptor antagonists

(H2RAs) in suppressing acid, it is intuitive that they may not result in as great a benefit in symptom relief as PPIs if GERD is the cause of patients' presenting NCCP. H2RAs have shown a limited response in this group of patients. In a small uncontrolled study by Stahl and colleagues,[49] 13 patient with NCCP were treated with ranitidine 150 mg orally four times a day. Seven of the 13 patients did not respond but increasing the dose resulted in a clinical response in all patients. This study highlights the need for aggressive acid suppression initially in this group of patients. In addition to less aggressive acid suppression by H2RAs, tolerance usually develops with these agents after 2–3 weeks of repeated use resulting in decline in efficacy. Therefore, the initial use of PPIs in NCCP is the preferred initial approach.

The role of pH and/or impedance monitoring in those unresponsive to aggressive acid suppression is to often document normality rather than abnormal results. One important clinical question in the management of patients unresponsive to a PPI trial is if pH monitoring should be performed on or off PPI therapy. The answer to this question is currently controversial but the most recent study using impedance monitoring on therapy and wireless pH monitoring off therapy suggests that a combined approach may be necessary.[50] Pritchett and colleagues[50] studied 39 patients with refractory extraesophageal symptoms with impedance/pH monitoring on twice daily PPIs, and then the same patients were evaluated with wireless pH monitoring off acid suppressive therapy. The study showed that on-therapy impedance testing was normal in 64% of patients, whereas off PPI therapy resulted in normal pH findings in only 28% of patients (**Fig. 1**). Thus, in most patients with persistent throat symptoms, on-therapy testing is more likely to exclude GERD as the cause than off-therapy pH testing. If impedance/pH testing is negative in these patients, diagnosis other than reflux should be considered.

An algorithm for the treatment of patients with NCCP is presented in **Fig. 2**. Given the beneficial response and more aggressive acid suppression with PPIs and that PPIs are also used as a diagnostic test to determine the cause of NCCP, an initial trial of 1 to 2 months of PPI therapy is a reasonable approach (see **Fig. 2**). In patients who respond to PPI therapy, tapering the dose to minimal acid suppression should be attempted. If patients do not improve after 2 months of therapy with PPIs, diagnostic testing such as pH monitoring or impedance pH monitoring may be useful in assessing if the patient's acid or nonacid reflux is controlled while on therapy. Impedance/pH monitoring (if available) or pH monitoring should be used while patients are on therapy to assess for continued reflux. If this test is normal then a search for causes other than

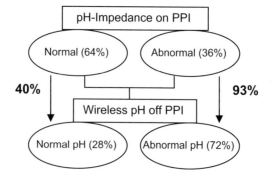

Fig. 1. The likelihood of abnormal pH off therapy if abnormal impedance on therapy was present. Efficacy of esophageal impedance/pH monitoring in patients with refractory GERD, on and off therapy.

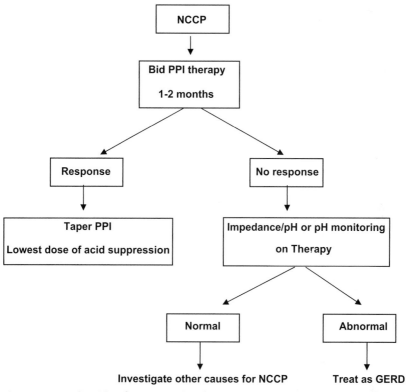

Fig. 2. Treatment algorithm for GERD-related NCCP.

GERD should be initiated. pH testing off PPI therapy will only assess the presence of acid reflux at baseline but does not suggest a causal link between GERD and NCCP. Surgical fundoplication cannot be recommended if patients do not respond to PPI therapy. In a selected population of patients (those responsive to PPI therapy) surgical success is to be expected similar to typical GERD.[51]

SUMMARY

In patients with NCCP the most important clinical consideration is to rule out a cardiac cause given its life-threatening nature. Because many patients with NCCP may not present with the classic symptom of GERD, an empiric trial with PPI therapy can be used as a diagnostic test and as therapy. Twice daily PPI therapy is recommended for 1 to 2 months. Diagnostic testing such as EGD, pH, or impedance monitoring is predominately used for those unresponsive to PPI therapy. Response to PPI therapy can suggest a possible causal link between GERD and NCCP and lack of response should prompt a search for other causes of NCCP.

REFERENCES

1. Eslick GE. Non-cardiac chest pain: epidemiology and natural history, health care seeking and quality of life. Gastroenterol Clin North Am 2004;33:1–23.
2. Richter JE. Chest pain and gastroesophageal reflux disease. J Clin Gastroenterol 2000;30:S39–41.

3. Fass R, Hyun JG, Sewell JL. Pathophysiology of non-cardiac chest pain. In: Fass R, Eslick G, editors. Non cardiac chest pain, a growing medical problem. San Diego (CA): Plural Publishing; 2007. p. 25–37.

4. Lawrence L, National Center for Health Statistics. Detailed diagnoses and procedures for patients discharged from short stay hospitals, United States, 1984. Hyattsville (MD): US Department of Health and Human Services, Public Health Services; 1986. Vital and Health Statistics, Series 13:86.

5. Richter JE, Bradley LA, Castell DO. Esophageal chest pain: current controversies in pathogenenesis, diagnosis and therapy. Ann Intern Med 1989;110:68–78.

6. Richter JE. Approach to the patient with non-cardiac chest pain. In: Yamada T, editor. Textbook of gastroenterology. 2nd edition. Philadelphia: JB Lippincott; 1995. p. 648–76.

7. Lock G, Talley NJ, Fett SI, et al. Prevalence and clinical spectrum of gastroesophageal reflux: a population based study in Olmstead County, Minnesota. Gastroenterology 1997;112:1448–56.

8. Mousavi S, Tosi J, Eskandarian R, et al. Role of clinical presentation in diagnosing reflux related non-cardiac chest pain. J Gastroenterol Hepatol 2007;22:218–21.

9. Fass R, Tougas G. Functional heartburn: the stimulus, the pain and the brain. Gut 2002;51:885–92.

10. Orlando RC. Current understanding of the mechanisms of gastro-oesophageal reflux disease. Drugs 2006;66(Suppl 1):1–5.

11. Orlando RC. Esophageal perception and non-cardiac chest pain. Gastroenterol Clin North Am 2004;33:25–33.

12. Chauhan A, Petch MC, Schofield PM. Cardio-esophageal reflex in humans as a mechanism for "linked angina". Eur Heart J 1996;17:407–13.

13. Rosztoczy A, Vass A, Izbeki F, et al. The evaluation of gastroesophageal reflux and esophagocardiac reflex in patients with angina-like chest pain following cardiologic investigations. Int J Cardiol 2007;118:62–8.

14. Hu WH, Martin CJ, Talley NJ. Intra-esophageal acid perfusion sensitizes the esophagus to mechanical distension: a barostat study. Am J Gastroenterol 2000;95:2189–94.

15. Sarkar S, Aziz Q, Woolf CJ, et al. Contribution of central sensitization to the development of non-cardiac chest pain. Lancet 2000;356:1154–9.

16. Tougas G, Spaziani R, Hollerback S, et al. Cardiac autonomic function and esophageal acid sensitivity in patients with non-cardiac chest pain. Gut 2001;49:706–12.

17. Patel S, Rao S. Biomechanical and sensory parameters of the human esophagus at four levels. Am J Physiol Gastrointest Liver Physiol 1998;275:G187–91.

18. Fass R, Naliboff B, Higa L, et al. Differential effect of long-term esophageal acid exposure on mechanosensitivity and chemosensitivity in humans. Gastroenterology 1998;115:1363–73.

19. DeVault KR. Acid infusion does not affect intra-esophageal balloon distension induced sensory and pain thresholds. Am J Gastroenterol 1997;92:947–9.

20. Mehta AJ, De Caestecker JS, Camm AJ, et al. Sensitization to painful distension and abnormal sensory perception in the esophagus. Gastroenterology 1995;108:311–9.

21. Peghini PL, Johnston BT, Leite LP, et al. Mucosal acid exposure sensitizes a subset of normal subjects to intra-oesophageal balloon distension. Eur J Gastroenterol Hepatol 1996;8:979–83.

22. Sarkar S, Hobson AR, Furlong PL, et al. Central neural mechanisms mediating human visceral hypersensitivity. Am J Physiol Gastrointest Liver Physiol 2001;281:G1196–202.

23. Balaban DH, Yamamoto Y, Liu J, et al. Sustained esophageal contraction: a marker of esophageal chest pain identified by intraluminal ultrasonography. Gastroenterology 1999;116:29–37.
24. Siddiqui A, Rodriguez-Stanley S, Zubaidi S, et al. Esophageal visceral sensitivity to bile salts in patients with functional heartburn and in healthy control subjects. Dig Dis Sci 2005;50:81–5.
25. Johnston BT, Troshinksy MB, Catell JA, et al. Comparison of barium radiology with esophageal pH monitoring in the diagnosis of gastroesophageal reflux disease. Am J Gastroenterol 1996;91:1181–5.
26. Joseph S, Hirano I. Gastroesophageal reflux disease: diagnosis. In: Fass R, editor. GERD/dyspepsia: hot topics. Philadelphia: Hanley & Belfus; 2004. p. 41–54.
27. Wu W. Ancillary tests in the diagnosis of gastroesophageal reflux disease. Gastroenterol Clin North Am 1990;19:671–82.
28. Fang J, Bjorkman D. A critical approach to non-cardiac chest pain: pathophysiology, diagnosis and treatment. Am J Gastroenterol 2001;96:958–68.
29. Euler A, Byrne W. Twenty-four-hour esophageal intraluminal pH probe testing: a comparative analysis. Gastroenterology 1981;80:957–61.
30. Richter J, Castell DO. Gastroesophageal reflux. Pathogenesis, diagnosis, and therapy. Ann Intern Med 1982;97:93–103.
31. Behar J, Biancani P, Sheahan D. Evaluation of esophageal tests in the diagnosis of reflux esophagitis. Gastroenterology 1976;71:9–15.
32. Fass R, Fennerty M, Ofman J, et al. The clinical and economic value of a short course of omeprazole in patients with non-cardiac chest pain. Gastroenterology 1998;115:42–9.
33. Schenk B, Kuipers E, Klinkenberg-Knol E, et al. Omeprazole as a diagnostic tool in gastroesophageal reflux disease. Am J Gastroenterol 1997;92:1997–2000.
34. Martinez S, Malagon I, Garewal HS, et al. Non-erosive reflux disease (NERD)-acid reflux and symptom patterns. Aliment Pharmacol Ther 2003;17:537–45.
35. Des Varannes SB, Mion F, Ducrotté P, et al. Simultaneous recording of oesophageal acid exposure with conventional pH monitoring and a wireless system (Bravo). Gut 2005;54:1682–6.
36. Hewson EG, Sinclari JW, Dalton CB, et al. Twenty-four hour esophageal pH monitoring: the most useful test for evaluating non cardiac chest pain. Am J Med 1991;90:576–83.
37. Dekel R, Martinex-Hawthorne SD, Guillen RJ, et al. Evaluation of symptom index in identifying gastroesophageal reflux disease related non cardiac chest pain. J Clin Gastroenterol 2004;38:24–9.
38. Vela MF, Camacho-Lobato L, Srinivasan R, et al. Simultaneous intra-esophageal impedance and pH measurement of acid and nonacid gastroesophageal reflux: effect of omeprazole. Gastroenterology 2001;120:1599–606.
39. Young M, Sanowski R, Talbert G, et al. Omeprazole administration as a test for gastroesophageal reflux. Gastroenterology 1992;102:A192.
40. Squillace S, Young M, Sanowski R. Single dose omeprazole as test for non cardiac chest pain. Gastroenterology 1993;107:A197.
41. Xia H, Lai K, Lam KF, et al. Symptomatic response to lansoprazole predicts abnormal acid reflux in endoscopy negative patients with non cardiac chest pain. Aliment Pharmacol Ther 2003;17:369–77.
42. Pandak W, Arezo S, Everett S, et al. Short course of omeprazole: a better first diagnostic approach to non-cardiac chest pain than endoscopy, manometry or 24-hour esophageal pH monitoring. J Clin Gastroenterol 2002;35:307–14.
43. Fass R, Pulliam G, Haden C. Patients with non cardiac chest pain receiving an empirical trial of high dose lansoprazole, demonstrate early symptom

response – a double blind, placebo controlled trial. Gastroenterology 2001; 120(A221):1162.

44. Fass R, Fullerton H, Hayden C, et al. Patients with non cardiac chest pain receiving an empiric trial of high dose rabeprazole, demonstrate early symptom response – a double blind placebo controlled trial. Gastroenterology 2002;122: A580–1 W1175.

45. Cremonini F, Wise J, Moayyedi P, et al. Meta-analysis: diagnostic and therapeutic use of proton pump inhibitors in on-cardiac chest pain. Am J Gastroenterol 2005; 100:1226–32.

46. Wang W, Huang J, Zheng G. Is proton pump inhibitor testing an effective approach to diagnose gastroesophageal reflux disease in patients with non-cardiac chest pain? A meta analysis. Arch Intern Med 2005;165:1222–8.

47. Ofman J, Grlnek IM, Udani J. The cost effectiveness of the omeprazole test in non-cardiac chest pain. Am J Med 1999;107:219–27.

48. Kahrilas P, Shaheen N, Vaezi MF. AGA medical position statement on the management of gastroesophageal reflux disease. Gastroenterology 2008;135: 1383–91.

49. Stahl WG, Beton RR, Johnson CS, et al. Diagnosis and treatment of patients with gastroesophageal reflux and non-cardiac chest pain. South Med J 1994;87: 739–42.

50. Pritchett JM, Aslam M, Slaughter JC, et al. Efficacy of esophageal impedance/pH monitoring in patients with refractory gastroesophageal reflux disease, on and off therapy. Clin Gastroenterol Hepatol 2009;7(7):743–8.

51. Farrell TM, Richardson WS, Trus TL, et al. Response of atypical symptoms of gastroesophageal reflux to antireflux surgery. Br J Surg 2001;88:1649–52.

Dysphagia as a Cause of Chest Pain: An Otolaryngologist's View

Julia Vent, MD, PhD[a], Simon F. Preuss, MD, PhD[a],
Guy D. Eslick, PhD, MMedSc (Clin Epi), MMedStat[b,c,d],*

KEYWORDS

- Dysphagia • Chest pain • Differential diagnosis
- Esophagoscopy

Dysphagia is an important alarm symptom, as is chest pain. The combination of the two can pose difficulties in terms of diagnosis due to the causal relationship between the two conditions (**Fig. 1**). The main diagnosis to rule out in a patient presenting with retrosternal chest pain is a myocardial infarction, a medical emergency usually treated in the emergency department, for which no time may be wasted or lost. Patients presenting with dysphagia, that is, difficulty and pain when swallowing, must undergo a thorough clinical and diagnostic evaluation. When presenting to an otolaryngologist, the physical examination includes direct and indirect laryngoscopy in the awake and cooperative patient. Further, a rigid hypopharyngoscopy and esophagoscopy must be performed under general anesthesia, if all other possible causes for dysphagia, such as neurologic or cardiac causes, are ruled out. Dysphagia is an alarm signal, because (eg, in the case of a foreign body aspiration) it can result in the perforation of the hypopharynx, with consequent mediastinitis or pneumonia and lethal sepsis.

EPIDEMIOLOGY
Prevalence

There is a lack of studies documenting the epidemiology of dysphagia.[1] There are of course numerous patient-based reports of dysphagia being associated with

[a] Department of Otorhinolaryngology, Head and Neck Surgery, University of Hospital Cologne, Kerpener Street 62, Cologne 50924, Germany
[b] School of Public Health, The University of Sydney, New South Wales, Australia
[c] Department of Gastroenterology, Nepean Clinical School, The University of Sydney, New South Wales, Australia
[d] Program in Molecular and Genetic Epidemiology, Harvard School of Public Health, 677 Huntington Avenue, Building 2, 2nd Floor, Room 209, Boston, MA 02115, USA
* Corresponding author. Program in Molecular and Genetic Epidemiology, Harvard School of Public Health, 677 Huntington Avenue, Building 2, 2nd Floor, Room 209, Boston, MA 02115.
E-mail address: geslick@hsph.harvard.edu

Med Clin N Am 94 (2010) 243–257
doi:10.1016/j.mcna.2010.01.009
0025-7125/10/$ – see front matter Crown Copyright © 2010 Published by Elsevier Inc. All rights reserved.

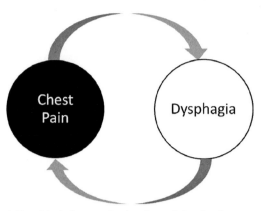

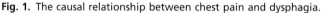

Fig. 1. The causal relationship between chest pain and dysphagia.

cerebrovascular accidents, Parkinson disease, and esophageal malignancy, to mention a few.[2,3] Population-based studies are rare, with only a few currently published.[4–8] Moreover, the estimated prevalence of dysphagia in these studies was between 6% and 22%, which is somewhat high.

A Swedish study of 2329 individuals older than 55 years found that almost one-third (27%) had esophageal dysfunction and 13% with normal esophageal function had dysphagia. No mention was made of differences in prevalence by gender, but the overall prevalence was reported as 22.3%.[4] Bloem and colleagues[5] conducted a study of 130 elderly individuals (aged >87 years) from the Netherlands and observed that 16% had symptoms of dysphagia, but that these symptoms were not associated with age, gender, or mental status. A larger study (n = 556) of 50- to 79-year-old individuals in the community reported that a very small number (1.6%) had obstructive symptoms and just over one-fifth (20.9%) had globus sensation that increased slightly with increasing age.[6] In a United States study of 1021 individuals aged 30 to 64 years, functional gastrointestinal symptoms were determined and 6% of individuals reported trouble swallowing more than a quarter of the time.[7] A Japanese study of elderly people (aged >65 years; n = 1313) living at home reported that 13.8% had symptoms of dysphagia.[8]

In a more recent population-based study that focused on dysphagia, it was determined that among an adult population 18 years and older the prevalence of dysphagia was 17%, showing a positively skewed distribution (**Fig. 2**) with high rates among younger age groups, with a peak in the 40- to 49-year age group for both males (28%) and females (34%).[9] This study was the first to assess dysphagia among younger adults in a community sample. All previous studies had assessed dysphagia among older adults, usually older than 50 years, due to the belief that it was more common in this age range; however, this finding highlighted that dysphagia is prevalent among younger individuals in the community.

Risk Factors

Risk factors associated with dysphagia have been largely unexplored. There have only been 7 studies looking at risk factors related to dysphagia, with all of these published after 2003. The main focus of these studies was spinal surgery (n = 3),[10–12] stroke (n = 1),[13] pediatrics (n = 1),[14] geriatrics (n = 1),[15] chemoradiotherapy (n = 1),[16] and dysphagia (n = 1).[9] Risk factors identified from these studies included larger radiation

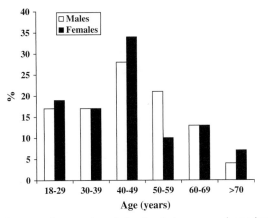

Fig. 2. The population prevalence rates of dysphagia by age and gender. (*From* Eslick GD, Talley NJ. Dysphagia: epidemiology, risk factors and impact on quality of life—a population-based study. Aliment Pharmacol Ther 2008;27(10):971–9; with permission.)

portal field,[16] stroke, esophageal reflux, chronic obstructive pulmonary disease,[15] advanced age, diabetes mellitus, large infarcts,[13] unexplained respiratory problems,[14] duration of pain and number of vertebral levels, gender, revision surgeries, and multi-level surgeries.[10–12]

A recent population-based study reported that hypertension was a risk factor for dysphagia (odds ratio [OR] = 2.58, 95% confidence interval [CI]: 1.22–5.44),[9] while it is known that dysphagia has been reported as a complication of stroke.[13] However, hypertension per se has not been previously reported, and it must be noted that some potential confounders (ie, body mass index, diet, alcohol intake, nonsteroidal anti-inflammatory drug use) could not be adjusted for in this study. In addition, this study reported several other independent risk factors including odynophagia with gastro-esophageal reflux (OR = 3.41, 95% CI: 1.16–10.04), intermittent dysphagia with gastroesophageal reflux (OR = 2.96, 95% CI: 1.76–4.98), anxiety (OR = 1.09, 95% CI: 1.01–1.19), and a reduction in the "role physical" subscale (OR = 0.98, 95% CI: 0.97–0.99), while progressive dysphagia was associated with depression (OR = 1.34, 95% CI: 1.07–1.67) and reduced "general health" (OR = 0.95, 95% CI: 0.90–0.99).

Dysphagia and Chest Pain

Dysphagia has been reported as a risk factor for noncardiac chest pain in the community.[17] This study consisted of 1000 adult (>18 years old) individuals randomly selected from the Sydney population. The analysis revealed that dysphagia was associated with an almost 2.5-fold increased risk of chest pain (OR = 2.43, 95% CI: 1.54–3.84). Moreover, individuals experiencing an increased frequency of dysphagia (OR = 2.52, 95% CI: 1.63–3.89) and increased severity of dysphagia (OR = 1.95, 95% CI: 1.03–3.67) were more likely to have chest pain. It must be borne in mind that whereas chest pain is a common symptom that is very heterogeneous, (Guy D. Eslick, unpublished data, 2009) suggest that dysphagia is more common among patients with noncardiac chest pain (OR = 2.16, 95% CI: 1.02–4.73) than those with cardiac chest pain (OR = 0.73, 95% CI: 0.33–1.63) and even angiographically proven coronary heart disease (OR = 0.43, 95% CI: 0.23–0.94).

ANATOMY OF THE UPPER DIGESTIVE TRACT AND UPPER AIRWAYS

The upper digestive tract starts with lips, teeth, hard and soft palate including uvula, mandible, and maxilla. The floor of mouth and tongue are constructed of multiple muscles and connective tissue, as well as the palatine tonsils, and are covered by non-keratinizing, squamous cell epithelium. The pharynx consists of 3 pharyngeal constrictor muscles forming the superior pharyngeal constrictor, which causes elevation and contraction of the velum. This process achieves complete closure of the velo-pharyngeal port, and is facilitated by the contraction of the superior pharyngeal constrictor, which narrows the pharynx.

The medial and inferior pharyngeal constrictors initiate the pharyngeal peristalsis. The food bolus and saliva are carried by sequential peristaltic action of the middle and inferior pharyngeal constrictors into and through the pharynx to the cricopharyngeal sphincter.

The esophagus consists of 3 major narrowings, the first one being the cricopharyngeal sphincter, the second at the height of the aortic arch (with proximity of the right ventricle), and the third at the sphincter and entrance to the stomach.

The larynx is made up of thyroid cartilage, where fibers of the inferior constrictor attach to the sides of the thyroid cartilage anteriorly. Lateral of the thyroid cartilage are the piriform sinuses, which end inferiorly at the cricopharyngeus muscle, the most inferior structure of the pharynx, which serves as the valve at the top of the esophagus. The pharyngeal constrictors insert into the thyroid cartilage anteriorly to form the piriform sinuses. The uppermost structure of the larynx is the epiglottis, which rests against the base of the tongue. A wedge-shaped space called the vallecula is formed between the base of the tongue and epiglottis bilaterally. The valleculae and the piriform sinuses are known as the pharyngeal recesses or side pockets, into which food may fall and reside before or after the swallowing reflex is triggered. This area comprises the space where tumors can originate from or foreign bodies may get stuck.

On contraction, the pharyngoesophageal sphincter or juncture (P-E segment) prevents air from entering the esophagus during respiration and material from refluxing back up the esophagus and into the pharynx. The esophagus is a 23- to 25-cm long, hollow muscular tube.

PHYSIOLOGY OF THE SWALLOWING PROCESS

The swallowing process transports saliva or ingested material from the mouth to the stomach. The preparatory phase consists of taking material into the mouth; the food is chewed, mixed with saliva, and usually positioned on top of the anterior tongue in anticipation of a swallow. At the onset of a normal swallowing act, the tip of the tongue is pushed against the superior incisors or maxillary alveolar ridge. A semisolid or liquid bolus is cupped within a depression of the anterior one- to two-thirds of the tongue.[18] During the oral phase of swallowing, the tongue elevates and rolls posteriorly in a peristaltic motion, making sequential contact with the hard and soft palate, thereby propelling the bolus into the pharynx.[19] Entry of the bolus into the pharynx occurs simultaneously with elevation of the soft palate against the posterior pharyngeal wall, sealing the nasopharynx from regurgitation. The pharyngeal phase of swallowing starts as the moving wave of glossopalatal opposition crosses the fauces. Pharyngeal peristalsis continues as the posterior third of the tongue makes sequential descending contact with the posterior wall of the pharynx. Along with this, the pharyngeal constrictors contract in a descending sequence.[20] In the hypopharynx, peristaltic obliteration of the pharyngeal lumen is achieved by opposition of the closed larynx and the inferior pharyngeal constrictor. During the swallow sequence, the upper esophageal sphincter (UES), also termed the pharyngoesophageal sphincter, relaxes for about 0.5 seconds during which transsphincteric flow of a swallowed bolus occurs.[21,22] The transiently relaxed UES, formed mainly by the cricopharyngeus, is opened by anterior traction exerted by the superior-anterior excursion of the hyoid and also by pulsion forces imparted by a swallowed bolus.[23] During the oral and pharyngeal phases of swallowing, the larynx is lifted substantially upward and forward by the combined contraction of the suprahyoid muscles, thyrohyoids, and pharyngeal elevators. This superior-anterior excursion of the larynx not only serves to open the UES by traction but also enlarges the pharynx to receive the bolus, engulfs the bolus, and acts as an ancillary mechanism to protect the larynx against aspiration. The major mechanism preventing aspiration of swallowed material into the larynx is contraction of the intrinsic laryngeal muscles, which approximate the arytenoids and epiglottis, close the false cords, and adduct the vocal cords.[24] Passage of the pharyngeal peristaltic contraction wave through the cricopharyngeus terminates UES relaxation and marks the transition between the pharyngeal and esophageal phases of swallowing.

NOMENCLATURE

Dysphagia is defined by difficulty in swallowing, which can commonly occur, for example, due to a cold or following a stroke, or be caused by reflux disease or a tumor. Dysphagia compromises nutrition and hydration, and may lead to aspiration pneumonia and dehydration.

Aphagia is the inability to swallow. Patients present with drooling, as even their own saliva cannot be swallowed.

DIAGNOSTIC WORKUP

- A patient presenting to the Ear/Nose/Throat (ENT) Department or ENT specialist undergoes a thorough history taking. When did the symptom first occur, for how long does it persist, is the peroral food intake compromised? What is the location or lateralization of the dysphagia? Is it sudden onset or slow progression? Is there regurgitation of digested or undigested food or acid?
- The patient then undergoes a clinical physical examination including indirect laryngoscopy and loupe laryngoscopy. If no saliva remnants or foreign bodies are seen, radiologic examinations are initiated. Methylene blue and food swallow videography via transnasal flexible endoscopy are then performed.
- The radiologic examinations include static imaging of neck and chest (computed tomography [CT]/magnetic resonance), as well as dynamic investigation: A barium swallow (**Fig. 3**) examination and a videocinematograph show the peristalsis of the hypopharynx and esophagus, and may give hints to hypertrophic sphincter foreign bodies and tumors.
- Rigid esophagoscopy and hypopharyngoscopy (panendoscopy) are performed under general anesthesia in cases of suspected foreign body or tumor to facilitate extraction/biopsy.

DIFFERENTIAL DIAGNOSES AND TREATMENT SUGGESTIONS

As inflammatory causes of dysphagia, gastroesophageal reflux disease (GERD) must be primarily mentioned. The reader is referred to the article on GERD elsewhere in this issue.

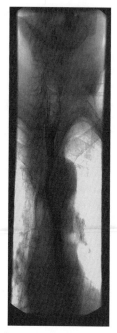

Fig. 3. Example of a physiologic barium swallow examination, showing the physiologic narrowing at the height of the aortic arch.

An underlying infectious cause of esophagitis with chest pain and dysphagia may be Candida esophagitis in the immunosuppressed, but cases of other viral or bacterial infection of the digestive tract are known also in the immunocompetent host.[25] Cardiac causes such as myocardial infarction or right heart hypertrophy can furthermore be the underlying cause of chest pain; however, one assumes that the patient has had a full cardiologic workup (including electrocardiograph, chest radiograph, and echocardiograph) before presenting to the otorhinolaryngologist. A mediastinal mass, such as a thymus tumor (most often a thymoma, lymphoma, or thymus tumor) is ruled out by a chest radiograph. The authors recently reported a patient with a cervical neurofibroma who had presented with progressive chest pain and globus sensation.[26] A recent case report of a rare perforation of the esophagus due to an osteophyte[27] must also be taken into consideration, and is easily diagnosed with a barium swallow and radiograph, as well as rigid panendoscopy. A Zenker diverticulum is diagnosed by a barium swallow radiograph, and usually presents with dysphagia and chest pain, as well as regurgitation of undigested food. Zenker diverticulum is best treated with a myotomy of the cricopharyngeal muscle, which may be performed transorally by laser (**Fig. 4**),[28] or by endoscopic stapler diverticulostomy.[29,30] In specific cases, an open approach via lateral collotomy is performed.

Cancer of the Hypopharynx

Unlike many other cancers of the head and neck area, carcinoma of the hypopharynx is rarely found early when it is small and localized to the site of the primary lesion. More frequently, the patient is not aware of the problem until the tumor is large, obstructive symptoms or pain occurs, and the cancer extends to the adjacent structures and the cervical lymph nodes. The extensive lymphatic drainage of the hypopharynx

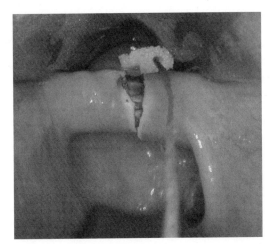

Fig. 4. Intraoperative view of a laser resection of the cricopharyngeal muscle in a Zenker diverticulum. The string gauze protects the esophageal mucosa from injury by a laser beam.

and the cervical esophagus and the long interval during which the tumor is asymptomatic account for the extensive involvement of lymph nodes and adjacent structures at the time of diagnosis.[31] Therefore, hypopharynx tumors often present with dysphagia and aspiration due to infiltration of the arytenoid cartilage and the pharyngoesophageal sphincter. Hypopharyngeal carcinomas metastasize early into the cervical lymph nodes (**Fig. 5**). Specific diagnostic procedures for a staging examination include CT scans of the neck and rigid endoscopy under general anesthesia to facilitate biopsy of the suspected cancer tissues. Staging examinations should include a CT scan of the chest to exclude pulmonary metastases that are seen in about 10% of all cases. Surgery, usually in combination with postoperative radiotherapy/chemotherapy, is

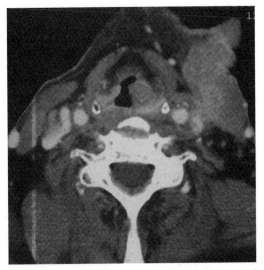

Fig. 5. CT scan of a hypopharyngeal cancer on the left piriform sinus, showing the narrowing of the glottic lumen and a large metastatic cervical lymph node ipsilateral.

believed to provide the highest cure and local control rates in patients with cancer of the hypopharynx.[32–35] Even more important, surgery may immediately provide successful and long-lasting palliation for airway obstruction, obstructive dysphagia, and aspiration because local control is frequently achieved even in locally advanced cancer.[36–40]

Cancer of the Esophagus

In the United States in 2008, the American Cancer Society estimates an incidence of 16,470 new cases (12,970 men and 3500 women) of esophageal cancer; 14,280 persons (11,250 men and 3030 women) are expected to die of the disease. The age-adjusted incidence is 5.8 cases per 100,000 persons.[41] Adenocarcinoma of the esophagus has the fastest growing incidence rate of all cancers in the United States. The prevalence is increasing by approximately 10% per year, which is faster than any other malignancy.[42,43] This increase is largely secondary to the well-established association between gastroesophageal reflux disease, Barrett esophagus, and esophageal adenocarcinoma. Three studies have shown a relationship between frequency of reflux symptoms and risk of adenocarcinoma. The constant acid reflux will irritate the lining of the esophagus, and complications can occur, such as Barrett esophagus. Individuals who develop Barrett esophagus are about 40 times more likely to develop esophageal cancer than individuals in the general population. In Western countries, esophageal cancer has undergone an epidemiologic shift, from predominantly squamous cell carcinoma (SCC) seen in association with tobacco and alcohol abuse to adenocarcinoma associated with Barrett metaplasia, seen almost exclusively in middle-aged Caucasian men with gastroesophageal reflux disease.[44] Symptoms of esophageal cancer include heartburn, pain or discomfort in the chest area, pain in the throat or between the shoulder blade, dysphagia with the inability to swallow solid foods, and regurgitation of undigested food, as well as severe weight loss. If esophageal carcinoma is suspected following characteristic clinical symptoms, a systematic approach to preoperative staging should include esophago-gastroduodenoscopy to obtain the histologic diagnosis of esophageal carcinoma, CT scan of the chest and abdomen, and endoscopic ultrasonography to evaluate the depth of tumor penetration.[45] Surgical resection is the current standard of care for the treatment of patients with resectable esophageal carcinoma, with primary combined-modality therapy reserved for prohibitive surgical candidates. Earlier detection combined with complete surgical extirpation of disease and lower postoperative mortality have all contributed to improved survival, but survival rates still are poor, with an average 5-year overall survival rate of 20% to 25%.[46–49]

Foreign Body of the Hypopharynx or Esophagus

Aspiration of a foreign body or a large bolus of food commonly occurs in children, the elderly, demented people, and patients with esophageal stenoses. The most common foreign body is a fish bone, seen frequently in the ENT clinic. The fish bone is usually stuck in a tonsil or at the base of the tongue, but it may also get stuck in the hypopharynx and especially piriform sinus. In these locations, it is best extracted via rigid endoscopy under general anesthesia. All foreign bodies must be immediately extracted, as they may cause perforation of the mucosa with subsequent perforation of the pharynx or esophagus.

Neurologic Causes of Dysphagia

Neurologic causes of dysphagia include central causes such as stroke, Parkinson disease, or disseminated encephalitis. The diagnoses include electromyography

(EMG), and treatment options include botulinum toxin injection.[50,51] Further, multiple system atrophy (such as amyotrophic lateral sclerosis) may be the disease underlying dysphagia and can be the first presenting symptom, so a neurologic workup is vital.[52]

Motor disorders are characterized by a delayed peristalsis of the esophagus, with consequent slow emptying into the stomach. Achalasia is an esophageal motility disorder characterized by the failure to relax the lower esophagus sphincter in response to swallowing. Primary achalasia, the most common form, has no known underlying cause. Achalasia can also be due to esophageal cancer or Chagas disease (an infectious disease common in South America). Achalasia affects about 1 person in 100,000 per year. Achalasia typically presents in the barium swallow radiograph with a dilated esophagus with a retained column of barium and a tight sphincter known as "bird's beak." Achalasia needs to be treated with a myotomy of the lower esophageal sphincter.[53–55] Functional esophagogastric junction (EGJ) obstruction is characterized by pressure topography metrics demonstrating EGJ outflow obstruction of a magnitude comparable to that seen with post-fundoplication dysphagia. Affected patients experience dysphagia or chest pain. In some cases, functional EGJ obstruction may represent an incomplete achalasia syndrome.[56]

Psychogenic Dysphagia

Last but not least, a globus sensation with concomitant dysphagia can be of psychogenic cause. If after the thorough diagnostic workup no pathologies are found, and the patient complains of a persistent dysphagia (which may not always be painful), an underlying psychogenic disease must be ruled out. The patient should then be referred to a psychiatrist who specializes in psychosomatic disorders for further diagnostics and therapy. Vaiman and colleagues[57,58] studied the EMG examinations of such patients extensively. These investigators showed that psychogenic/hysteria-conversion dysphagia has no pathologic EMG patterns associated with deglutition. Skeletal muscle tension during deglutition, observed in some cases, has no connection with the act of swallowing itself.

SPECIFIC METHODS OF DIAGNOSIS

In all cases, a thorough and interdisciplinary approach can help to optimize diagnosis and treatment. The functional aspects of diagnostics are best shown by a videocinematograph, which is a barium swallow examination recorded as a movie, so that the

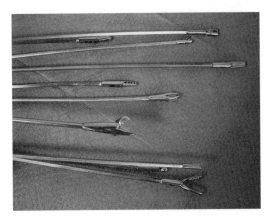

Fig. 6. Various instrument tips for biopsies and extraction of foreign bodies.

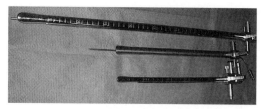

Fig. 7. Rigid esophagoscopes with inserted suction devices and length gradation in centimeters.

treating physicians can slowly, repeatedly, and thoroughly envision the swallowing act of the patient. The radiologist may help identify the origin of the symptoms by interpreting the various radiographic findings in normal and abnormal states of the pharynx.[59]

The surgical equipment and specific otorhinolaryngologic instruments are shown in **Figs. 6–8**. Rigid esophagoscopes are available in different diameters and lengths, depending on the physical size of the patient. Direct laryngoscopes can be fixed during laryngoscopy, so the surgeon can operate bimanually under the operating microscope (**Fig. 9**). It is preferable to perform a rigid panendoscopy rather than a flexible endoscopy in particular cases. The benefits of using rigid instruments include the better unfolding of the mucosa in the hypopharyngeal region, which is additionally more effective in diagnosing a cancerous lesion; moreover, large and pointed foreign bodies (see Clinical Case 1) are more safely and readily extracted. There are numerous instruments specifically designed for the extraction of distinctive foreign bodies and biopsies in rigid endoscopy (see **Fig. 6**). The significance of rigid endoscopy is highlighted by a report on a failed extraction of a sharp esophageal foreign body with a flexible endoscope.[60] Emphysema of the mediastinum and neck can be caused by a perforation of the hypopharynx or trachea as a complication of panendoscopy or,

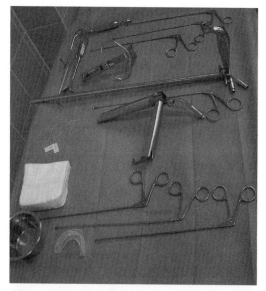

Fig. 8. Instrument table showing all instruments needed for a panendoscopy: silicone tooth guarder, laryngoscope, multiple forceps, esophagoscope, McIvor tongue depressor.

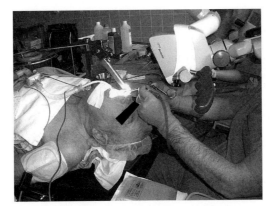

Fig. 9. Direct laryngoscopy allows bimanual, microscopic surgery.

as seen here, by a sharp foreign body aspiration, for example, dentures (**Fig. 10** and Clinical Case 2). The choice of endoscope (rigid vs flexible) should therefore be dictated by the type of foreign body being removed and the location of the foreign body within the esophagus, as well as the experience of the surgeon.[60]

Clinical Case 1

A demented 84-year-old man had been denying any food intake for 2 weeks. This refusal was initially attributed to his dementia and diminished will for life. When he presented with fevers and drooling saliva, chest radiography was performed and revealed a boney mass at the height of the second esophageal sphincter. Rigid panendoscopy evacuated a 2 × 2-cm large chicken bone (**Fig. 11**). This bone had caused necrotic mucositis with perforation into the mediastinum.

Clinical Case 2

A 79-year-old woman presented from a nursing home with chest pain and aphagia that had been persisting for at least 24 hours. She was demented and had denied any food intake, with a progressive loss of the ability to swallow her saliva. Chest radiography was performed because of her rising temperature. The radiograph revealed a metallic mass in the hypopharynx. Rigid esophagoscopy was performed and showed partial dentures in the left piriform sinus, which were extracted by rigid pharyngoscopy without perforation of the hypopharynx. A nasogastric tube was placed and intravenous antibiotics were administered to prevent mediastinitis.

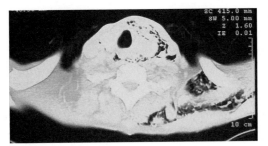

Fig. 10. Emphysema of the neck and mediastinum after perforation of the hypopharynx by a foreign body, with lateroposition of the trachea.

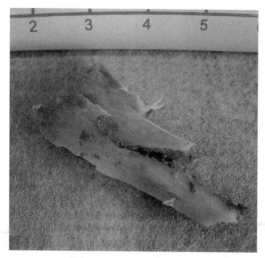

Fig. 11. Chicken bone evacuated from the esophagus in an elderly man. Note the sharp edges. The scale indicates centimeters.

SUMMARY

The various, at times life-threatening conditions causing dysphagia need to be ruled out in a patient presenting with this main symptom. It is thus crucial to perform a thorough history taking, physical examination, and radiologic diagnostic workup. A rigid panendoscopy under general anesthesia is used to diagnose and treat foreign bodies, and to facilitate staging and biopsy in suspected hypopharyngeal or esophageal cancer.

REFERENCES

1. Kuhlemeier KV. Epidemiology and dysphagia. Dysphagia 1994;9(4):209–17.
2. Cook IJ. Oropharyngeal dysphagia. Gastroenterol Clin North Am 2009;38(3): 411–31.
3. Lind CD. Dysphagia: evaluation and treatment. Gastroenterol Clin North Am 2003;32(2):553–75.
4. Kjellen G, Tibbling L. Manometric oesophageal function, acid perfusion test and symptomatology in a 55-year-old general population. Clin Physiol 1981;1(4): 405–15.
5. Bloem BR, Lagaay AM, van BW, et al. Prevalence of subjective dysphagia in community residents aged over 87. BMJ 1990;300(6726):721–2.
6. Lindgren S, Janzon L. Prevalence of swallowing complaints and clinical findings among 50-79-year-old men and women in an urban population. Dysphagia 1991; 6(4):187–92.
7. Talley NJ, Weaver AL, Zinsmeister AR, et al. Onset and disappearance of gastrointestinal symptoms and functional gastrointestinal disorders. Am J Epidemiol 1992;136(2):165–77.
8. Kawashima K, Motohashi Y, Fujishima I. Prevalence of dysphagia among community-dwelling elderly individuals as estimated using a questionnaire for dysphagia screening. Dysphagia 2004;19(4):266–71.

9. Eslick GD, Talley NJ. Dysphagia: epidemiology, risk factors and impact on quality of life—a population-based study. Aliment Pharmacol Ther 2008;27(10):971–9.

10. Smith-Hammond CA, New KC, Pietrobon R, et al. Prospective analysis of incidence and risk factors of dysphagia in spine surgery patients: comparison of anterior cervical, posterior cervical, and lumbar procedures. Spine (Phila Pa 1976) 2004;29(13):1441–6.

11. Riley LH III, Skolasky RL, Albert TJ, et al. Dysphagia after anterior cervical decompression and fusion: prevalence and risk factors from a longitudinal cohort study. Spine (Phila Pa 1976) 2005;30(22):2564–9.

12. Lee MJ, Bazaz R, Furey CG, et al. Risk factors for dysphagia after anterior cervical spine surgery: a two-year prospective cohort study. Spine J 2007;7(2): 141–7.

13. Hamidon BB, Nabil I, Raymond AA. Risk factors and outcome of dysphagia after an acute ischaemic stroke. Med J Malaysia 2006;61(5):553–7.

14. Lefton-Greif MA, Carroll JL, Loughlin GM. Long-term follow-up of oropharyngeal dysphagia in children without apparent risk factors. Pediatr Pulmonol 2006; 41(11):1040–8.

15. Roy N, Stemple J, Merrill RM, et al. Dysphagia in the elderly: preliminary evidence of prevalence, risk factors, and socioemotional effects. Ann Otol Rhinol Laryngol 2007;116(11):858–65.

16. Koiwai K, Shikama N, Sasaki S, et al. Risk factors for severe dysphagia after concurrent chemoradiotherapy for head and neck cancers. Jpn J Clin Oncol 2009;39(7):413–7.

17. Eslick GD, Jones MP, Talley NJ. Non-cardiac chest pain: prevalence, risk factors, impact and consulting—a population-based study. Aliment Pharmacol Ther 2003; 17(9):1115–24.

18. Larson C. Neurophysiology of speech and swallowing. Semin Speech Lang 1985; 6:275–91.

19. Ramsey G, Watson J, Gramiak R, et al. Cinefluorographic analysis of the mechanism of swallowing. Radiology 1955;64:498–518.

20. Doty R, Bosma J. An electromyographic analysis of reflex deglutition. J Neurophysiol 1956;19:44–60.

21. Kahrilas PJ, Dodds WJ, Dent J, et al. Upper esophageal sphincter function during deglutition. Gastroenterology 1988;95(1):52–62.

22. Kahrilas PJ, Dodds WJ, Dent J, et al. Upper esophageal sphincter function during belching. Gastroenterology 1986;91(1):133–40.

23. Cook IJ, Dodds WJ, Dantas RO, et al. Opening mechanisms of the human upper esophageal sphincter. Am J Physiol 1989;257(5 Pt 1):G748–59.

24. Logemann JA. Evaluation and treatment of swallowing disorders. San Diego (CA): College Hill Press; 1983.

25. Geraci G, Pisello F, Modica G, et al. Herpes simplex esophagitis in immunocompetent host: a case report. Diagn Ther Endosc 2009;2009:717183.

26. Vent J, Quante G, Markert E, et al. [Dysphagia as a presenting symptom of a cervical neurofibroma]. HNO 2009;57(6):625–8 [in German].

27. Rathinam S, Makarawo T, Norton R, et al. Thoracic osteophyte: rare cause of esophageal perforation. Dis Esophagus 2010;23:E5–E8.

28. Kos MP, David EF, Mahieu HF. Endoscopic carbon dioxide laser Zenker's diverticulotomy revisited. Ann Otol Rhinol Laryngol 2009;118(7):512–8.

29. Lang RA, Spelsberg FW, Naumann A, et al. [Zenker's diverticulum treated by transoral diverticulostomy: technique and results]. Zentralbl Chir 2007;132(5): 451–6 [in German].

30. Lang RA, Spelsberg FW, Winter H, et al. Transoral diverticulostomy with a modified Endo-GIA stapler: results after 4 years of experience. Surg Endosc 2007; 21(4):532–6.
31. Deleyiannis FW, Piccirillo JF, Kirchner JA. Relative prognostic importance of histologic invasion of the laryngeal framework by hypopharyngeal cancer. Ann Otol Rhinol Laryngol 1996;105(2):101–8.
32. Kleinsasser O, Glanz H, Kimmich T. [Treatment of carcinoma of the piriform sinus]. HNO 1989;37(11):460–4 [in German].
33. Axon PR, Woolford TJ, Hargreaves SP, et al. A comparison of surgery and radiotherapy in the management of post-cricoid carcinoma. Clin Otolaryngol Allied Sci 1997;22(4):370–4.
34. Pingree TF, Davis RK, Reichman O, et al. Treatment of hypopharyngeal carcinoma: a 10-year review of 1,362 cases. Laryngoscope 1987;97(8 Pt 1):901–4.
35. Hoffman HT, Karnell LH, Shah JP, et al. Hypopharyngeal cancer patient care evaluation. Laryngoscope 1997;107(8):1005–17.
36. de Vries EJ, Stein DW, Johnson JT, et al. Hypopharyngeal reconstruction: a comparison of two alternatives. Laryngoscope 1989;99(6 Pt 1):614–7.
37. Julieron M, Germain MA, Schwaab G, et al. Reconstruction with free jejunal autograft after circumferential pharyngolaryngectomy: eighty-three cases. Ann Otol Rhinol Laryngol 1998;107(7):581–7.
38. Schuller DE, Mountain RE, Nicholson RE, et al. One-stage reconstruction of partial laryngopharyngeal defects. Laryngoscope 1997;107(2):247–53.
39. Jones AS, Roland NJ, Husband D, et al. Free revascularized jejunal loop repair following total pharyngolaryngectomy for carcinoma of the hypopharynx: report of 90 patients. Br J Surg 1996;83(9):1279–83.
40. Chevalier D, Triboulet JP, Patenotre P, et al. Free jejunal graft reconstruction after total pharyngolaryngeal resection for hypopharyngeal cancer. Clin Otolaryngol Allied Sci 1997;22(1):41–3.
41. Holmes RS, Vaughan TL. Epidemiology and pathogenesis of esophageal cancer. Semin Radiat Oncol 2007;17(1):2–9.
42. Pera M, Cameron AJ, Trastek VF, et al. Increasing incidence of adenocarcinoma of the esophagus and esophagogastric junction. Gastroenterology 1993;104(2): 510–3.
43. Devesa SS, Shaw GL, Blot WJ. Changing patterns of lung cancer incidence by histological type. Cancer Epidemiol Biomarkers Prev 1991;1(1):29–34.
44. Lagergren J, Bergstrom R, Lindgren A, et al. Symptomatic gastroesophageal reflux as a risk factor for esophageal adenocarcinoma. N Engl J Med 1999;340(11): 825–31.
45. Greenlee RT, Hill-Harmon MB, Murray T, et al. Cancer statistics, 2001. CA Cancer J Clin 2001;51(1):15–36.
46. Altorki NK, Girardi L, Skinner DB. En bloc esophagectomy improves survival for stage III esophageal cancer. J Thorac Cardiovasc Surg 1997;114(6):948–55.
47. Lerut T, De LP, Coosemans W, et al. Surgical strategies in esophageal carcinoma with emphasis on radical lymphadenectomy. Ann Surg 1992;216(5):583–90.
48. Lerut T, Coosemans W, Van RD, et al. Surgical treatment of Barrett's carcinoma. Correlations between morphologic findings and prognosis. J Thorac Cardiovasc Surg 1994;107(4):1059–65.
49. Steup WH, De LP, Deneffe G, et al. Tumors of the esophagogastric junction. Long-term survival in relation to the pattern of lymph node metastasis and a critical analysis of the accuracy or inaccuracy of pTNM classification. J Thorac Cardiovasc Surg 1996;111(1):85–94.

50. Alfonsi E, Merlo IM, Ponzio M, et al. An electrophysiological approach to the diagnosis of neurogenic dysphagia; implications for botulinum toxin treatment. J Neurol Neurosurg Psychiatry 2010;81:54–60.
51. Alfonsi E, Versino M, Merlo IM, et al. Electrophysiologic patterns of oral-pharyngeal swallowing in parkinsonian syndromes. Neurology 2007;68(8):583–9.
52. Merlo IM, Occhini A, Pacchetti C, et al. Not paralysis, but dystonia causes stridor in multiple system atrophy. Neurology 2002;58(4):649–52.
53. Kilic A, Schuchert MJ, Pennathur A, et al. Long-term outcomes of laparoscopic Heller myotomy for achalasia. Surgery 2009;146(4):826–31.
54. Schuchert MJ, Luketich JD, Landreneau RJ, et al. Minimally invasive surgical treatment of sigmoidal esophagus in achalasia. J Gastrointest Surg 2009;13(6): 1029–35.
55. Kilic A, Schuchert MJ, Pennathur A, et al. Minimally invasive myotomy for achalasia in the elderly. Surg Endosc 2008;22(4):862–5.
56. Scherer JR, Kwiatek MA, Soper NJ, et al. Functional esophagogastric junction obstruction with intact peristalsis: a heterogeneous syndrome sometimes akin to achalasia. J Gastrointest Surg 2009;13(12):2219–25.
57. Vaiman M, Shoval G, Gavriel H. Malingering dysphagia and odynophagia electromyographic assessment. Am J Otolaryngol 2009;30(5):318–23.
58. Vaiman M, Shoval G, Gavriel H. The electrodiagnostic examination of psychogenic swallowing disorders. Eur Arch Otorhinolaryngol 2008;265(6): 663–8.
59. Grant PD, Morgan DE, Scholz FJ, et al. Pharyngeal dysphagia: what the radiologist needs to know. Curr Probl Diagn Radiol 2009;38(1):17–32.
60. Roffman E, Jalisi S, Hybels R, et al. Failed extraction of a sharp esophageal foreign body with a flexible endoscope: a case report and review of the literature. Arch Otolaryngol Head Neck Surg 2002;128(9):1096–8.

Chest Pain in Focal Musculoskeletal Disorders

Mette Jensen Stochkendahl, MSc[a,b,*],
Henrik Wulff Christensen, DC, MD, PhD[b]

KEYWORDS
- Chest pain • Noncardiac chest pain • Musculoskeletal pain
- Physical examination • Cervical spine • Thoracic spine

Primary health care providers play an important role in the initial evaluation and treatment of patients with acute or chronic chest pain. As chest pain may have benign and life-threatening causes, it is imperative that clinicians have a thorough and structured approach to the evaluation of the patient with chest pain. The musculoskeletal system is recognized as a benign cause, but is sometimes not given the same systematic approach as when a more serious condition is suspected.

In patients with chest pain, the first priority for clinicians is to consider potentially life-threatening causes, but in primary care, the cause of pain may be benign in approximately 80% of cases, of which musculoskeletal chest pain accounts for almost 50%.[1–3] In patients with noncardiac chest pain, a sizeable minority are never diagnosed or given a plan for follow-up.[4–7] Nevertheless, as many as 75% experience persistent or recurrent symptoms,[8,9] and the lack of a diagnosis may result in depression,[10] anxiety[11] and a decrease in daily activity.[8,10,12] In addition, noncardiac chest pain may lead to inappropriate and unnecessary investigations and management with associated further anxiety and time lost from work.[6,13] In patients with noncardiac chest pain, conflicting evidence exists regarding mortality. Some studies have indicated an excellent prognosis for survival and a future risk of cardiac morbidity similar to that reported in the background population,[14–16] whereas others have indicated much poorer outcomes.[17–19] Therefore, it is imperative that the clinician has a current knowledge of the diagnostic approaches to patients with chest pain, especially musculoskeletal chest pain, to expedite diagnosis and appropriate management,

[a] Institute of Sports Science and Clinical Biomechanics, University of Southern Denmark, Campusvej 55, DK-5230 Odense M, Denmark
[b] Research Department, Nordic Institute of Chiropractic and Clinical Biomechanics, Forskerparken 10 A, DK-5230 Odense M, Denmark
* Corresponding author. Research Department, Nordic Institute of Chiropractic and Clinical Biomechanics, Forskerparken 10 A, DK-5230 Odense M, Denmark.
E-mail address: m.jensen@nikkb.dk

Med Clin N Am 94 (2010) 259–273
doi:10.1016/j.mcna.2010.01.007
0025-7125/10/$ – see front matter © 2010 Elsevier Inc. All rights reserved.

thereby reducing unnecessary referrals to expensive clinical investigations and unnecessary patient anxiety.

PREVALENCE
General Population

The prevalence of musculoskeletal chest pain in the general population has recently been evaluated by 2 cross-sectional surveys. In Australia (2003), Eslick and colleagues[9] defined musculoskeletal-like chest pain as chest pain worse on movement. Using self-report questionnaires, 35% (n = 76) of those reporting noncardiac chest pain also described pain that could be musculoskeletal in origin, equally distributed between female and male responders. In 2007, in a cross-sectional survey of more than 34,000 Danish twins by Leboeuf-Yde and colleagues[20] the 1-year prevalence estimate of radiating pain from the thoracic spine to the chest wall was 5%. Women were more often affected, especially when they were in their late 40s and late 60s.

In the Copenhagen Heart Study (1978), questionnaire responders from an urban cohort with suspected stable angina pectoris (**Box 1**) were invited to a clinical examination.[21] Of those accepting, 18% (n = 81) had musculoskeletal chest pain, more commonly seen in women than men (24% vs 11%, respectively).

Primary Care

In primary care, the prevalence of thoracic pain has been estimated to account for 1% to 3% of all contacts with general physicians, with musculoskeletal chest pain ranking as the most common diagnosis accounting for 21% to 49% of those patients with chest pain.[1–3,22] The prevalence of musculoskeletal chest pain peaked at ages 21 to 40 years. Women were more often found to be affected than men.[2]

Coronary Care Units and Emergency Departments

Several studies have looked at the prevalence of musculoskeletal chest pain in coronary care units and emergency department in patients with suspected acute coronary syndrome. In those patients without acute coronary syndrome, a nonspecific diagnosis of musculoskeletal chest pain has been evaluated in 4 studies.[6,14,23,24] Musculoskeletal chest pain ranked from the most prevalent cause at 23%[6] to the fourth most prevalent cause at 3%, following chest pain of cardiac undetermined origin, gastrointestinal origin, and pulmonary disease.[14]

In addition, 3 studies have specifically defined subgroups and diagnostic procedures that result in higher prevalence of musculoskeletal chest pain (almost 30% in patients without acute myocardial infarction).[5,25,26]

Outpatient Settings and Patients with Suspected Stable Angina Pectoris

In patients referred for coronary angiography, 11% to 18% have been classified as having musculoskeletal chest pain.[27,28] In patients with normal coronary arteriography these figures increase to 23% to 35%.[29,30]

Box 1
Definition stable angina pectoris

A clinical syndrome characterized by discomfort in the chest, jaw, shoulder, back or arm. It is typically aggravated by exertion or emotional stress and relieved by rest or nitroglycerine.

Data from Diamond GA, Forrester JS. Analysis of probability as an aid in the clinical diagnosis of coronary-artery disease. N Engl J Med 1979;300:1350–8.

DEFINITIONS

The musculoskeletal system is recognized as a possible source of pain in patients with chest pain.[8,31–34] However, a confident diagnosis of musculoskeletal chest pain can be difficult to establish because no reference standard exists to verify this diagnosis. The broad term musculoskeletal chest pain encompasses pain from many different musculoskeletal sources and with many proposed mechanisms, including traumatic, nontraumatic, inflammatory, and noninflammatory origins, but definitions and terms overlap (**Box 2**). To complicate matters there are only a few Medline subheadings (MeSH) that adequately differentiate aspects of musculoskeletal chest pain to guide clinicians and researchers in efforts to gain knowledge in this area.

For all of these conditions, with the exception of degenerative pathology of the spine, psoriatic arthritis, spondyloarthropathies, and stress fracture, the diagnosis is essentially based on history and clinical examination findings with the use of investigations to exclude other conditions, rather than to confirm the diagnosis. This article focuses on the clinical features of the focal musculoskeletal disorders most commonly diagnosed as causes of musculoskeletal chest pain. However, only segmental dysfunction has been evaluated in prospective clinical trials by chiropractors. The generalized pain syndromes of fibromyalgia and fibrositis are addressed elsewhere in this issue.

Box 2
Subgroups of musculoskeletal chest pain

Cervicothoracic angina

Intercostal myalgia

Segmental thoracic dysfunction

Pectoral myalgia

Costovertebral dysfunctions

Fibrositis

Degenerative pathology of the spine

Stress fracture

Cervical angina

Costochondritis

Thoracic outlet

Tietze syndrome

Chest wall tenderness

Fibromyalgia

Chest wall syndrome

Sternoclavicluar disease

Slipping rib

Seronegative spondyloarthropathies

Myositis

Psoriatic arthritis

Tietze Syndrome

Tietze syndrome was first described in 1921 by the German surgeon Alexander Tietze (1864–1927).[35] Although the syndrome has frequently been described in the literature, true Tietze syndrome is probably rare. Tietze syndrome is characterized by the presence of painful swelling of the costal cartilages caused by a benign inflammation. Although similar, Tietze syndrome is not identical to costochondritis, which also affects the costal cartilages. The inflammation and swelling of the costal cartilages seen in Tietze syndrome are absent in costochondritis. Tietze syndrome affects younger people of either gender with a predilection for the upper ribs, particularly second and third costochondral junctions. Lesions are unilateral and single in 70% to 80% of cases.[35–37] If multiple, lesions usually affect neighboring articulations on the same side. Onset may be insidious, and heat and erythema may be present. It is now recognized that in Tietze syndrome the presence or absence of swelling is only an indicator of the severity of the condition. Although the true causes of Tietze syndrome are not well understood,[35] it often results from a physical strain or minor injury, such as excessive coughing, vomiting, or impacts to the chest.[36] The syndrome was at one time believed to be associated with, or caused by, a viral infection acquired during surgery, but this is now known not to be the case. Diagnosis is based on clinical grounds after exclusion of other conditions. Routine investigations do not show any abnormalities,[36] but bone scintigraphy and ultrasound are suggested as screening procedures.[37,38] Pain usually has a self-limited course within weeks to months, but may in cases become more chronic.[36] Suggested treatments consist of reassurance, local application of heat and use of nonsteroidal antiinflammatory drugs (NSAIDS).[35,36] Local steroid or lidocaine injections may be indicated in refractory cases,[35,37] but there are no formal studies to support the evidence of a potential treatment effect of any of the suggested therapies.

Costochondritis

Costochondritis is used interchangeably with costosternal syndrome and chest wall syndrome, and definitions are not consistent.[35,36,39] These syndromes are all characterized by pain and local tenderness at costochondral or chondrosternal articulations, or even at the xiphoid process, but without the inflammation and swelling seen in Tietze syndrome. It is presumably a much more common cause of chest pain affecting as many as 30% of presentations in emergency departments.[39] In primary care, costochondritis has been reported in 42% of patients with musculoskeletal chest pain,[3] but as with Tietze syndrome, reports of prevalence are mostly based on cases,[39–41] and the exact prevalence is difficult to evaluate. Little is known of the pathogenesis, but in a subgroup of patients with costochondritis, an association with seronegative spondylarthropathies has been recognized, and costochondritis has been seen as the presenting feature in such conditions.[40] In others, repetitive physical activity has been reported as a precipitating factor.[38] Pain may be provoked at rest, during movement of the ribcage or related to breathing.[36] It most often has a self-limited course, but recurrences are common as are prolonged cases. Treatment includes reassurance, and manual therapy has been shown to be beneficial in some cases.[42] Injections with local anesthetics for immediate response and sulfasalazine for prolonged effect have been suggested as beneficial treatment options.[40]

Muscular Tenderness

Along with costochondritis, muscular tenderness of the intercostal and pectoral muscles may be one of the most common causes of musculoskeletal chest pain. In primary care, intercostal tenderness has been reported to be the most common origin of pain, comprising almost 50% of all patients with chest pain.[2] Others have reported pectoral tenderness to be the second most common cause of musculoskeletal chest pain accounting for approximately 25% of cases and intercostal tenderness accounting for only 9%.[3] Another study in a hospital setting examining patients referred for coronary angiography with stable angina pectoris found up to 98% of all patients with an overall diagnosis of chest pain from the musculoskeletal system to have chest wall tenderness.[27]

The cause has been attributed to a history of unaccustomed or excessive activity, such as lifting, painting a ceiling, chopping wood, coughing or exertion of undertrained muscles. Similarly a state of tension or anxiety can produce excessive tension. Onset may be either gradual or sudden. The patients will report localized pain and tenderness over the strained muscles. Pain is made worse by maneuvers that tense or stretch the muscles.[35]

Within different clinical disciplines (eg, rheumatology, cardiology, or chiropractic), these clinical conditions of muscular tenderness are diagnosed with manual palpation (**Figs. 1** and **2**). However, the manual palpation methods have rarely been evaluated in clinical settings. Only 1 study, to our knowledge, has evaluated the reliability of palpation for tenderness of the chest wall and found great variation between examiners when palpating for tenderness.[27] This may hamper clinicians' ability to diagnose and classify part of the potential muscular component of chest pain.

Segmental Dysfunction of the Neck and Thoracic Spine

Coming from the posterior aspect of the chest wall or neck, segmental dysfunction of the spine is perhaps one of the most under-diagnosed causes of musculoskeletal chest pain.[43] The term "segmental dysfunction" refers to a disturbance of function affecting quality and range of motion of spinal segments without structural change. The definition embodies disturbances in function that can be represented by decreased or aberrant motion.[44] Segmental dysfunction in the lower cervical (C4 to C7) and upper thoracic spine (Th1 to Th8) may cause pain referred to the anterior aspects of the chest wall.[27,45] This is because dysfunctional spinal segments tend to refer pain to a zone corresponding to the distribution of the segmental innervations of the deep structures.[46] Excessive strain in the spinal joints after trauma, effort, or false movement may lead to this abnormal firing of nociceptive structures.[43] Segmental dysfunction may be present with or without degenerative pathologies of the spine.

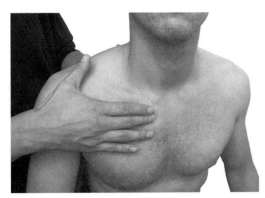

Fig. 1. Manual palpation of the anterior chest wall using soft contact with the index or middle finger contact and with the clinician placed behind the patient.

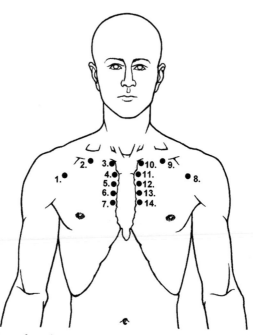

Fig. 2. Potential points of tenderness on the anterior chest wall. Pectoralis major points are located at the anterior axillary lines 3 cm caudal to the clavicles (points 1 and 8). Pectoralis minor points are located at the medioclavicular lines just caudal to the clavicles (points 2 and 9). The intercostals muscles are palpated lateral to the sternum at the intercostals space between II/III and VI/VII (points 3–7 and 10–14).

Segmental dysfunction has been reported to account for between 14% of patients with musculoskeletal chest pain[5] and 29% of all patients admitted with acute chest pain suspected of acute myocardial infarction.[26] In a population with chronic chest pain admitted for coronary angiography at a cardiology department, 18% of the population was found to have a clinical syndrome of chest discomfort originating from the cervicothoracic spine and thorax, called cervicothoracic angina (CTA).[27] Using the same definition in a population of patients with acute chest pain and no clear diagnosis at initial presentation, the prevalence is currently being evaluated in a PhD thesis, the results of which will be communicated elsewhere.[47]

The prospective clinical study of patients with chronic chest pain by Christensen and colleagues[27] has been able to establish a few clinical characteristics that could differentiate patients with CTA and patients without (**Box 3**). The different pain descriptors appeared with similar frequencies in the 2 groups, except for sharp pain, which was more frequent in the patients positive for CTA, who also had their symptoms for a shorter time and with less frequent episodes. Physical activity provoking pain was significantly less frequent in the CTA-positive group, and they suffered more often from self-reported neck pain, thoracic spine pain, and shoulder-arm pain.[27] In contrast to common beliefs, movement of the thorax was seldom found to provoke the chest pain in patients with chronic chest pain (8%, $P = .06$).[27] In the study by Christensen and colleagues[27] systematic classification of patients according to international guidelines for type and severity of angina pectoris appeared to be an important indicator for distinguishing patients with and without CTA. Type of angina pectoris was classified according to Diamond and Forrester[48] into classes of typical, atypical,

Box 3
Clinical features with significant differences in frequency between CTA-positive patients and CTA-negative patients with chronic chest pain

CTA-positive patients are more likely to have

    Sharp pain

    Shorter duration of pain

    Neck pain

    Thoracic spinal pain

    Shoulder-arm pain

    Noncardiac pain and atypical angina[25]

CTA-negative patients are more likely to have

    More frequent episodes of pain

    Pain related to physical activity

    Typical angina[48]

    Higher CCS class of angina severity[49]

Data from Christensen HW, Vach W, Gichangi A, et al. Cervicothoracic angina identified by case history and palpation findings in patients with stable angina pectoris. J Manipulative Physiol Ther 2005;28:303–11.

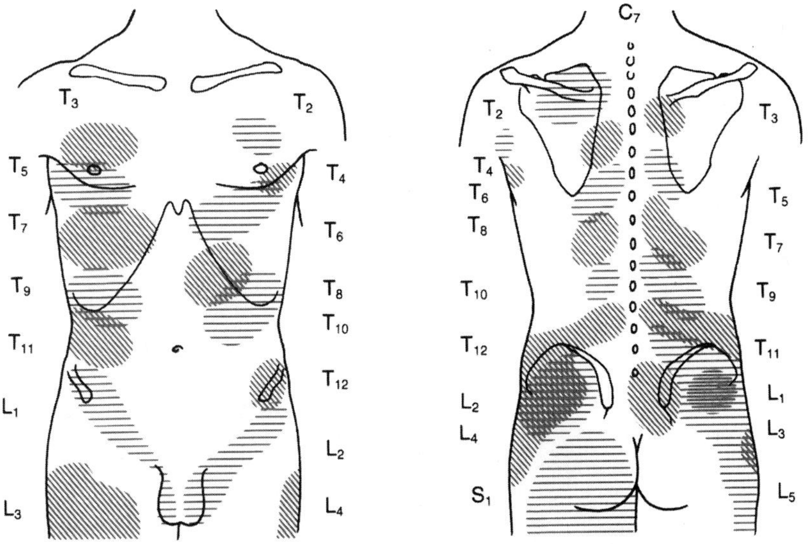

Fig. 3. Patterns of referred pain from deep somatic structures of the thoracic and lumbar spinal segments based on experiments by Kellgren et al[46] and Feinstein et al[67] in which spinal and paraspinal structures were injected with hypertonic saline. (*From* Dvorak J, Dvorak V. Manual medicine diagnostics. Stuttgart (NY): Georg Thieme Verlag; 1990; with permission.)

and noncardiac chest pain, whereas severity was graded in 4 categories in accordance with the Canadian Cardiovascular Society (CCS).[49] Noncardiac pain and atypical angina pectoris were significantly more frequent in the CTA-positive group. In addition, there was a significant trend for generally higher CCS class in the CTA-negative group.

Pain caused by segmental dysfunction has been reported to be worst at rest or after prolonged sitting and with spinal rotation[43,50]; but pain worst at rest has only been reported in approximately one-third of patients with chronic chest pain and does not seem to be a discriminatory factor.[27] Unlike in ischemic heart disease, activity may relieve pain.[43] However, the opposite scenario with pain on physical activity and relief by rest may also be the case in up to 50% of patients with CTA.[27] Paraspinal muscular tenderness is often present together with spinal joint dysfunction,[50] and sometimes pain may be reproduced by palpation of the spinal joints and related structures (**Fig. 4**).[43] Excessive strain (acute or repeated) in such joints after trauma, effort, or false movement may lead to this abnormal firing of nociceptive structures.[43]

Benefits of spinal manipulative treatment (SMT) have been evaluated in a nonrandomized clinical trial comparing patients with CTA and treated with SMT with untreated patients without CTA.[51] Approximately 75% of patients with CTA reported improvement in pain and in general health after treatment, compared with a statistically significant smaller proportion of 22% and 25% of patients without CTA. However, the design of this nonrandomized trial had several limitations and the value of SMT was not fully elucidated.

Cervical Angina

Cervical angina has been defined as chest pain that resembles true cardiac angina but originates from cervical discopathy with nerve root compression.[52] Cervical angina has been described by different investigators in the past 70 years.[53–58] Patients with cervical angina may be considered in an end stage of a progressing pathology in which degenerative changes of the spine have led to discopathy. Unlike most other focal musculoskeletal chest pain syndromes, the diagnosis can be confirmed by magnetic resonance imaging or radiographic findings. The patients require specialist attention for further evaluation and management.

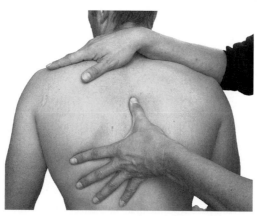

Fig. 4. Manual palpation of thoracic spine motion. The patient is guided by the clinician through movements of rotation and/or side bending by a gentle push of the forearm of the clinician's indifferent hand. At the end of range of motion, the clinician's palpating hand gently applies extra force over the spinal joints to assess joint movement.

Slipping Rib

Slipping rib, also called rib-tip-syndrome, is a less known source of mechanical rib pain, accounting for approximately 5% of musculoskeletal chest pain cases in primary care.[3,35,36] Slipping rib is attributed to loosening of the fibrous attachments binding the lower costal cartilages to one another allowing a rib tip to curl upwards and over-ride the inner aspect of the rib above, causing pressure on the intercostal nerve between. The disorder is most likely traumatic in origin, as many patients recall past injury to the affected side. Onset is insidious, with intermittent unilateral pain in the lower margin of the ribcage. A painful click is sometimes felt over the tip of the costal cartilage involved with certain movements. The costal cartilage involved is tender and moves more freely than normal on palpation. Remission is slow and pain may linger for several months. Beneficial therapies include reassurance and mild analgesics.

Mechanisms of Visceral and Somatic Chest Pain

Chest pain may be broadly categorized as visceral or somatic in origin. Visceral pain includes pain from structures including the heart, esophagus, stomach, and so forth. whereas somatic pain includes pain from the musculoskeletal structures, dermal tissues, and the coverings of major organs. The depth of the tissue in somatic pain tends to determine if it is superficial somatic (skin, tendon sheaths, periosteum, superficial fasciae) or deep somatic (muscle, fasciae, tendons, joint capsules, ligaments, periosteum).[59]

Using cardiac pain as illustrative of the mechanisms of visceral pain, cardiac pain is transmitted by afferent sympathetic nerve fibers and vagal nerve fibers.[59] This visceral type of pain is mediated by free nerve endings that have receptors located in the mucosa, muscle, and serosa of the heart and can be stimulated chemically or mechanically.[60–62] The sympathetic nerves have cell bodies in the dorsal root ganglia and synapse on the interneurons in the dorsal horn of the spinal cord. Interneurons that receive visceral pain are called viscerosomatic neurons. They also receive somatic afferent input from skin, tendons, and muscles. The visceral pain from the heart is transmitted via the 4 to 5 upper thoracic spinal segments as well as some cervical segments. The sensory impulses from the viscera of the thorax and from the body wall (muscles, skin, joints), however, share the same spinal segments, making the differentiation of causes and diagnosis of chest pain difficult in some cases.[63,64] The convergence of visceral and somatic pain fibers on the same interneurons in the spinal cord might explain why visceral pain is often referred, that is, why it is often perceived in somatic areas remote from the involved organ.

Therefore, pain arising from different organs, such as the chest wall, esophagus, or the heart may be indistinguishable as may pain arising from the spine.[64] The ascending pathways to the brain project through the anterolateral system of the spinal cord to the medulla, midbrain, and thalamus. In the medulla, visceral pain pathways interact with the reticular formation, mediating arousal and autonomic responses to pain. In the midbrain, projections to the periaqueductal gray matter are important for descending modulation. From the thalamus, visceral pain input is relayed to areas of the cortex, as demonstrated in man using positron emission tomography, where it is decoded as a painful sensation.[65]

Using musculoskeletal pain as illustrative of the mechanisms of somatic pain, sensory receptors in musculoskeletal structures are characterized by an ability to respond to a particular stimulus with a relative insensitivity to certain other stimuli.

Nociceptors are sensitive to stimuli that are potential noxious. Mechanical, chemical, and thermal stimuli may cause nociception. The nociceptors can be sensitized by a wide variety of mechanisms that can lower the threshold from nociceptive stimuli and make it possible for nonnociceptive stimuli to be registered as pain-producing stimuli. The pain impulses are mediated by afferent nerve fibers linking the peripheral nociceptor with the spinal cord. The primary afferent fibers enter the dorsal horn of the spinal cord and synapse with second-order neurons.[66] The ascending pathways have been described previously.

Different musculoskeletal structures of the spinal region have been characterized as pain producing in human studies from the mid-twentieth century using irritant injection solutions. Kellgren[46] outlined the distribution of pain from ligaments, which was different from the well-known dermatomes. He found that fascia, periosteum, and tendons give rise to pain of segmental distribution. Feinstein[67] outlined the distribution for pain and tenderness when the interspinous ligament is irritated (**Fig. 3**). Several spinal segments referred pain to the anterior chest wall. Furthermore, the thoracic zygapophyseal joints at segments T3 to T9 can cause intense areas of provoked pain one segment inferiorly and slightly lateral to the joint injected and similar pain referred toward the anterior chest wall.[68] Large and more recent studies of patterns of musculoskeletal referred pain do not exist.

DIAGNOSTIC METHODS

Most musculoskeletal chest pain syndromes are essentially clinically diagnosed without reference standards to verify the diagnoses. The cornerstone to diagnosis is manual palpation of pain and motion of muscles and joints of the chest wall and cervicothoracic spine. As a result, the syndrome is difficult to confirm and susceptible to interobserver variation. The interobserver variation of manual palpation of the spine has been evaluated several times.[69,70] Results indicate that although there is a high degree of interobserver variability in palpation of spinal motion and of anterior muscular tenderness of the chest wall,[71] the degree of interobserver variability in palpation of tenderness and assessment of patients based on full clinical evaluation is limited to a clinically acceptable level.[69,72]

The issue of verifying clinical diagnosis, especially spinal motion and pain, without reference standards has been addressed through various indirect measures.[73–77] Results lend support to the validity of palpation in detecting spinal segmental dysfunction. One study has used myocardial perfusion scintigraphy as a proxy measure in patients with suspected stable angina pectoris referred for coronary angiography.[27] The results suggest that an experienced clinician can fairly convincingly identify a subset of patients with suspected angina pectoris as having segmental dysfunction. Diagnosis was based on a 4-step approach encompassing a combination of palpation of the chest wall, neck and thoracic spin (see **Figs. 1, 2** and **4**), classification of type (more common among noncardiac chest pain), and severity of angina (more frequent with a CCS grade 1), the presence of neck pain, sharp pain, and pain relived by rest. Additional indirect support for the diagnosis of segmental dysfunction in this patient subset came from improvements in pain and general health with a trial of manual therapy.[51]

IMPLICATIONS FOR CLINICAL PRACTICE

The implications of the material discussed in this article for clinical practice are summarized in **Box 4**.

Box 4
What can the clinician do?

- Take a systematic case history to identify cases of excessive strain (acute or repeated) that may indicate a musculoskeletal origin of pain; pay attention to traumatic origin of the chest pain

- Use internationally accepted classification systems of angina pectoris (ie, according to CCS and Diamond and Forrester) to identify those patients with low risk of ischemic heart disease

- Do a systematic and structured palpation of the cervical and thoracic spine and the anterior and posterior aspect of the thorax to identify signs of inflammation, and to identify segmental dysfunction and muscular tenderness

- Perform a clinical examination including neurologic examination for sensory disturbances, muscular strength, and peripheral reflexes of the upper and lower extremities to rule out nerve root compression. Look for swelling, heat, and erythema of the costosternal joints

- Possible referral for manual assessment (chiropractor) if the clinician does not have the palpation and treatment skills to clarify a musculoskeletal diagnosis

---

SUMMARY

Despite being a recognized and frequent source of chest pain, focal musculoskeletal disorders remain poorly understood. Nevertheless, the small amount of available research indicates that a detailed case history with emphasis on pain characteristics, precipitating, provoking and relieving factors, and classification of patients according to international guidelines of angina pectoris should be used in combination with a systematic, manual palpation of the spine and chest wall to positively diagnose a focal musculoskeletal cause of chest pain. Appropriate conservative treatment approaches, including manual therapy and mild analgesics, can be initiated to treat the sometimes disabling cause of the disorders.

REFERENCES

1. Klinkman MS, Stevens D, Gorenflo DW. Episodes of care for chest pain: a preliminary report from MIRNET. Michigan Research Network. J Fam Pract 1994;38: 345–52.
2. Svavarsdottir AE, Jonasson MR, Gudmundsson GH, et al. Chest pain in family practice. Diagnosis and long-term outcome in a community setting. Can Fam Physician 1996;42:1122–8.
3. Verdon F, Herzig L, Burnand B, et al. Chest pain in daily practice: occurrence, causes and management. Swiss Med Wkly 2008;138:340–7.
4. Capewell S, McMurray J. "Chest pain-please admit": is there an alternative? A rapid cardiological assessment service may prevent unnecessary admissions. BMJ 2000;320:951–2.
5. How J, Volz G, Doe S, et al. The causes of musculoskeletal chest pain in patients admitted to hospital with suspected myocardial infarction. Eur J Intern Med 2005; 16:432–6.
6. Spalding L, Reay E, Kelly C. Cause and outcome of atypical chest pain in patients admitted to hospital. J R Soc Med 2003;96:122–5.
7. Adamek RJ, Roth B, Zymanski CH, et al. Esophageal motility patterns in patients with and without coronary heart disease and healthy controls. Hepatogastroenterology 1999;46:1759–64.
8. Chambers J, Bass C. Chest pain with normal coronary anatomy: a review of natural history and possible etiologic factors. Prog Cardiovasc Dis 1990;33:161–84.

9. Eslick GD, Jones MP, Talley NJ. Non-cardiac chest pain: prevalence, risk factors, impact and consulting–a population-based study. Aliment Pharmacol Ther 2003; 17:1115–24.

10. Fagring AJ, Gaston-Johansson F, Danielson E. Description of unexplained chest pain and its influence on daily life in men and women. Eur J Cardiovasc Nurs 2005;4:337–44.

11. Chambers J, Bass C. Atypical chest pain: looking beyond the heart. QJM 1998; 91:239–44.

12. Jerlock M, Kjellgren KI, Gaston-Johansson F, et al. Psychosocial profile in men and women with unexplained chest pain. J Intern Med 2008;264:265–74.

13. Henderson RD, Wigle ED, Sample K, et al. Atypical chest pain of cardiac and esophageal origin. Chest 1978;73:24–7.

14. Prina LD, Decker WW, Weaver AL, et al. Outcome of patients with a final diagnosis of chest pain of undetermined origin admitted under the suspicion of acute coronary syndrome: a report from the Rochester Epidemiology Project. Ann Emerg Med 2004;43:59–67.

15. Berman DS, Germano G, Shaw LJ. The role of nuclear cardiology in clinical decision making. Semin Nucl Med 1999;29:280–97.

16. Klocke FJ, Baird MG, Lorell BH, et al. ACC/AHA/ASNC guidelines for the clinical use of cardiac radionuclide imaging–executive summary: a report of the American College of Cardiology/American Heart Association Task Force on Practice Guidelines (ACC/AHA/ASNC Committee to revise the 1995 guidelines for the clinical use of cardiac radionuclide imaging). Circulation 2003;108:1404–18.

17. Eslick GD, Talley NJ. Natural history and predictors of outcome for non-cardiac chest pain: a prospective 4-year cohort study. Neurogastroenterol Motil 2008; 20:989–97.

18. Wilhelmsen L, Rosengren A, Hagman M, et al. "Nonspecific" chest pain associated with high long-term mortality: results from the primary prevention study in Goteborg, Sweden. Clin Cardiol 1998;21:477–82.

19. Sekhri N, Feder GS, Junghans C, et al. How effective are rapid access chest pain clinics? Prognosis of incident angina and non-cardiac chest pain in 8762 consecutive patients. Heart 2007;93:458–63.

20. Leboeuf-Yde C, Nielsen J, Kyvik KO, et al. Pain in the lumbar, thoracic or cervical regions: do age and gender matter? A population-based study of 34,902 Danish twins 20–71 years of age. BMC Musculoskelet Disord 2009;10:39.

21. Jensen G. [Angina pectoris-epidemiology and need for treatment]. Nord Med 1982;97:99–101 [in Danish].

22. Buntinx F, Knockaert D, Bruyninckx R, et al. Chest pain in general practice or in the hospital emergency department: is it the same? Fam Pract 2001;18:586–9.

23. Knockaert DC, Buntinx F, Stoens N, et al. Chest pain in the emergency department: the broad spectrum of causes. Eur J Emerg Med 2002;9:25–30.

24. Herlitz J, Karlson BW, Lindqvist J, et al. Characteristics and long-term outcome of patients with acute chest pain or other symptoms raising suspicion of acute myocardial infarction in relation to whether they were hospitalized or directly discharged from the emergency department. Coron Artery Dis 2002;13:37–43.

25. Fruergaard P, Launbjerg J, Hesse B, et al. The diagnoses of patients admitted with acute chest pain but without myocardial infarction. Eur Heart J 1996;17: 1028–34.

26. Bechgaard P. [Segmentally thoracic pain in patients admitted to a coronary care unit]. Ugeskr Laeger 1982;144:13–5 [in Danish].

27. Christensen HW, Vach W, Gichangi A, et al. Cervicothoracic angina identified by case history and palpation findings in patients with stable angina pectoris. J Manipulative Physiol Ther 2005;28:303–11.

28. Levine PR, Mascette AM. Musculoskeletal chest pain in patients with "angina": a prospective study. South Med J 1989;82:580–5, 591.

29. Ockene IS, Shay MJ, Alpert JS, et al. Unexplained chest pain in patients with normal coronary arteriograms: a follow-up study of functional status. N Engl J Med 1980;303:1249–52.

30. Wise CM, Semble EL, Dalton CB. Musculoskeletal chest wall syndromes in patients with noncardiac chest pain: a study of 100 patients. Arch Phys Med Rehabil 1992;73:147–9.

31. Braunwald E. Part I: examination of the patient: the history. In: Braunwald E, editor. Heart disease. 6th edition. Philadelphia (PA): WB Saunders Company; 2001. p. 27–45.

32. Best RA. Non-cardiac chest pain: a useful physical sign? Heart 1999;81:450.

33. Chambers J, Bass C, Mayou R. Non-cardiac chest pain: assessment and management. Heart 1999;82:656–7.

34. Kryger P. [Medicinsk Kompendium]. 15th edition. Copenhagen (Denmark): Nyt Nordisk Forlag Arnold Busch; 1999.

35. Fam AG, Smythe HA. Musculoskeletal chest wall pain. CMAJ 1985;133:379–89.

36. Semble EL, Wise CM. Chest pain: a rheumatologist's perspective. South Med J 1988;81:64–8.

37. Kamel M, Kotob H. Ultrasonographic assessment of local steroid injection in Tietze's syndrome. Br J Rheumatol 1997;36:547–50.

38. Habib PA, Huang GS, Mendiola JA, et al. Anterior chest pain: musculoskeletal considerations. Emerg Radiol 2004;11:37–45.

39. Disla E, Rhim HR, Reddy A, et al. Costochondritis. A prospective analysis in an emergency department setting. Arch Intern Med 1994;154:2466–9.

40. Freeston J, Karim Z, Lindsay K, et al. Can early diagnosis and management of costochondritis reduce acute chest pain admissions? J Rheumatol 2004;31:2269–71.

41. Wolf E, Stern S. Costosternal syndrome – its frequency and importance in differential diagnosis of coronary heart disease. Arch Intern Med 1976;136:189–91.

42. Rabey MI. Costochondritis: are the symptoms and signs due to neurogenic inflammation. Two cases that responded to manual therapy directed towards posterior spinal structures. Man Ther 2008;13:82–6.

43. Arroyo JF, Jolliet P, Junod AF. Costovertebral joint dysfunction: another misdiagnosed cause of atypical chest pain. Postgrad Med J 1992;68:655–9.

44. Bergmann TF, Petersen DH, Lawrence DJ. Chiropractic technique: principles and procedures. Philadelphia (PA): Churchill Livingstone Inc; 1993.

45. Dwyer A, Aprill C, Bogduk N. Cervical zygapophyseal joint pain patterns. I: a study in normal volunteers. Spine 1990;15:453–7.

46. Kellgren JH. On the distribution of pain arising from deep somatic structures with charts of segmental pain areas. Clin Sci 1939;4:35–46.

47. Stochkendahl MJ. Musculoskeletal chest pain in patients with acute chest pain – diagnosis and manual treatment. PhD Thesis, Faculty of Health Sciences, University of Southern Denmark. Submitted.

48. Diamond GA, Forrester JS. Analysis of probability as an aid in the clinical diagnosis of coronary-artery disease. N Engl J Med 1979;300:1350–8.

49. Campeau L. Letter: grading of angina pectoris. Circulation 1976;54:522–3.

50. Hamberg J, Lindahl O. Angina pectoris symptoms caused by thoracic spine disorders. Clinical examination and treatment. Acta Med Scand Suppl 1981; 644:84–6.

51. Christensen HW, Vach W, Gichangi A, et al. Manual therapy for patients with stable angina pectoris: a nonrandomized open prospective trial. J Manipulative Physiol Ther 2005;28:654–61.

52. Wells P. Cervical angina. Am Fam Physician 1997;55:2262–4.

53. Brodsky AE. Cervical angina. A correlative study with emphasis on the use of coronary arteriography. Spine 1985;10(8):699–709.

54. Nachlas IW. Pseudo-angina pectoris originating in the cervical spine. JAMA 1934;103:323–5.

55. LeBan MM, Meerschaert JR, Taylor RS. Breast pain: a symptom of cervical radiculopathy. Arch Phys Med Rehabil 1979;60:315–7.

56. Davis D, Ritvo M. Osteoarthritis of the cervicodorsal spine (radiculitis) simulating coronary-artery disease. Clinical and roentgenologic findings. N Engl J Med 1948;238(25):857–66.

57. Davis D. Spinal nerve root pain (radiculitis) simulating coronary occlusion: a common syndrome. Am Heart J 1948;35:70–80.

58. Booth RE, Rothstein RD. Cervical angina. Spine 1976;1(1):28–32.

59. Procacci P, Zoppi M, Maresca M. Heart, vascular and haemophilic pain. In: Wall PD, Melzack R, editors. Textbook of pain. 4th edition. London (UK): Churchill Livingstone; 1999.

60. Sylven C. Angina pectoris. Clinical characteristics, neurophysiological and molecular mechanisms. Pain 1989;36:145–67.

61. Tomai F, Crea F, Gaspardone A, et al. Mechanisms of cardiac pain during coronary angioplasty. J Am Coll Cardiol 1993;22:1892–6.

62. Crea F, Pupita G, Galassi AR, et al. Role of adenosine in pathogenesis of anginal pain. Circulation 1990;81:164–72.

63. Souza TA. Differentiating mechanical pain from visceral pain. Top Clin Chiro 1994; 1(1):1–12.

64. Ness TJ, Gebhart GF. Visceral pain: a review of experimental studies. Pain 1990; 41:167–234.

65. Rosen SD, Paulesu E, Frith CD, et al. Central nervous pathways mediating angina pectoris [comments]. Lancet 1994;344:147–50.

66. Harford WV. Southwestern internal medicine conference: the syndrome of angina pectoris: role of visceral pain perception. Am J Med Sci 1994;307:305–15.

67. Feinstein B, Langton JNK, Jameson RM, et al. Experiments on pain referred from deep somatic tissues. J Bone Joint Surg 1954;36(5):981–97.

68. Dreyfuss P, Tibiletti C, Dreyer SJ. Thoracic zygapophyseal joint pain patterns. A study in normal volunteers. Spine 1994;19:807–11.

69. Stochkendahl MJ, Christensen HW, Hartvigsen J, et al. Manual examination of the spine: a systematic critical literature review of reproducibility. J Manipulative Physiol Ther 2006;29:475–85, 485.

70. Christensen HW, Vach W, Manniche C, et al. Palpation of the upper thoracic spine: an observer reliability study. J Manipulative Physiol Ther 2002;25(5):285–92.

71. Christensen HW, Vach W, Manniche C, et al. Palpation for muscular tenderness in the anterior chest wall: an observer reliability study. J Manipulative Physiol Ther 2003;26:469–75.

72. Brunse MH, Stochkendahl M, Vach W, et al. Examination of musculoskeletal chest pain – an inter-observer reliability study. Manl Ther 2009. DOI:10.1016/j.math.2009.10.003.

73. Harvey D, Byfield D. Preliminary studies with a mechanical model for the evaluation of spinal motion palpation. Clin Biomech 1991;6:79–82.
74. Macfadyen N, Maher CG, Adams R. Number of sampling movements and manual stiffness judgments. J Manipulative Physiol Ther 1998;21:604–10.
75. Haas M, Panzer D, Peterson D, et al. Short-term responsiveness of manual thoracic end-play assessment to spinal manipulation: a randomized trial of construct validity. J Manipulative Physiol Ther 1995;18(9):582–9.
76. Humphreys BK, Delahaye M, Peterson CK. An investigation into the validity of cervical spine motion palpation using subjects with congenital block vertebrae as a 'gold standard'. BMC Musculoskelet Disord 2004;5:19.
77. Jull G, Bogduk N, Marsland A. The accuracy of manual diagnosis for cervical zygapophysial joint pain syndromes. Med J Aust 1988;148:233–6.

Noncardiac Chest Pain and Fibromyalgia

Cristina Almansa, MD, PhD[a],*, Benjamin Wang, MD, FRCPC[b],
Sami R. Achem, MD[a]

KEYWORDS

- Noncardiac chest pain • Fibromyalgia
- Visceral hypersensitivity • Somatic hypersensitivity
- Central pain sensitization

Chronic widespread pain syndromes have been known for several centuries but the recognition of fibromyalgia as a distinct disorder is recent. The first description of fibromyalgia, then called *fibrositis* was published in 1904 by Sir William Gowers who described a syndrome of muscular regional pain, fatigue, and sleep disturbances that was characterized by the presence of increased tenderness at palpation or with the movement of affected areas, and was attributed to inflammatory patchy hyperplasia of the connective muscular fibrous tissue.[1] In the 1930s and 1940s several studies reported the location and nature of the tender points.[2,3] In the meantime, others focused on understanding the relationship between visceral pain and fibrositis.[4] Patton and Williamson[5] were the first to report a case of chest pain related to fibrositis, in a 52-year-old obese woman complaining of constricting pain in the left chest and left arm, who despite being initially managed as a myocardial infarction showed a normal electrocardiogram; the investigators later identified muscle spasm and tenderness of left erector spinae group and left trapezius as the cause of the angina-type pain. They called this entity "pseudovisceral pain," because it was identical to referred visceral pain but differed in origin.

In the 1970s, Moldofsky and colleagues[6] and Smythe and Moldofsky[7] were the first to change the term fibrositis to fibromyalgia (FM), to denominate a syndrome characterized by chronic musculoskeletal pain and tender points associated with non–rapid eye movement (REM) sleep disturbance. In 1990, the American College of Rheumatology (ACR) published the current accepted classification criteria for this entity, based on the results of a multicenter study comparing 293 patients diagnosed with fibromyalgia and 265 patients with other causes of chronic pain.[8] The World Health

[a] Division of Gastroenterology and Hepatology, Mayo College of Medicine, Mayo Clinic Florida, 4500 San Pablo Road, Jacksonville, FL 32224, USA
[b] Division of Rheumatology, Mayo Clinic Florida, 4500 San Pablo Road, Jacksonville, FL 32224, USA
* Corresponding author.
E-mail address: almansa.cristina@mayo.edu

Med Clin N Am 94 (2010) 275–289
doi:10.1016/j.mcna.2010.01.002
0025-7125/10/$ – see front matter © 2010 Elsevier Inc. All rights reserved.

Organization acknowledged fibromyalgia as an independent entity with the Copenhagen declaration in 1992.[9]

Recently, the diagnostic criteria for FM have been reconsidered, especially because the diagnosis may often be made in the absence of the requisite number of tender points.[10–12] It has been argued that existing tender point criteria bias prevalence statistics toward female patients.[12] Thus, Wolfe and colleagues[13] have undertaken to revise the diagnostic and severity criteria for FM, particularly to reconsider the usefulness of the tender point examination and to include other clinical features that better capture the complexity of this condition.

EPIDEMIOLOGY

To date, descriptive epidemiologic data for FM have largely relied on the established 1990 ACR classification criteria. The ancillary population-based study performed by Wolfe and colleagues[14] in Wichita (USA) estimated an overall prevalence of FM of 2% for both genders, 3.4% for women and 0.5% for men. According to a more recent study, FM is the third most common rheumatic disease after low back pain and osteoarthritis, affecting up to 5% of women in the United States.[15] Studies throughout the world report variable prevalence data: from 0.05% in China,[16] 0.22% in Cuba,[17] 1.4% in Mexico[18] and France,[19] 2.4% in Spain,[20] 3.3% in Canada[21] to 4.4% in Bangladesh.[22] FM more commonly affects middle-aged (usually more than 50 years old) women, living in rural areas, divorced with reduced household income, and lower educational level.[14,20] If the criteria are broadened, however, the prevalence certainly increases. Estimates of chronic widespread pain in the United Kingdom indicate a prevalence rate of 11% at any given time,[23] confirming that these conditions are common in the general population.

Coexistence of Fibromyalgia and Noncardiac Chest Pain

Functional chest pain

Patients with FM usually present symptoms of other unexplained medical conditions, such as chronic fatigue, bowel dysfunction, or mood disorders, leading to the proposal that FM is just 1 member of a broader family of conditions, the central sensitization syndromes, all of which may share a common underlying pathophysiology (**Fig. 1**).[24] This family of syndromes may include, but is not limited to, regional pain disorders such as myofascial pain syndrome and chronic fatigue syndrome, The relationship between FM and functional gastrointestinal disorders (FGID) is believed to be strong according to the increased number of digestive complaints referred by FM patients[25,26] but also by the number of studies documenting such association.[25–30]

FGID is a heterogeneous group of gastrointestinal diseases characterized by the absence of any structural or biochemical abnormality that could explain the symptoms.[31,32] According to the last consensus definition of FGID, functional chest pain is characterized by episodes of unexplained chest pain that are usually midline in location and of visceral quality, and easily confused with cardiac angina and pain from other esophageal disorders.[33] To our knowledge, there is only 1 study assessing the prevalence of functional chest pain in patients with FM.[25] In this study, the investigators compared a randomly selected sample of 100 patients with FM and 100 matched controls from the Spanish population. Patients and controls completed the Rome II Integrative Questionnaire for Functional Gastrointestinal Disorders to evaluate the prevalence of gastrointestinal symptoms and functional syndromes and the Symptom Checklist-90 Revised (SCL-90R) to evaluate psychological distress; patients also completed the Fibromyalgia Impact Questionnaire (FIQ) to assess the

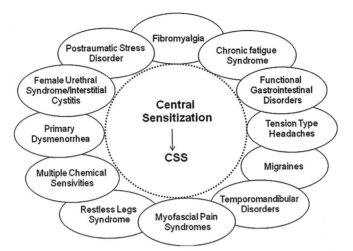

Fig. 1. Central sensitization syndromes share a common etiologic mechanism of central sensitization and frequently present with overlapping epidemiologic, clinical, and psychological features. (*Adapted from* Yunus MB. Role of central sensitization in symptoms beyond muscle pain, and the evaluation of a patient with widespread pain. Best Pract Res Clin Rheumatol 2007;21:481–97; with permission.)

overall impact of the disease. All gastrointestinal symptoms except vomiting were more often reported in FM; chest pain as an individual symptom was significantly more frequent in patients (55%, 95% confidence interval [CI] 45.2–64.8) than in controls (8%, 95% CI 2.7–10.3) (P<.05); on the other hand, the prevalence of functional chest pain was not significantly different between both groups (3%, 95% CI 0–6.3 in patients vs 1%, 95% CI 0–3 in controls). Patients with FM had higher scores for psychological distress, although the presence of functional chest pain did not correlate with additional distress in patients with FM. Moreover, those with coexisting functional chest pain and FM showed lower scores in the Positive Symptom Distress Index (PSDI), which measures the perceived intensity of symptoms, than those with FM but without functional chest pain (P<.05). These data should be interpreted with caution, given the small number of patients that were diagnosed with functional chest pain (n = 3). An additional limitation of this survey is the lack of formal testing, thus, it is possible that a proportion of patients complaining of chest pain may have had cardiac disorders, organic esophageal diseases such as gastroesophageal reflux, or musculoskeletal pain.

Musculoskeletal chest pain

Several studies have reported the prevalence of FM in patients with NCCP. In 1992, Wise and colleagues[34] described a 5% prevalence of FM in patients with NCCP (n = 100). In 1995, Mukerji and colleagues[35] reported a prevalence rate of FM of 30% in a sample of 40 consecutive NCCP patients attending an internal medicine clinic after complete rheumatologic evaluation.

Ho and colleagues[36] evaluated if the presence of chest wall tenderness or FM might help to distinguish between cardiac and noncardiac chest pain, comparing 2 groups of patients with chest pain who previously underwent coronary arteriography. Seven (6 women, 1 man) of 36 patients (19%) were diagnosed with FM according to the ACR criteria in the group of subjects with normal coronary angiograms, whereas only 1 (a man) of 35 (3%) was diagnosed with FM among those with abnormal coronary angiograms ($P = .027$). Commonly, FM associated disorders (Raynaud disease, irritable bowel syndrome, and chronic headache) and tenderness at different body sites were also significantly more frequent in the normal angiogram group. However, the differences previously found between patients with normal and abnormal angiograms were not later confirmed when the results were analyzed by gender, which led the investigators to conclude that the presence of chest wall tenderness and FM was not helpful to distinguish between cardiac and noncardiac chest pain and the differences observed were related to a higher predominance of women in the group with normal coronary angiograms.

In 2004, Dammen and colleagues[37] compared medical comorbidities in patients with chest pain of cardiac (n = 32) and noncardiac origin (n = 167), Based on the patient's self-reported diagnosis of a previous history of FM, the investigators did not find significant differences between groups in the rate of FM diagnosis (7.2% in NCCP vs 3.1% in cardiac patients) or other rheumatologic conditions (25.3% vs 34.4%).

How and colleagues[38] investigated the causes of musculoskeletal chest pain leading to hospital admission in 50 consecutive patients with chest pain without evidence of ischemic heart disease, respiratory disease, or gastrointestinal disease. Patients were included only when they were tender on anteroposterior chest compression, thoracic spine rotation, or firm sternal pressure. Thirteen patients (26%) had FM, 12 (24%) had inflammatory joint disease, and 25 (50%) had other regional painful conditions. Individuals with FM presented the highest scores of pain, anxiety, and depression.

Recently, Husser and colleagues[39] prospectively studied 37 consecutive patients with recurrent NCCP. Patients underwent psychiatric evaluation and completed the SCL-90R questionnaire to exclude psychiatric comorbidity; physical examination was done by an orthopedist to diagnose musculoskeletal abnormalities and a 7-day trial of a proton pump inhibitor (esomeprazole 40 mg daily) was also done to exclude pain related to gastroesophageal reflux. Twenty-one were found to have various psychiatric disorders (57%) including anxiety and depression (n = 10), depression (n = 5), panic disorder (n = 3), and somatization (n = 3). Six patients had musculoskeletal abnormalities (15%), 4 had chostochondritis (10.8%), 1 had thoracic spondylodynia (2.7%), and 1 had FM (2.7%). Sixteen patients (43%) responded to the proton pump inhibitor trial; 6 of these patients had multiple conditions (3 depression, 2 chostochondritis, and 1 FM). **Table 1** summarizes the studies evaluating the prevalence of FM in patients with NCCP.

PATHOGENESIS
Abnormal Pain Processing

Work to elucidate the pathophysiology of FM and related pain syndromes has historically focused on abnormalities in muscle metabolism and joint and soft tissue structure. These investigations have not yielded adequate explanation about the cause and perpetuation of the clinical syndromes, although undoubtedly they may be valid sources of pain. Pain signals, however, seem to be misprocessed at a more central level,[40] a pathophysiologic model that has gained increasing support in recent years. The pathogenesis of these conditions seems to involve dysregulation of pain pathways, leading to central sensitization. In addition to the hallmark pain manifestations of these syndromes, it is recognized that the frequently occurring concomitant symptoms are associated with abnormalities in the physiology of central neurotransmitters, neurohormones, and sleep.[40,41]

Although the pathogenesis of FM and NCCP is not yet completely understood, both disorders seem to share a common longstanding pain hypersensitivity manifested as

Table 1
Summary of studies evaluating the prevalence of FM in NCCP

Author, Year	NCCP (N)	Fibromyalgia Prevalence (%)	FM Diagnostic Criteria
Wise et al,[43] 1992	100	5	ACR criteria
Mukerji et al,[44] 1995	40	30	At least 8 paired tender points
Ho et al,[45] 2001	36	25	ACR criteria
Dammen et al,[46] 2004	167	7.2	Self-reported diagnosis
How et al,[47] 2005[a]	50[a]	26[a]	History and physical examination (multiple tender areas, poor sleep patterns, anxiety, and depression)
Husser et al,[34] 2006	37	2.7	Orthopedist evaluation

[a] Prevalence estimated only for NCCP of musculoskeletal origin.

allodynia (a non-noxious stimuli induces pain) and hyperalgesia (the painful response to a noxious stimuli lasts longer and has higher intensity than normal) present not only at the site of injury (primary) but also at distant or generalized sites (secondary).[42] In FM, hyperalgesia and allodynia are indicated by the painful stimulation of tender points with a pressure of 4 kg/cm^2 or less, a stimulus usually non-noxious in healthy patients.[43]

In patients with NCCP the presence of allodynia has been reported in several studies. Richter and colleagues[44] showed that balloon distension of the distal esophagus, up to a maximum of 10 mL, induces pain more likely in patients with NCCP than in healthy controls (60% vs 20%); furthermore NCCP patients developed chest pain at lower volumes ($\leq$8 mL) compared with controls ($\geq$9 mL).

Sarkar and colleagues[45] compared sensory responses to electrical stimulation after acid infusion in the lower esophagus of NCCP patients (n = 7) and healthy controls (n = 19). Sensory responses were monitored in acid-exposed areas (distal esophagus), non–acid-exposed areas (proximal esophagus), and the cutaneous area of pain referral before and after acid and saline infusion. In the distal esophagus of healthy controls, acid infusion but not saline infusion decreased the pain threshold in the proximal esophagus and chest wall. Moreover, pain thresholds in the proximal esophagus of NCCP patients fell further and responses to acid infusion were significantly longer compared with healthy controls, although no differences were found in both groups after saline infusion. This study showed not only the presence of secondary allodynia in patients with NCCP but also the concurrence of visceral and somatic hypersensitivity.

Studies comparing the effect of thermal stimulus on the chest wall and electrically induced esophageal pain have shown that visceral and somatic stimuli activate similar brain areas.[46] However, there are some differences in the central processing of somatic and visceral pain that may explain the differences in perception, behavior, and vagal response to noxious stimulation of the viscera or somatic structures.[47] Indeed, both stimuli activate secondary somatosensory and parietal cortices, thalamus, basal ganglia, and cerebellum; somatic pain produces greater activation in the anterior insula and ventrolateral prefrontal cortex, whereas visceral stimulation results in activation of bilateral inferior primary somatosensory cortex, bilateral primary motor cortex, and a more rostral region of the dorsal anterior cingular cortex.[47]

Syndromes of widespread pain, including FM, all share neuropathophysiologic features that result in heightened pain sensitivity. Although these disorders are aptly described as central sensitivity syndromes, mechanisms that involve abnormalities in peripheral nerve transmission, central sensory processing in the spinal cord, supraspinal mechanisms, and autonomic responses have all been described to account for many of the symptoms experienced by patients.

At the peripheral nerve level, work focusing on the role of ion-sensing channels in primary afferent neurons has elucidated the potential of certain channel species as points of pharmacologic intervention. Sluka and colleages[48] describes how secondary mechanical hyperalgesia fails to develop in mice knocked out for the membrane protein acid-sensing ion channel 3 (ASIC3), yet re-expression of ASIC3 in muscle tissue of ASIC3 knockout mice restores the development of hyperalgesia.[49] The calcium channel subunit $\alpha 2$-δ is abnormally up-regulated in chronic pain syndromes, and serves as a binding site for drugs such as gabapentin and pregabalin.[50] This secondary pain hypersensitivity also results from an increase in excitability of spinal cord neurons induced by activation of nociceptive C-fibers at the site of injury, leading to central sensitization. Central sensitization is also mediated by the phosphorylation of N-methyl-D-aspartate (NMDA) receptors located at dorsal horn neurons in the spinal cord by the release of neurotransmitters such as glutamate, neurokinin A, or substance P by the nociceptive presynaptic receptors. Activation of NMDA channels through the exchange of magnesium by calcium ions depolarizes the neural membrane, which increases the excitability (hyperalgesia) of neurons and amplifies the received stimulus (allodynia).[51–53] This observation has been experimentally reproduced in visceral and somatic tissues in humans to generate the phenomenon of temporal summation, or wind-up, by which nociceptive signals are amplified and perpetuated at the spinal cord level (**Fig. 2**).[54]

Pain hyper-responsiveness has also been reported at the supraspinal level in nociceptive and affective aspects. Imaging techniques such as functional magnetic resonance imaging (fMRI) have been used to demonstrate hyperactivity in thalamic pain centers and its common projections, such as the insular cortex, which have interconnections with the amygdala, prefrontal cortex, and anterior cingulate cortex.[55] Furthermore, relative decreases in the activity of central pain inhibitory centers, such as the rostral anterior cingulate cortex, are seen.[56] There is, therefore, a situation of extremes whereby pain responses are permitted to be heightened and perpetuated.

In addition, hypothalamic-pituitary-adrenal axis abnormalities and autonomic dysfunction have been well described in FM, NCCP, and other related conditions, and may explain some of the accompanying visceral functional disturbances.[57–61]

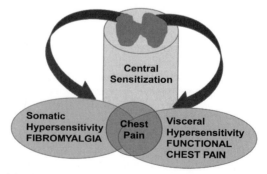

Fig. 2. Central sensitization and NCCP. The pathogenesis of NCCP in patients with FM may be caused by a mechanism of central sensitization via visceral or somatic hypersensitivity.

Increases in sympathetic outflow with decreases in parasympathetic tone result in visceral hyperactivity, which can be manifest as irritable bowel-like symptoms in the gastrointestinal tract, functional bladder abnormalities (in such syndromes as interstitial cystitis), peripheral vasospasm, interstitial peripheral edema, and inappropriate postural cardiovascular responses, among others. Decreases in central norepinephrine release with decreased sympathetic tone reduce pain inhibition in descending pathways of the central nervous system.

Total sleep time, sleep efficiency, and REM sleep are decreased and arousals are increased in patients with fibromyalgia.[62] The α-δ pattern is often observed in polysomnographic studies: intrusion of α (wakeful) brain activity into δ states (stage 3, or deep sleep). α-δ sleep can be seen in patients with chronic pain of any cause, and is clinically associated with nonrestorative symptomatology, which in turn is associated with higher perceived levels of pain.[63]

Psychological Comorbidity

Psychological conditions, such as anxiety, depression, and somatization, are common in patients with NCCP and FM,[14,64–66] although the role of psychological distress in the pathogenesis of these diseases is complex.

Different theories have been postulated to explain the increased relationship between psychological abnormalities and certain functional or medically unexplained diseases: first, psychological factors may cause these disorders; second, psychological distress is the result of having a chronic and painful condition; and third, that certain abnormal psychological profiles increase health care seeking.[67] The current trend is to understand these syndromes as a process, resulting in different stimuli over time; thus, psychological, social, and biologic factors would be interrelated and implied in the origin, perpetuation, and expression of the patient's symptom, a hypothesis already known as the biopsychosocial model (**Fig. 3**).[67,68]

DIAGNOSIS

The diagnostic algorithm of chest pain in a patient with FM is initially identical to that in a patient without FM: first exclude cardiac origin and then evaluate other potential causes of chest pain (see corresponding article in this issue).

However, once disorders of cardiovascular origin and common upper gastrointestinal conditions, such as gastroesphageal reflux or an esophageal motility disorder, have been ruled out, a well-structured and systematic anamnesis and psychological assessment should be conducted bearing in mind the possibility of FM.

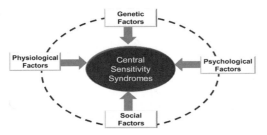

Fig. 3. Biopsychosocial model in central sensitivity syndromes. Genetic, physiologic, psychological and social factors are all related and implied in the origin, perpetuation, and expression of symptoms in patients with central sensitization syndromes.

FM is a complex syndrome characterized not only by the presence of chronic widespread pain but also by its frequent association with unexplained symptoms from other organ systems, such as fatigue, nonrestorative sleep or insomnia, a sensation of swelling, dysesthesias, cognitive difficulties, dizziness, syncope, Raynaud phenomenon, dry mouth, headaches, digestive complaints, anxiety, or depression, among others.[69] The overlap of these symptoms with FM is so important that some investigators have considered them as auxiliary in the diagnosis.[8]

The classification criteria of FM established in 1990 by the ACR require the presence of chronic widespread pain and tenderness at 11 of 18 body sites[8]; chronic widespread pain is considered as the presence of pain in the upper and lower body, axial skeletal and left and right sides, for at least 3 months, without any history of lesion or trauma that can explain the symptoms.[14]

Systematic palpation of tender points is the most relevant physical examination maneuver of a patient with suspected FM. This examination must be performed with an approximate force of 4 kg/cm^2, which is equivalent to the moment when blanching of the examiner's nail bed occurs. The 18 tender points are at 9 symmetric paired locations (**Fig. 4**).[8]

In a patient with FM and coexisting chest pain, the physical examination is of special interest, because it is common, although not specific, to find chest wall tenderness (especially at the tender points located in the anterior chest wall as the midpoint of the upper border of the trapezius and the second rib lateral to the chostochondral junction) and in some cases reproduction of the pain on palpation.[34–36,70]

Although the ACR criteria for the diagnosis of FM are used in most clinical trials and research studies, in practice they are not easy to apply, and many clinicians make a diagnosis without the formal tender point examination.[10] There is a belief that these points represent a marker of severity and distress, and that FM constitutes the extreme of the chronic widespread pain continuum.[71,72]

In 2006, Katz and colleagues,[73] aware of this situation, designed a study to determine the concordance among ACR criteria, clinician diagnosis, and survey criteria in 206 consecutive patients. The survey criteria were previously proposed by the investigators and were based in a score of 8 or higher in a Regional Pain Scale (RPS) and a fatigue score of 6 or higher on a visual analog scale.[74] Among the 206 patients, 101 (49%) were diagnosed clinically with FM, 60 (29%) according to the ACR criteria and 83 (40.3%) based on survey criteria. Clinical and survey criteria were concordant in 74.8% of cases; clinical and ACR criteria in 75.2% of cases and survey criteria and ACR criteria in 72.3%. Of the patients who were diagnosed as having FM by at least 1 method, only 33% would be diagnosed by the 3 methods; 17% would be diagnosed clinically only, 12% by the survey criteria, and 2% by the ACR criteria only. The investigators concluded that given that there is no gold standard for FM and the concordance rates were moderately in agreement, all these methods might be useful in the diagnosis of FM.[73]

Recently, the ACR has begun the task of revising the diagnostic and severity criteria for FM, appreciating the fact that the tender point examination may not be necessary to assign a diagnosis. Wolfe and colleagues[13] recently proposed novel criteria that largely exclude the need for tender points, although at the same time generally adhering to the concept of FM presented in the 1990 criteria. These new criteria are based largely on an index of widespread pain (WPI) and a symptom severity score (SSS), which comprises the presence of fatigue, nonrestorative sleep, cognitive disturbances, and other somatic symptoms. These criteria offer better face validity by capturing the concept of FM as a disorder of central sensitization with frequent nonmusculoskeletal and constitutional symptoms. Although validation studies have yet to

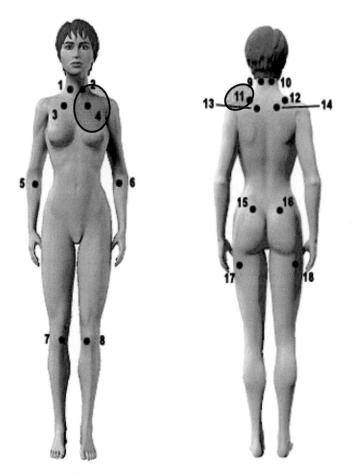

Fig. 4. Tender points in fibromyalgia. The authors have highlighted those tender points of special interest in the diagnosis of NCCP in patients with FM. (*Adapted from* Villanueva VL, Valiá JC, Cerdá G, et al. Fibromyalgia diagnosis and treatment. Current knowledge. Rev Soc Esp Dolor 2004;11:430–43; with permission.) 1, 2, low cervical region: (front neck area) at the anterior aspect of the interspaces between the transverse processes of C5 to C7; 3, 4, second rib: (front chest area) at second costochondral junctions; 5, 6, lateral epicondyle (elbow area) 2 cm distal to the lateral epicondyle; 7, 8, knee (knee area) at the medial fat pad proximal to the joint line; 9, 10, occiput (back of the neck) at the suboccipital muscle insertions; 11, 12, trapezius muscle (back shoulder area) at the midpoint of the upper border; 13, 14, supraspinatus muscle (shoulder blade area) above the medial border of the scapular spine; 15, 16, gluteal (rear end) at the upper outer quadrant of the buttocks; 17, 18, greater trochanter (rear hip) posterior to the greater trochanteric prominence.

be conducted, these new criteria will likely offer greater sensitivity and place the patient in the correct diagnostic arena where the principles of treatment would apply.

As the diagnosis of FM is based solely on clinical and exploratory data without clinically available biologic diagnostic markers, the value of laboratory and diagnostic tests in FM is low.[70] The only tests recommended are a complete blood count and basic chemistry panels including thyroid hormones and those indicated based on the symptoms and physical examination findings.[70] Markers of systemic autoimmunity and infectious agents are generally unfruitful. See **Fig. 5** for a proposed management algorithm in patients with NCCP and suspected FM.

TREATMENT

Various pharmacologic and nonpharmacologic treatments have been shown to have short-term positive effects on individual symptoms of FM: antidepressant such as amitryptiline, cyclobenzaprine, fluoxetine, duloxetine, milnacipran[75,76]; opiates such as tramadol and other central nervous system acting agents such as gabapentin and pregabalin (approved by the US Food and Drug Administration)[75,77]; aerobic exercise,[78] cognitive behavioral therapy,[78] and even alternative treatments such as homeopathy, hydrotherapy, or acupuncture.[79,80] However, to date the results of several meta-analysis show that none of these therapeutic interventions have been effective to control all the symptoms related to the FM syndrome or change the natural history of the disease.[75] Given the heterogeneity of patients with FM, the better approach seems to be to individualize the treatment for every patient according to their main complaints.[75]

Data suggest that a multimodality approach that addresses the issues of pain, fatigue, and sleep and mood disorders, and includes cognitive behavioral therapy, produces the greatest benefit in the long-term.[78] This approach includes the use of analgesics such as nonsteroidal antiinflammatory drugs and tramadol for pain relief (but avoiding moderate to potent opiate analgesics), antidepressants, sleep aids, and atypical neuroactive agents such as pregabalin, usually in a carefully titrated, stepwise approach as chemical and drug sensitivities are common.[75–78]

Exercise, often with the initial assistance of a physical therapist familiar with the precepts of FM treatment, should be gradual and graded to avoid over-exhaustion and more pain, and to promote sustainability.[78] A formal sleep evaluation, including polysomnography, is often required to diagnose treatable disorders of sleep such as obstructive apnea, restless leg syndrome, or sleep disordered breathing.[79]

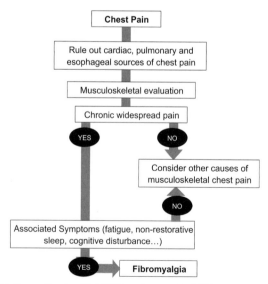

Fig. 5. Approach to the patient with NCCP and suspected FM.

Table 2	
Potential therapeutic approach in NCCP and FM	
Pharmacologic: Pain Control	**Nonpharmacologic: Adjuvant Therapy**
Tramadol	Physical therapy (gradual supervised exercise programs)
Cyclobenzaprine	Sleep evaluation and therapy
Tricyclic antidepressants	Cognitive behavioral therapy
Pregabaline Duloxetine Milnacipran	Treatment of other coexisting conditions (psychological, gastrointestinal, and so forth)

Cognitive behavioral therapy may be incorporated to treat dysfunctional pain attitudes and behaviors and promote lifestyle adjustments such as goal-setting, prioritization, pacing, and building support systems.[78] More and more specialized centers for treatment of FM using a comprehensive paradigm are being established. Referral of the patient should be considered. **Table 2** summarizes current therapeutic approach in patients with NCCP and FM.

SUMMARY

FM remains an enigmatic and challenging clinical entity to manage, given its wide spectrum of symptoms, chronicity, associated psychopathology, and lack of clinically available diagnostic tests. However, recent insights into the pathophysiology of FM offer hope that this condition, and all central sensitization syndromes, can be more readily diagnosed, measured, and treated. Among the manifestations of FM, NCCP seems to be frequent. The clinician should be vigilant to the possibility of FM and its important attendant comorbidities as an important contributor in these clinical situations.

REFERENCES

1. Gowers WR. A lesson on lumbago: its lessons and analogues. Br Med J 1904;1: 117–21.
2. Pugh LG, Christie TA. A study of rheumatism in a group of soldiers with reference to the incidence of trigger points and fibrositic nodules. Ann Rheum Dis 1945; 5(1):8–10.
3. Steindler A, Luck JV. Differential diagnosis of pain in the low back: allocation of the source of pain by the procaine hydrochloride method. JAMA 1938;110: 106–13.
4. Kelly M. The nature of fibrositis III: multiple lesions and the neural hypothesis. Ann Rheum Dis 1946;5(5):161–7.
5. Patton IJ, Williamson JA. Fibrositis as a factor in the differential diagnosis of visceral pain. Can Med Assoc J 1948;58(2):162–6.
6. Moldofsky H, Scarisbrick P, England R, et al. Musculoskeletal symptoms and non-REM sleep disturbance in patients with "fibrositis syndrome" and healthy subjects. Psychosom Med 1975;37:341–51.
7. Smythe HA, Moldofsky H. Two contributions to understanding of the "fibrositis" syndrome. Bull Rheum Dis 1977–1978;28(1):928–31.
8. Wolfe F, Smythe HA, Yunus MB, et al. The American College of Rheumatology 1990 criteria for the classification of fibromyalgia. Report of the multicenter criteria committee. Arthritis Rheum 1990;33:160–72.

9. Quintner J. Fibromyalgia: the Copenhagen declaration. Lancet 1992;340(8827):1103.

10. Fitzcharles MA, Boulos P. Inaccuracy in the diagnosis of fibromyalgia syndrome: analysis of referrals. Rheumatology (Oxford) 2003;42:263–7.

11. Clauw DJ, Crofford LJ. Chronic widespread pain and fibromyalgia: what we know, and what we need to know. Best Pract Res Clin Rheumatol 2003;17:685–701.

12. Crofford LJ, Clauw DJ. Fibromyalgia: where are we a decade after the American College of Rheumatology classification criteria were developed? Arthritis Rheum 2002;46:1136–8.

13. Wolfe F, Clauw D, Fitzcharles MA, et al. Clinical diagnostic and severity criteria for fibromyalgia [abstract]. Arthritis Rheum 2009;60(10 Suppl):S210.

14. Wolfe F, Ross K, Anderson J, et al. The prevalence and characteristics of fibromyalgia in the general population. Arthritis Rheum 1995;38(1):19–28.

15. Berger A, Dukes E, Martin S, et al. Characteristics and healthcare costs of patients with fibromyalgia syndrome. Int J Clin Pract 2007;61:1498–508.

16. Zeng QY, Chen R, Darmawan J, et al. Rheumatic diseases in China. Arthritis Res Ther 2008;10(1):R17.

17. Reyes-Llerena GA, Guibert-Toledano M, Penedo-Coello A, et al. Community-based study to estimate prevalence and burden of illness of rheumatic diseases in Cuba: a COPCORD study. J Clin Rheumatol 2009;15(2):51–5.

18. Cardiel MH, Rojas-Serrano J. Community based study to estimate prevalence, burden of illness and help seeking behavior in rheumatic diseases in Mexico City. A COPCORD study. Clin Exp Rheumatol 2002;20(5):617–24.

19. Bannwarth B, Blotman F, Roué-Le Lay K. Fibromyalgia syndrome in the general population of France: a prevalence study. Joint Bone Spine 2009;76(2):184–7.

20. Mas AJ, Carmona L, Valverde M, et al. Prevalence and impact of fibromyalgia on function and quality of life in individuals from the general population: results from a nationwide study in Spain. Clin Exp Rheumatol 2008;26(4):519–26.

21. White KP, Speechley M, Harth M. The London Fibromyalgia Epidemiology Study: the prevalence of fibromyalgia syndrome in London, Ontario. J Rheumatol 1999; 26(7):1570–6.

22. Haq SA, Darmawan J, Islam MN, et al. Prevalence of rheumatic diseases and associated outcomes in rural and urban communities in Bangladesh: a COPCORD study. J Rheumatol 2005;32(2):348–53.

23. Croft P, Rigby AS, Boswell R, et al. The prevalence of chronic widespread pain in the general population. J Rheumatol 1993;20:710–3.

24. Yunus MB. Role of central sensitization in symptoms beyond muscle pain, and the evaluation of a patient with widespread pain. Best Pract Res Clin Rheumatol 2007;21:481–97.

25. Almansa C, Rey E, García R, et al. Prevalence of functional gastrointestinal disorders in patients with fibromyalgia and the role of psychological distress. Clin Gastroenterol Hepatol 2009;7:438–45.

26. Triadafilopoulos G, Simms RW, Goldenberg DL. Bowel dysfunction in fibromyalgia syndrome. Dig Dis Sci 1991;36(1):59–64.

27. Romano TJ. Coexistence of irritable bowel syndrome and fibromyalgia. W V Med J 1988;84:16–8.

28. Yunus MB, Masi AT, Aldag JC, et al. A controlled study of primary fibromyalgia syndrome: clinical features and association with other functional syndromes. J Rheumatol Suppl 1989;19:62–71.

29. Veale D, Kavanagh G, Fielding JF, et al. Primary fibromyalgia and the irritable bowel syndrome: different expressions of a common pathogenetic process. Br J Rheumatol 1991;30(3):220–2.

30. Sivri A, Cindas A, Dincer F, et al. Bowel dysfunction and irritable bowel syndrome in fibromyalgia patients. Clin Rheumatol 1996;15:236–83.

31. Longstreet GF, Thompson WG, Chey WD, et al. Functional bowel disorders. Gastroenterology 2006;130:1480–91.

32. Thompson WG. The road to Rome. Gastroenterology 2006;130:1550–6.

33. Galmiche JP, Clouse RE, Balint A, et al. Functional esophageal disorders. Gastroenterology 2006;130:1459–65.

34. Wise CM, Semble EL, Dalton CB. Musculoskeletal chest wall syndromes in patients with noncardiac chest pain: a study of 100 patients. Arch Phys Med Rehabil 1992;73(2):147–9.

35. Mukerji B, Mukerji V, Alpert MA, et al. The prevalence of rheumatologic disorders in patients with chest pain and angiographically normal coronary arteries. Angiology 1995;46(5):425–30.

36. Ho M, Walker S, McGarry F, et al. Chest wall tenderness is unhelpful in the diagnosis of recurrent chest pain. QJM 2001;94:267–70.

37. Dammen T, Arnesen H, Ekeberg O, et al. Psychological factors, pain attribution and medical morbidity in chest pain with and without coronary artery disease. Gen Hosp Psychiatry 2004;26:463–9.

38. How J, Volz G, Doe S, et al. The cause of musculoskeletal chest pain in patients admitted to hospital with suspected myocardial infarction. Eur J Intern Med 2005; 16:432–6.

39. Husser D, Bollmann A, Kühne C, et al. Evaluation of noncardiac chest pain: diagnostic approach, coping strategies and quality of life. Eur J Pain 2006;10: 51–5.

40. Bennett RM. Emerging concepts in the neurobiology of chronic pain: evidence of abnormal sensory processing in fibromyalgia. Mayo Clin Proc 1999;74:385–98.

41. Pillemer SR, Bradley LA, Crofford LJ, et al. The neuroscience and endocrinology of fibromyalgia. Arthritis Rheum 1997;40:1928–39.

42. Nielsen LA, Henriksson KG. Pathophysiological mechanisms in chronic musculoskeletal pain (fibromyalgia): the role of central and peripheral sensitization and pain disinhibition. Best Pract Res Clin Rheumatol 2007;21(3):465–80.

43. Russell IJ, Larson AA. Neurophysiopathogenesis of fibromyalgia syndrome: a unified hypothesis. Rheum Dis Clin North Am 2009;35:421–35.

44. Richter JE, Barish CF, Castell DO. Abnormal sensory perception in patients with esophageal chest pain. Gastroenterology 1986;91:845–52.

45. Sarkar S, Aziz Q, Woolf CJ, et al. Contribution of central sensitization to the development of noncardiac chest pain. Lancet 2000;356:1154–9.

46. Hobson AR, Chizh B, Hicks K, et al. Neurophysiological evaluation of convergent afferents innervating the human esophagus and area of referred pain on the anterior chest wall. Am J Physiol Gastrointest Liver Physiol 2010;298(1):G31–6.

47. Mayer EA, Aziz Q, Coen S, et al. Brain imaging approaches to the study of functional GI disorders: a Rome working team report. Neurogastroenterol Motil 2009; 21:579–96.

48. Sluka KA, Radhakrishnan R, Benson CJ, et al. ASIC3 in muscle mediates mechanical, but not heat, hyperalgesia associated with muscle inflammation. Pain 2007;129:102–12.

49. Ikeuchi M, Kolker SJ, Burnes LA, et al. Role of ASIC3 in the primary and secondary hyperalgesia produced by joint inflammation in mice. Pain 2008; 137(3):662–9.

50. Finnerup NB, Jensen TS. Clinical use of pregabalin in the management of central neuropathic pain. Neuropsychiatr Dis Treat 2007;3(6):885–91.

51. Staud R, Domingo M. Evidence for abnormal pain processing in fibromyalgia syndrome. Pain Med 2001;2:208–15.
52. Woolf CJ, Thompson SW. The induction and maintenance of central sensitization is dependent on N-methyl-D-aspartic acid receptor activation; implications for treatment of post-injury hypersensitivity states. Pain 1991;44:293–9.
53. Orlando RC. Esophageal perception and noncardiac chest pain. Gastroenterol Clin North Am 2004;33:25–33.
54. Sarkar S, Woolf CJ, Hobson AR, et al. Perceptual wind-up in the human oesophagus is enhanced by central sensitization. Gut 2006;55:920–5.
55. Guedj E, Cammilleri S, Niboyet J. Clinical correlate of brain SPECT perfusion abnormalities in fibromyalgia. J Nucl Med 2008;49:1798–803.
56. Jenson KB, Kosek E, Petzke F, et al. Evidence of dysfunctional pain inhibition in fibromyalgia reflected in rACC during provoked pain. Pain 2009;144(1–2): 95–100.
57. Crofford LJ, Pillemer SR, Kalogeras KT, et al. Hypothalamic-pituitary-adrenal axis perturbations in patients with fibromyalgia. Arthritis Rheum 1994;37:1583–92.
58. Dinan TG, Quigley EMM, Ahmed S, et al. Hypothalamic-pituitary-gut axis dysregulation in irritable bowel syndrome: plasma cytokines as a potential biomarker? Gastroenterology 2006;130:304–11.
59. Martinez-Lavin M, Hermosillo AG, Rosas M, et al. Circadian studies of autonomic nervous balance in patients with fibromyalgia: a heart rate variability analysis. Arthritis Rheum 1998;41:1966–71.
60. Hollerbach S, Bulat R, May A, et al. Abnormal processing of esophageal stimuli in patients with noncardiac chest pain (NCCP). Neurogastroenterol Motil 2001; 12(6):555–65.
61. Tougas G, Spaziani R, Hollerbach S, et al. Cardiac autonomic function and oesophageal acid sensitivity in patients with non-cardiac chest pain. Gut 2001;49(5): 706–12.
62. Molony RR, MacPeek DM, Schiffman PL, et al. Sleep, sleep apnea and the fibromyalgia syndrome. J Rheumatol 1986;13(4):797–800.
63. Moldofsky H. The significance of dysfunctions of the sleeping/waking brain to the pathogenesis and treatment of fibromyalgia syndrome. Rheum Dis Clin North Am 2009;35(2):275–83.
64. Clouse R, Carney RM. The psychological profile of non-cardiac chest pain patients. Eur J Gastroenterol Hepatol 1995;7:1160–5.
65. Song CW, lee SL, Jeen YT, et al. Inconsistent association of esophageal symptoms, psychometric abnormalities and dismotility. Am J Gastroenterol 2001;96:2312–6.
66. McBeth J, Macfarlane GJ, Benjamin S, et al. Features of somatization predict the onset of chronic widespread pain: results of a large population-based study. Arthritis Rheum 2001;44(4):940–6.
67. Drossman DA. Psychosocial factors and the disorders of GI function: what is the link? Am J Gastroenterol 2004;99(2):358–60.
68. Ferrari R. The biopsychosocial model: a tool for rheumatologists. Baillieres Best Pract Res Clin Rheumatol 2000;14:787–95.
69. Bennett RM. Clinical manifestations and diagnosis of fibromyalgia. Rheum Dis Clin North Am 2009;35:215–32.
70. Yunus MB. A comprehensive medical evaluation of patients with fibromyalgia syndrome. Rheum Dis Clin North Am 2002;28:201–7.
71. Aaron LA, Buchwald D. Chronic diffuse musculoskeletal pain, fibromyalgia and co-morbid unexplained clinical conditions. Best Pract Res Clin Rheumatol 2003;17(4):563–74.

72. Wolfe F. The relation between tender points and fibromyalgia symptom variables: evidence that fibromyalgia is not a discrete disorder in the clinic. Ann Rheum Dis 1997;56:268–71.
73. Katz RS, Wolfe R, Michaud K. Fibromyalgia diagnosis. A comparison of clinical, survey and American College Rheumatology criteria. Arthritis Rheum 2006;54(1): 169–76.
74. Wolfe F. Pain extent and diagnosis: development and validation of the regional pain scale in 12,799 patients with rheumatic disease. J Rheumatol 2003;30: 369–78.
75. Abeles M, Solitar BM, Philinger MH, et al. Update of fibromyalgia therapy. Am J Med 2008;121(7):555–61.
76. Häuser W, Bernardy K, Uçeyler N, et al. Treatment of fibromyalgia syndrome with antidepressants: a meta-analysis. JAMA 2009;301(2):198–209.
77. Häuser W, Bernardy K, Uçeyler N, et al. Treatment of fibromyalgia syndrome with gabapentin and pregabalin—a meta-analysis of randomized controlled trials. Pain 2009;145(1–2):69–81.
78. Goldenberg DL, Burckhardt C, Crofford L. Management of fibromyalgia syndrome. JAMA 2004;292(19):2388–95.
79. Gold AR, Dipalo F, Gold MS, et al. Inspiratory airflow dynamics during sleep in women with fibromyalgia. Sleep 2004;27(3):459–66.
80. Villanueva VL, Valiá JC, Cerdá G, et al. Fibromyalgia diagnosis and treatment. Current knowledge. Rev Soc Esp Dolor 2004;11:430–43.

Assessment and Treatment of Psychological Causes of Chest Pain

Kamila S. White, PhD

KEYWORDS

- Chest pain • Coronary artery disease
- Noncardiac chest pain • Nonanginal
- Anxiety • Depression • Cognitive behavior therapy

Because it sometimes indicates acute, life-threatening events in patients with or without known heart disease, the experience of chest pain can be frightening. Chest pain prompts an estimated 4.6 million people in the United States to seek emergency medical care each year.[1] Some of these individuals receive an organic explanation for their chest pain (eg, coronary artery disease [CAD], myocardial infarction). CAD is the leading cause of death in men and women in developed nations, particularly among ethnic minorities.[2,3] Chest pain is common in CAD, particularly among patients with chronic refractory angina.[4] In contrast to patients with cardiac disease, some patients experience chest pain but are free of obstructive CAD or other cardiac causes for their chest pain. These patients are often determined to suffer from noncardiac chest pain (NCCP). At least half of all patients referred for cardiac evaluations do not have ischemic heart disease or another serious medical disorder to account for their chest symptoms.[5,6] In fact, the total economic burden of medical care for patients who are admitted with suspected ischemic symptoms but who do not sustain acute myocardial infarction has been estimated at 10 to 13 billion dollars annually.[7] In either case, organic or nonorganic, the assessment and treatment of psychological factors may be important to for the patient with chest pain.

Psychological assessment and treatment may clinically aid the patient with chest pain in ways that may influence disease onset and progression. Psychological interventions can promote behavior changes, and aid adherence and compliance with medical treatments. Treatments aimed at emotional disorders (eg, depression, anxiety) can ease the burden of pain and disease through biobehavioral pathways (ie, behavioral, pathophysiological) and help patients cope with disease-related issues. This article highlights factors important for psychological assessment and

Department of Psychology, University of Missouri-St. Louis, 212 Stadler Hall, One University Boulevard, St. Louis, MO 63121, USA
E-mail address: whiteks@umsl.edu

Med Clin N Am 94 (2010) 291–318
doi:10.1016/j.mcna.2010.01.005
0025-7125/10/$ – see front matter © 2010 Elsevier Inc. All rights reserved.

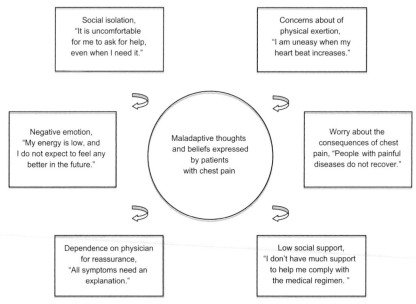

Fig. 1. Maladaptive cognitions expressed by patients with chest pain that may augment pain and emotional distress.

treatment of the chest pain patient. First, practical guidelines for an integrated cognitive, affective, and behavioral assessment are presented that include diagnostic evaluation of clinical disorders, assessment of psychological problems, and appraisal of health behaviors for primary or secondary prevention. Included in this is a discussion of the benefits of a functional behavioral analysis. Second, an overview of psychological treatments is presented, with an emphasis on empirically supported psychological treatments for the reduction of negative emotion and its association with chest pain.

PSYCHOLOGICAL ASSESSMENT

Psychological assessment with the chest pain patient involves an integration of cognitive, affective, and behavioral functioning in relation to medical health and disease. This approach is often central out of necessity. Personal medical history is often the first target of assessment partly because patients are often more at ease discussing medical history than the influence of it on their lives and their coping responses. Assessment of the patient's knowledge about their disease, their perception of the treatment regimen, and factors that have influenced their adherence and compliance are important factors to assess. Treatment nonadherence is one of the primary reasons for referral to psychologists. Treatment nonadherence is consistently poor among patients with CAD. For example, in a recent longitudinal study conducted over 7 years, almost half of the CAD patients reported that they did not consistently adhere to secondary prevention medications.[8] Discerning the cause of nonadherence may be a goal of psychological assessment. Sources of nonadherence may be financial (eg, economic hardship, poverty), cognitive (eg, memory, confusion, dementia), affective (eg, depression, anxiety), or other psychological factors (eg, denial). As a result, an account of all medications prescribed and taken including those taken without a prescription (eg, herbal, over-the-counter) is recommended. Clinicians may find that approaching patients with an empathic, nonjudgmental concern to engage them in the assessment may increase the likelihood of sincere responses, in light of the possible factors that may guide their reporting of treatment adherence and compliance.

Consultation and liaison activities are often central to assessment and treatment planning. In outpatient settings, for example, it is customary to discuss the boundaries of the consult with the patient and to obtain informed consent to contact the physician (ie, verbal permission and a signed release form) at the outset of the assessment. This release of information is central to patient care for a couple of reasons.

First, collaborating with the referring physician and other medical team members is important for the patient's health and safety. For referrals to clinical psychologists and other practitioners who work with chest pain patients or patients with cardiac conditions, ongoing assessment of the patient's health and safety is vital. In addition to common psychological risks (eg, suicidal), clinicians need to be aware of risks associated with medication noncompliance, avoidance of follow-up medical visits, and further physical symptoms (eg, increased shortness of breath, unexplained worsening of chest symptoms). It is important to consult the patient's physician when new symptoms develop or when persistent symptoms worsen. Successful communication and ongoing collaboration with the multidisciplinary team are important for the patient's health and safety.

Second, obtaining the referral question can be important to address any patient misunderstandings or misinterpretations. Psychological referrals for chest pain patients generally involve (1) management of cardiovascular risk factors (eg, smoking, eating habits, exercise), (2) adherence to medical treatment and cardiac rehabilitation, and (3) treatment of clinical disorders or adjustment and coping difficulties.[9] Although these are the most common referral questions, the patient's perceptions of the reasons for the referral may differ. For instance, anxious heart patients may misperceive a psychological referral from their physician as an indication that their chest symptoms are not genuine or that the physician believes they have a mental illness causing the symptoms. For these reasons, an optimal referral and evaluation bolstered by the support and clarity from the referring physician is important. Patients may be most receptive to psychological referrals that are introduced by physicians as part of routine care essential for health outcomes. This referral may be especially helpful for older CAD patients, many of whom are less typical of conventional psychotherapy populations, being apt to diminish emotional problems or resist recommendations for psychological care.[9,10]

A functional behavioral analysis can be an efficient guide for the psychological assessment process. The functional analysis is a method of gathering and incorporating clinical information that may include information from the personal medical history, medical record, clinical interview, self-report questionnaires, self-monitoring, behavioral tests, psychophysiologic tests, and structured diagnostic interview. The analysis will help guide a complete understanding of the cognitive, behavioral, and physiologic components of the patient's chest pain experience and accompanying emotional distress. Several important factors may be particularly relevant for the patient with chest pain. The characterization of the chest pain episodes including the frequency, intensity, duration, and quality of the pain and discomfort may be important. The situational antecedents (eg, exertion, being alone, driving on highways), the internal antecedents (ie, interoceptive fears, heart rate fluctuations, hunger feelings, thoughts about a cardiac event that might happen) that precipitate the chest pain episodes, and the factors that alleviate the pain (eg, rest, medication) are assessed. The patient's cognitive appraisals or possible misappraisals about the chest symptoms (eg, beliefs that the chest pain may not stop, fears of incapacitation or death) are assessed. His or her behavioral reactions include cardioprotective behavior (eg, avoidance of exertion, changes in alcohol use, sedentary behavior) and escape behavior (leaving or avoiding work, social isolation, avoidance of being alone, use of medication) (**Fig. 1**). An evaluation is made of the social consequences of these behaviors and the possible negative affects, personal quality of life, and the patient's family and supportive others. Involvement of supportive others may be useful in the assessment and treatment process. **Box 1** summarizes a select group of relatively brief instruments that may be useful for screening and assessing cognitive and psychological factors in patients with chest pain, as appropriate.

Psychosocial Influences

Psychosocial factors often influence the course and prognosis for patients with chest pain. Among the psychosocial factors that have been found to influence CAD and chest pain outcomes are social factors (ie, low social support, social isolation), job strain, stress (ie, stressful life events, financial stress), temperament characteristics influences ("type D" personality [similar to neuroticism], a hostile temperament), and the negative emotions (ie, depression, anxiety). The negative emotions, for example, exert a harmful influence on CAD outcomes and quality of life. A sizeable, persuasive literature links depression to CAD morbidity and mortality; for a review see Carney and Friedland.[11] In the year following initial CAD diagnosis, the presence of depression doubles the risk for cardiac events, including cardiac mortality.[12,13] A growing body of literature points to the role of anxiety (particularly phobic anxiety) as a risk factor for CAD morbidity and mortality; for a review see White.[14] Sudden, strong emotion is one of the two most common precipitating events experienced before sudden cardiac death (SCD); exercise is the other event.[15] Perhaps the most compelling support for a link between anxiety and CAD has arisen from longitudinal studies conducted with initially healthy samples that have controlled for the effects of known cardiovascular risk factors in the prediction of subsequent disease. In the past 2 decades, large-scale community-based studies have established a significant relationship between anxiety and subsequent death due to cardiac pathology in men[16-18] and women.[19]

Diagnostic Evaluation of Psychiatric Disorders

Systematic evaluation of psychiatric disorders for chest pain patients may be beneficial to identify clinical problems that may be causal or comorbid with chest pain. As others have wisely pointed out,[20] it can be challenging to discern whether a medical condition is a cause, correlate, or complicating factor in patients with co-occurring emotional disorders. In the case of panic attacks, for example, the physical symptoms of panic can mimic cardiorespiratory (eg, shortness of breath, chest pain, palpitations), gastrointestinal (eg, stomach upset, nausea), and otoneurological (eg, vertigo, disequilibrium) symptoms. Of course, the presence of a psychiatric disorder does not rule out the coexistence of medical disorder, and the necessity of treating both. Further, some psychiatric disorders (ie, anxiety and depression) are prospectively associated with an increased risk of cardiovascular morbidity and mortality (for reviews see Refs.[11,14]). The Structured Clinical Interview for DSM-IV (SCID-IV)[21] and the Anxiety Disorders Interview Schedule for the DSM-IV (ADIS-IV)[22] are among the most widely used structured interviews to assess current and lifetime Axis I disorders. Throughout the interview, the clinician can judiciously query to separate symptoms of the disease (eg, low energy, weakness) and natural reactions to a cardiac diagnosis from a clinically significant psychiatric disorder. Most DSM-IV disorders

Box 1
Useful instruments to screen and assess for cognitive and psychological factors in patients with chest pain

General psychiatric screening

    Brief symptom inventory (BSI)[184,185]

        Format: Self-report

        Length: 53 items

    Hospital Anxiety and Depression Scale (HADS)[186]

        Format: Self-report

        Length: 14 items

    Health-Related Quality of Life (Short Form SF-36)[187]

        Format: Self-report

        Length: 20 items

    Brief Psychiatric Rating Scale-Expanded (BPRS)[188]

        Format: Self-report, Interview

        Length: 18 items, variable

Brief cognitive screening

    Mini-mental state examination-modified[189]

        Format: Interview

        Length: 12 minutes

    Neurobehavioral Cognitive Status Examination (CSE)[190]

        Format: Interview

        Length: 45 minutes

Affective and anxiety disorders

    Beck anxiety inventory[191]

        Format: Self-report

        Length: 21 items

    Beck depression inventory-II[192]

        Format: Self-report

        Length: 25 items

    Primary Care Evaluation of Mental Disorders (PRIME-MD)[193,194]

        Format: Self-report, Interview

        Length: 10 minutes

    Anxiety Disorders Interview Schedule for DSM-IV (ADIS-IV)[195]

        Format: Interview

        Length: 60 minutes Variable

    Structured Clinical Interview for DSM-IV (SCID-IV)[196]

        Format: Interview

        Length: 60 minutes Variable

require clinically significant distress or require that the patient experience impaired social, occupational, or other functioning as a result.[23] Use of diagnostic clinical interviews ensures that clinically significant psychopathology is differentiated from symptoms that may reflect the disease itself, its treatment (eg, side effects from medications), or other adjustment issues related to a chronic illness. Inclusion of family members or other reporters (eg, adult children) may be useful to corroborate patient reports, particularly if family members are not good reporters. Indeed, some cases show signs of cognitive impairments and disorders (ie, dementia) or other disorders (eg, Axis II disorders) that may necessitate additional assessment and referral for dedicated care.

Prevention of Negative Health Behaviors

Health behaviors may be a focus of psychological assessment for the chest pain patient, and the costs and benefits to making lifestyle changes differs for primary, secondary, and tertiary prevention. For chest pain patients seeking primary prevention, lifestyle changes are made in the absence of heart disease or other cardiac problems (eg, noncardiac chest pain patients). On the other hand, lifestyle changes for a patient with established atherosclerosis who is symptomatic (eg, angina) is essential. Secondary prevention efforts may include a risk factor modification program to prevent unfavorable health outcomes linked with an advancing disease process.[24] Targets of health behavior change may include smoking behavior, unhealthy dietary patterns, physical inactivity, failure to adhere to medical regimen, or other lifestyle choices that are associated with the destructive metabolic syndrome (ie, abdominal obesity, hypertension, insulin resistance, low- and high-density lipoprotein cholesterol) (**Table 1**).[25]

Working with the patient to establish concrete, achievable health behavior goals in a specific time period can be practical and rewarding for the patient, the physician, and the health care team. Although patients and physicians often aim to achieve more goals in a shorter time, setting unrealistic goals at the outset of therapy can disappoint the patient and may detract from him or her making any health behavior changes. In the case of the chest pain patient with CAD, these patients are often overwhelmed by several interconnected, often multifaceted, negative health behaviors. Research and clinical experts have pointed to the benefits of ranking and prioritizing the medical problems and emotional needs (eg, depression, anxiety) of these patients to best meet their care.[24] As a clinical example, a 64-year-old male chest pain patient with CAD was referred for psychological services because of an inability to incorporate recommended lifestyle changes that included smoking cessation, increased physical activity, and dietary changes. Tackling all of these health behaviors together can be stressful for a CAD patient who may also be experiencing low energy, an inconsistent motivation for health behavior change, and real-world obstacles to accomplishing these tasks (eg, limited number of insurance sessions). Perhaps a successful set of treatment goals might be to enroll in a smoking cessation program, meet with a dietitian, and begin a daily physical activity routine in accord with physician recommendations. For patients that have difficulty making the prescribed health behavior changes recommended by their physician, they might benefit from an evaluation of the costs, barriers, and benefits to health behavior change. This evaluation may include the thoughts, emotions, behaviors, and physical factors that hinder them from making progress. For instance, a clinician may find that a patient may benefit from external social support to incorporate dietary changes in the home. As a result, enlisting the help of a supportive other (eg,

Table 1
Modifiable risk factors and psychosocial risk factors for chest pain and cardiac related syndromes

Modifiable health behaviors

  Smoking behavior
  Sedentary lifestyle
  Obesity (ie, 35% or more above ideal body weight)
  Hypertension
  Diabetes mellitus
  Unhealthy dietary patterns
  High overall or "bad" cholesterol (low-density lipoprotein [LDL])
  Low "good" cholesterol (high-density lipoprotein [HDL])

Psychosocial factors

  Depression
  Anxiety
  Reactive to stress
  Social isolation
  Anger expression
  Hostile temperament
  Vital exhaustion
  Low social support

Data from Cardiac related syndromes American Heart Association. Heart and stroke statistical update. Dallas, TX: AHA; 2009.

adult child, partner) to accomplish some of the treatment goals may be useful for some patients. Health behavior change can be demanding, and some patients are referred for psychological evaluation because they lack the motivation for health behavior change. Research incorporating motivational interviewing techniques has shown promise for some areas of health behavior change, including smoking cessation,[26] and holds promise with chest pain patients[27] (see section "Eliciting Behavior Change").

Psychological Factors and Noncardiac Chest Pain

The role of medical reassurance

Medical tests are a requisite first step for the chest pain patient, but for patients with NCCP whose pain is persistent in the absence of absence of myocardial ischemia, CAD, or other identifiable cardiac cause, the test results sometimes fail to alleviate their concerns.[28] Although studies in this area are fraught by sampling biases, psychological factors appear to play an influential role in exacerbation and persistence of chest pain and related symptoms in NCCP.[29] Extensive medical testing may be iatrogenic for some patients with NCCP. Patients may begin to worry that because follow-up testing is unable to uncover a cause for their pain, they may conclude that their illness is unusual, difficult to diagnose, and therefore unlikely to be treatable. Even after sometimes extensive testing, patients with NCCP often do not receive a definitive diagnosis[30] and are not offered treatment beyond medical reassurance that their chest pain does not suggest any abnormal functioning. Unfortunately, however, research has not supported the mainstream assumption that providing patients with test results indicating no abnormalities will reassure them that they do not have a medical problem.[31] Indeed, many NCCP patients develop negative ideas about their symptoms *before* they undergo testing.[32] Delays in the evaluation process may have a differential impact on patients who have established negative perceptions of their symptoms in advance of testing, and reassurance may be particularly ineffective in these cases.[33] Perhaps not surprisingly, providing more reassurance has not been found to be effective.[34] The timing and method of delivery, on the other hand, may be important factors to enhance the function of reassurance. A recent study showed that patients who were provided with information about the medical test itself and an explanation of a normal test result *prior to* testing was related to increased patient reassurance and reduced chest pain and medication use following exercise stress testing.[35] Replication of this work is needed. Nevertheless, it may be that providing patients with knowledge and explanations about the possible outcomes (including normal results) before testing may lessen patients' preconceived negative thoughts about the underlying causes of their chest pain and their illness in general.

Medical Course and Quality of Life

Some patients with NCCP are relieved; on the other hand, other patients experience persistent chest pain, decreased quality of life, and negative health consequences. Because chest pain can be upsetting, intrusive, and disruptive of daily activities, NCCP can impair functioning and reduce quality of life. With few exceptions,[36] most studies show that quality of life is more impaired in patients with NCCP than in healthy controls in both population-based[37] and treatment-seeking patient samples.[38] In some cases, the impairment in quality of life in NCCP is comparable to that experienced by patients with cardiac chest pain,[39,40] with NCCP patients showing higher negative affectivity and less social problem-solving ability than their matched CAD counterparts.[41] Even after negative coronary angiograms, approximately 50% of NCCP patients cannot exert themselves and are disabled by their condition.[42] In fact, when compared with cardiac patients, individuals with NCCP patients experience more physical symptoms and use more medical care than do cardiac patients.[40] Moreover, NCCP patients engage in more protective behaviors (eg, avoidance of exertion) than do patients with coronary artery disease.[40] Compared with healthy controls, NCCP patients have more impaired physical functioning, more role difficulties due to physical limitations, and poorer general health perceptions overall.[38] Qualitative interview data have also documented the negative impact of chest pain on patients' daily lives.[43] For many, quality of life impairment is often associated with chest pain impairment (ie, frequency, severity), and these impairments have been linked to social and occupational disruption (ie, work absenteeism).[39] Adding to its significance, if left untreated, patients with NCCP often show a chronic course,[44] and anxiety is associated with worsening chest pain[45] over time.[46] For instance, Tew and colleagues[46] found that 50% of NCCP patients with comorbid panic disorder visited the emergency department more than once per year for chest pain, and many continue to seek medical treatment.[47] Although NCCP patients are likely to receive repeated medical evaluations and prescriptions, often benzodiazepines, they are unlikely to receive psychological screening or assessment.[48]

The health care utilization of the NCCP patient can be costly. It has been estimated that the costs related to lack of a specific diagnosis in the presence of normal angiographic findings for United States patients alone is $750 million annually,[49] and the annual total economic burden of medical care for NCCP patients has been estimated at 10 to 13 billion dollars.[7] After excluding expensive cardiac explanations as the cause of chest pain, many patients are referred to other medical disciplines, most commonly gastroenterology. Estimates indicate that about 30% to 50% of NCCP patients are eventually diagnosed with gastroesophageal reflux disease (GERD)[50,51]; yet, only half of the NCCP patients who reported chest pain during the 24-hour pH diagnostic study showed corresponding increases in acid levels.[51] Other research has shown little temporal association between GERD symptoms and episodes of chest pain in NCCP samples.[52] Although a physical basis for NCCP is established for some patients (most often GERD),[53] the condition is generally not thought to be sufficient to account for the level of psychological distress and seeking health care for chest pain in many cases.[40,51,54] Other medical conditions that may instigate or co-occur with NCCP include musculoskeletal disorders (eg, osteoarthritis) and respiratory disorders (eg, bronchial spasms, asthma).

The prognosis for the NCCP patient is mixed. These data are mixed partly due to the diagnostic precision of the original cardiac assessments and the criteria examined across the different studies. Although the syndrome of NCCP is thought to be physiologically benign in the short term, emerging research shows a higher than expected long-term risk of cardiac events,[55–57] particularly among older women.[58] Rates of coronary events in NCCP patients over time have varied, depending on the duration of the study and the number of patients. Whereas some studies show a benign prognosis for NCCP patients following a negative coronary angiography,[59,60] others have shown that NCCP is associated with an increased risk for CAD events including nonfatal myocardial infarction,[58,61] a cardiac-cause mortality rate similar to patients with CAD,[55] and a higher mortality rate than the normal population.[62] These studies underscore the importance of thorough medical assessment. The diagnostic precision of each study differed; at present, coronary angiography is considered the "gold standard" for diagnosing CAD, which is accessible in most medical settings and is usually conducted with minimally invasive cardiac catheterization.[63,64] Many patients with NCCP are determined to have NCCP after a less invasive assessment (eg, normal exercise stress tests, normal echocardiogram, and a cardiologist's clinical evaluation); however, there is the potential for misclassification (ie, a false-negative finding of coronary artery disease). It is possible that NCCP patients undergoing catheterization may have undergone more testing and may be different from NCCP patients undergoing less invasive testing. In other words, it may be that the NCCP patient that undergoes less invasive testing is different (ie, more severe, more cardiac risk factors, less reassured, more anxious, or more determined) from the NCCP patient who undergoes coronary angiography. Relative to the other settings, however, the NCCP patient undergoing angiography is likely to be the one with the highest and most expensive health care utilization, and an important target for intervention.

Research suggests that traditional cardiovascular risk factors are elevated among patients with NCCP and that this risk is related to increased anxiety and chest pain.[65] Similar findings have been reported by others, including Dammen and colleagues[66] who found that the rates of traditional cardiovascular risk factors did not differ across samples of CAD and NCCP samples. Taken together, these data suggest that NCCP patients who experience chest pain and worry about their illness also possess elevated traditional cardiovascular risk factors. Longitudinal studies show that patients with NCCP experience chest pain from 1 to 11 years after the initial evaluation,[47,55,67] and nearly half of NCCP patients (44%–50%) continue to believe that they have a cardiac condition up to 1 year after negative evaluations.[68,69]

A thorough examination of the age and gender distribution of NCCP has been complicated by the selection parameters (ie, prescreening criteria) and referral patterns in past research. Overall, patients with NCCP tend to be somewhat younger than patients with cardiac disease.[46] Although some studies show a higher representation of females than males among patients with NCCP, studies without any preselection criteria (ie, in unselected or consecutive samples) show a nearly equal gender distribution[45] except for some possible differences for young females who show a higher rate of health care use. Patients often describe their chest pain with an assorted range of responses including sharp, tightness, aching, burning, pressure, dull, heavy, and include other associated symptoms (ie, shortness of breath).[70] Few studies have examined racial and ethnic similarities and differences in NCCP. Some data suggest that African American patients may be less apt to report symptoms of chest pain relative to white patients because they may be more likely to attribute their symptoms to noncardiac causes[71]; however, the extent that these data point to health care access or other factors related to health care seeking behavior remains uncertain.

Psychopathology

Consistent evidence points to an overrepresentation of psychological conditions among patients with NCCP, mostly heterogeneous anxiety and depressive disorders.[45,46,72,73] Specifically, a higher prevalence of generalized anxiety disorder (24%–70%), panic disorder (33%–50%), and major depressive disorder (11%–22%) have been found among NCCP patients, and still other patients who experience distress and impairment but who do not meet diagnostic criteria (ie, those termed "subclinical" or "subsyndromal"). As a result, theoretical conceptualizations of NCCP tend to incorporate this overlap with the anxiety and mood disorders.[74–76] Studies of the psychological characteristics of patients with NCCP highlight some distinguishing factors. NCCP patients tend to be interoceptively sensitive (particularly for cardiopulmonary sensations).[29,40,77] For instance, many patients tend to fear cardiac-congruent physical sensations (eg, palpitations, shortness of breath) more than cardiac-incongruent sensations (eg, gastrointestinal, cognitive dyscontrol, numbness).[29] Patients with NCCP may often show an exaggerated attention and sensitivity to bodily changes, and may engage in body scanning (mental or physical) or checking behaviors (eg, blood pressure monitoring, pulse checking) as a result. Some patients develop cardioprotective avoidance behavior; that is, they may be apt to avoid activities, substances, and strong emotional reactions that elicit sensations thought to be harmful to their heart (eg, avoid exercise, caffeine, anger, or stress). Relative to those with objective cardiac disease, patients with NCCP show a stronger disease conviction. Moreover, patients with NCCP have been shown to be less adept at managing stress, and often have fewer social resources to cope with stress.[78] The mechanisms underlying how psychological factors influence the onset and course of NCCP remain largely unexplored. It may be that these exaggerated responses in the patient with NCCP (ie, excessive vigilance, misdirected attention, and tendency to stay vigilant) are related to similar mechanisms implicated in emotion regulation.

Barriers to Psychological Referral

Despite the apparent health care costs and impact on patient functioning, health care providers may yet face challenges in the identification and referral of patients with NCCP for psychological services. Primary care clinics, emergency rooms, and cardiology and gastroenterology departments are estimated to have high percentages of patients reporting symptoms of the syndrome of NCCP. However, barriers influence proper diagnosis and referral for psychological evaluation. The diagnosis of the patient's chest symptoms as NCCP is often unhelpful from both a medical and psychological standpoint, primarily because it is a diagnosis of exclusion rather than inclusion. Patients who are determined to have NCCP often describe feeling most bothered by their noncardiac diagnosis because of all the possible medical conditions that might be causing their chest pain. The extent that psychiatric diagnoses in NCCP are distinct or overlapping and how these disorders influence the onset and clinical course of NCCP are relatively unknown. Much past research in this area has focused on panic and panic attacks. However, the experience of panic attacks is not a clinical diagnosis, and panic attacks often co-occur with anxiety or mood disorders, particularly among patients with NCCP.[29,45] Basic screening may increase recognition of patients in need of referral or additional assessment.

Summary

An integrated assessment is optimal to treatment planning with the chest pain patient. Obtaining informed consent for the referring physician is important for patient safety and improved communication. Systematic evaluation using diagnostic interviews can help to differentiate clinically significant psychopathology from other disease-related factors (eg, medication side effects, disease symptoms) or adjustment difficulties. Identifying concrete, achievable targets of change are best for the prevention of negative health behaviors (eg, smoking cessation, physical inactivity). Health care providers may find that basic screening for emotional disorders using short self-report inventories of anxiety and mood may facilitate the identification of patients who may benefit from additional psychological assessment in this population.

PSYCHOLOGICAL TREATMENT

In light of the potential medical risks linked with psychological interventions,[79] safety precautions are of chief significance in treatments implemented with the chest pain patient. Ongoing systematic assessment across treatment sessions to identify symptom changes over time (ie, showing both improvement and decline) is indispensable to safe, optimal psychological treatment. Psychological treatments for chest pain patients are often adapted from established therapies designed for persons who are medically well to meet the unique needs of chest pain patients. Managing CAD and living with the possibility of other fears including abrupt, unpredictable medical emergency (ie, heart attacks, chest pain episodes) can create wide-ranging psychosocial difficulties. As a result, the psychological and therapy goals and outcomes are taken into account as well as the possible physical health benefits at the outset of psychological treatment. Psychological interventions are frequently aimed at medical treatment adherence, risk factor management, coping with CAD, or psychopathology, and the treatment approach is customized to the target problems of the chest pain patient.

Management of Modifiable Risk Factors

Persuasive evidence has established the role of cardiac behavioral and physiologic risk factors in the development and progression of CAD. Modifiable cardiac behavioral risk factors include physical inactivity, obesity, and dietary patterns (ie, high fat, high cholesterol), and modifiable cardiac physiologic risk factors include serum dyslipidemia, high blood pressure, and being overweight.[80] CAD incidence and later morbidity and mortality have been linked to the dose, duration, and extent of hypertension, smoking, dyslipidemia, and physical inactivity across epidemiologic research studies.[81–86] Although risk factor modification is considered a chief objective of our modern cardiac rehabilitation programs, commencing and maintaining adherence and health behavior change for our patients is challenging and complex. The percentages of patients who have coexisting risk are high, and patients are often prescribed medications in combination with a regimen of physical activity, dietary changes, and smoking cessation, as applicable. Even though treatment adherence is coupled with improved cardiac outcomes,[87] the data on adherence are modest, with 25% to 40% adherence at short-term (6 months) follow-up.[88] Researchers have speculated that self-determined health behavior changes are more likely to be sustained than behavior changes persuaded by extrinsic pressures or situations,[89] perhaps partly because the patient is engaged in the process of internalizing and self-regulating the changes in behaviors.[90]

Eliciting Behavior Change

Some patients are uncertain, indifferent, or averse to changing a health behavior or to engaging in psychotherapy. The technique of motivational interviewing can be effective in eliciting readiness from individuals who are ambivalent toward change. Motivational interviewing encompasses both a set of techniques and a semidirective therapeutic style that is designed to increase an individual's intrinsic readiness to change by helping patients "explore and resolve ambivalence" by building a discrepancy between the current situation (eg, their life values, daily behaviors) and the desired life situation (ie, how they want their lives to be).[91] The interviewer helps the individual bring together discrepancies between current behaviors and long-term values and goals in an empathic manner, without confrontation. This theory-guided approach is collaborative, nonjudgmental, and nonadversarial. Clinicians balance helping patients increase their awareness of possible problems, costs, and risks associated with their current situation with helping them think differently about their behavior and the possible gains from behavior change, including a better future. To achieve decreased ambivalence and increased readiness for change, clinicians using motivational interviewing use an explicit instruction set[91] to help patients examine their reasons for and against change and to make more clear their priorities. This method of facilitating change via motivational interviewing, developed by Miller and Rollnick,[91] is supported by randomized controlled clinical trials across varied samples and a range of target behaviors, including substance abuse, smoking cessation,[92] physical activity, weight management,[93] medical adherence, and mental health issues.[94] For more detail, see Miller and Rollnick[91] and Rubak and colleagues.[95]

Treatment of DSM-IV Clinical Disorders

For many patients with chest pain, psychological care is aimed at the problems and stressors associated a DSM-IV (*Diagnostic and Statistical Manual of Mental Disorders* [Fourth Edition, Text Revised]) psychiatric disorder. Patients with CAD often experience comorbid depression and anxiety; however, there are few randomized clinical trials of the efficacy of psychotherapy for depression in this population, and there are no such trials aimed at anxiety. With regard to depression, extensive research conducted with medically well psychiatric samples has supported 2 psychotherapies in the treatment of depression: cognitive behavioral therapy (CBT), developed by Beck and colleagues,[96] and interpersonal psychotherapy (IPT), developed by Klerman.[97] CBT refers to a theory-based therapeutic approach with a wide-ranging set of techniques aimed at helping patients identifying and change problematic thoughts, sensations, and behaviors. More specifically, CBT for depression includes techniques designed to challenge maladaptive thought patterns, and help patients discover how their thoughts influence behaviors and mood and other patterns. Patients are also taught problem-solving skills and pleasant event scheduling.[96] Available evidence points to the efficacy of CBT for the treatment of depression in medically well psychiatric patients[98] and in patients with a chronic disease (eg, type II diabetes).[99] IPT describes an efficacious therapy using social problem solving as a method of overcoming depression. Primary interpersonal and social problems related to the mood difficulties are assessed, and skills are taught to develop and preserve relationships (eg, social skills) and social support. Evidence shows that IPT is effective for the treatment of depression in medically well psychiatric patients[100] and patients with a chronic disease[101]; however evidence suggests that IPT is not as effective as citalopram and is only equal to standard clinical care in the treatment of depression in patients with CAD.[102]

Combined Psychotherapy with Pharmacotherapy

Psychotropic medications are commonly prescribed to treat psychological problems in chest pain patients; however, the safety and efficacy of these medications in patients with CAD is limited. As researchers have noted, this is because most controlled clinical trials examining the efficacy of psychotropic medications rule out patients with chronic disease as part of the study inclusion criteria.[11,103] Psychologists working with patients prescribed psychotropic medications need to be familiar with the effects, side effects, and possible adverse effects of these medications. A review of the use psychotropic medications with cardiac patients is beyond the scope of this article, but the reader is encouraged to see Carney and Freedland[11] and Tabrizi and colleagues[104] for additional literature on this topic. By way of a synopsis, the selective serotonin reuptake inhibitors (SSRIs) are thought to have few adverse cardiac effects, but evidence has shown that drug-drug interactions are to be avoided in cardiac patients with depression.[105] Two placebo-controlled clinical trials provide some preliminary support for the use of SSRIs in patients with cardiac conditions.[102,106] Use of selective norepinephrine reuptake inhibitors (SNRIs) has also been supported, with few adverse events in the treatment of depression in patients with cardiac disease.[107] Tricyclic antidepressants are associated with tachycardia, orthostatic hypertension, and electrocardiographic changes. Although potentially useful for panic attacks and for sleep onset difficulties, withdrawal from benzodiazepines is associated with tachycardia. Other specific psychotropic medications are contraindicated in cardiac patients because of orthostatic hypertension (eg, trazodone) or because they are linked with potentially fatal arrhythmias including phenothiazine.[9] Finally, as part of the combined treatment approach of smoking cessation programs, the atypical antidepressant bupropion is prescribed. Research conducted with patients hospitalized with acute cardiovascular disease who were active smokers showed no impact of bupropion on safety (ie, patients in the medication group showed no differences in adverse events, cardiac events, or mortality relative to patients in the placebo group).[108]

In light of the potentially serious adverse events, a psychiatrist with expertise in both psychiatric and cardiac conditions may be ideally suited to best serve the needs of chest pain patients seeking pharmacotherapy for a psychiatric disorder. Similarly, psychologists working with cardiac patients who are taking psychotropic medications need to be attentive to the impact of medications on treatment, and they often need to take additional precautions beyond the customary clinical practices of medically well psychiatric patients. For example, clinicians working with older CAD patients prone to orthostatic hypertension because of a medication or medication change may require appropriate precautions during treatment to prevent falls and unintentional fall-related injuries (eg, head traumas, hip fractures). A recent study found that the risk of a single and recurrent fall for older adults was 3 times higher in the 2 days following a medication change.[109]

Psychological Treatments for Patients with NCCP

Despite the methodological challenges characterizing the syndrome of NCCP, biopsychosocial treatments for NCCP treatments are promising, and include psychopharmacotherapeutic and psychological treatments. Pharmacotherapy treatments have shown some success with NCCP.[110,111] Psychological treatments for NCCP have also shown promise, with few exceptions.[112] Some controlled clinical trials have demonstrated that psychological treatments are efficacious at reducing chest pain, functional impairment, and associated emotional distress. Some of the early studies on the psychological treatment of NCCP focused on teaching patients how to anticipate and control symptoms, modify ineffective health beliefs, and examine problems that may maintain the symptoms during 12 treatment sessions.[113,114] Outcome results showed significant reductions in chest pain, life disruption, and autonomic symptoms in the treatment group with no changes in the assessment-only group post treatment. These improvements were maintained at 4- and 6-month follow-up. In subsequent studies, other researchers demonstrated that CBT had a beneficial and differential effect on cognitive variables compared with usual care[115] in addition to improving chest pain frequency and intensity compared with usual care.[116] In fact, almost half (48%) of the patients receiving the CBT were pain-free at the 12-month follow-up compared with those receiving usual care (13%). In an effort to identify those NCCP patients who might be most interested in a treatment, Van Peski-Oosterbaan and colleagues[116] retrospectively assessed to what extent patients were interested in treatment from more than 1000 patients discharged with a diagnosis of "unexplained chest pain." Of note, chest pain characteristics (ie, frequency, duration) were not the best predictor of treatment interest. Patients who were most interested in a medical psychological treatment were younger, male, and had limitations in activities because of chest pain. Some research has shown that even a brief intervention to introduce patients to the physiologic arousal-reduction techniques (eg, breathing retraining) may be beneficial but not sufficient for some chest pain patients.[117] A small recent study examined the comparative benefits of relaxation and education for 22 patients with nonspecific chest pain, and the investigators found support for a functional relaxation group (eg, progressive relaxation training). This group showed fewer and less severe cardiovascular complaints, less somatization, and less anxiety than the control group.[118] Biofeedback has also shown some preliminary success in the treatment of NCCP compared with primary care visits, but attrition rates were higher for this treatment.[119] In addition, treatment of NCCP with hypnotherapy has been shown to reduce pain severity, improve well-being, and reduce medication use in patients compared with control condition patients (80% vs 23%), with quality of life improvements maintained for up to 2 years; of note, differences were not found for pain frequency, anxiety, or depression.[120]

The acceptability and effectiveness of psychological treatments for patients with NCCP has not been thoroughly evaluated. Some have suggested that previous treatments based on reattribution may not be sufficient, and that treatments with a broader biopsychosocial context may be preferable (eg, perhaps treatment programs offered need to be more analogous to a pain management service).[121] Others have urged a stepped-care approach in the treatment of NCCP.[112] Because anxiety and mood disorders are the most prevalent psychiatric disorders among patients with NCCP,[40,45,122,123] emerging transdiagnostic treatment approaches may be a good fit for the treatment of the anxious NCCP patient. This model of treating NCCP patients with comorbid emotional disorders might fit well within the context of Mayou's stepped-care approach. Patients with NCCP are nearly twice as likely as patients with CAD to experience psychiatric impairment,[124] and 2 to 3 times as likely to suffer from anxiety as patients with cardiac disease or the general population.[125,126] In a series of early studies, two-thirds of NCCP patients with normal and "near normal" coronary arteries (ie, $\leq$50% stenosis) met criteria for psychiatric disorders, most commonly anxiety neurosis.[127] Moreover, patients with Axis I psychiatric disorders report more frequent, more painful, and more persistent NCCP chest pain than patients without psychiatric disorders.[45]

Applicability of Transdiagnostic Treatments for Emotional Disorders

The emotional disorders are among the most treatable psychological conditions. Meta-analyses of pharmacologic and psychological treatments consistently show strong treatment effects. For the pharmacologic treatment of anxiety, for instance, patients can improve on treatment using medications including SSRIs, tricyclic antidepressants (TCAs), benzodiazepines, and monoamine oxidase inhibitors.[128,129] These medications likely attenuate the anxiety elicited by the fear cues associated with each disorder. This attenuation of anxiety lasts only as long as medication is continued,[129–131] and in some cases the medication management has been shown to be less durable than psychological treatments.[132] Moreover, pharmacotherapy for anxiety can increase cardiac risk factors, a particularly relevant factor in the context of NCCP patients, some of whom may have elevated cardiovascular risk profiles.[65,133] For example, TCAs are effective in panic disorder, but their cardiotoxicity precludes them as a first-line agent in the presence of cardiovascular disease. There is consistent evidence that CBT is an effective first-line strategy for the treatment of anxiety disorders. Several meta-analyses of anxiety disorder treatment-outcome studies support these assertions, showing strong treatment effects for CBT across the anxiety disorders; for meta-analytical reviews, see Refs.[134–136] Transdiagnostic approaches to the treatment of emotional disorders have emerged for 2 main reasons. First, consistent findings underscore the similarity among (and indistinguishability between) the emotional disorders.[137–139] Comorbidity studies using DSM-IV criteria indicate that at least 50% of patients with a principal anxiety disorder have one or more additional diagnoses at the time of assessment.[140] Studies like these may be conservative estimates of diagnostic co-occurrence stemming from various exclusion criteria (eg, cases with active suicidality, outpatient setting, and so forth). Nevertheless, comorbidity rates are somewhat high. Patients with a principal anxiety or mood disorder diagnosis at the time of assessment increased to 76% when lifetime diagnoses are considered.[141] A substantial body of literature supports the role of negative affect (ie, neuroticism, behavioral inhibition) and positive affect (ie, behavioral activation) in accounting for the onset, overlap, and maintenance of anxiety and depression.[142–144] For instance, in a sample of outpatients, Brown and colleagues[145] found that sizeable covariance among the latent factors corresponding to DSM-IV constructs of unipolar depression, panic disorder with agoraphobia, social phobia, generalized anxiety disorder, and obsessive-compulsive disorder was explained by the higher order dimensions of negative and positive affect; bipolar disorder was not included. Moreover, research emerging from the fields of neuroscience and functional psychopathology has begun to identify a higher order, common factor underlying the emotional disorders.[146–150] Second, single diagnosis treatments for anxiety disorders are comprised of common features, including psychoeducation, cognitive restructuring, prevention of avoidance, and exposure-based procedures.[151,152] Similar to single diagnosis treatments, transdiagnostic treatments have gained empirical support.[153–158]

Transdiagnostic treatments for emotional disorders are based on the fundamental principles of CBT,[156,157,159] and the application of these principles with the distressed chest pain patient may be efficacious. Fundamental principles of CBT for anxiety focus on reducing or eliminating exaggerated fears, identifying and altering cognitive misappraisals, and preventing the emotional and behavioral avoidance that serve to maintain the emotional disorder.[152,160,161] One particularly promising transdiagnostic CBT treatment is the Unified Treatment of Emotional Disorders.[157,162] In this treatment, the focus of extinction training extends to focus on interoceptive cues, including those associated with intense emotions, an extension of a concept first used in panic disorder.[163–165] This approach also emphasizes the adaptive, functional nature of emotions, helps facilitate greater tolerance of emotions, and seeks to identify and correct maladaptive attempts to regulate emotional experiences.[157,162] In transdiagnostic CBT, the exact core fear depends on the emotional disorder under treatment; and the cognitive biases and avoidance patterns that prevent disconfirmation of these fears are tailored to the individual. The treatment has in common the systematic attempts to provide conditions whereby patients can relearn a sense of safety in relation to feared cues, and has been efficacious in the treatment of anxiety.[152] In exposure-based procedures (ie, situational, interoceptive), patients repeatedly confront feared stimuli under controlled conditions, with the goal of extinguishing fears as patients acquire a sense of safety in the presence of the stimuli. For example, NCCP patients who avoid exertion because it increases heart rate and because it makes them fearful of harmful cardiac consequences would be encouraged to repeatedly engage in physically challenging situations without any safety signals (ie, no pulse checking). Cognitive-restructuring interventions aim to help patients reevaluate their automatic assumptions about their fears. For example, NCCP patients who fear that they must have a rare, serious disease because medical extensive testing has not been able to uncover its etiology would be encouraged to reevaluate the evidence about this assumption of medical testing. Self-monitoring and logical evaluation exercises encourage patients to test the accuracy of their assumptions compared with ongoing experiences. Testing out assumptions occurs as part of exposure interventions that help patients systematically relearn safety based on their new prospective experiences with feared cues.

There are several advantages for transdiagnostic CBT for the patient with NCCP. First, anxious NCCP patients are hypervigilant to somatic sensations, particularly cardiorespiratory cues,[29,77] and CBT focuses on extinction training to interoceptive cues (ie, chest sensations, hyperventilation), including those associated with intense emotions. The rationale is that anxiety is associated with hypersensitivity and vigilance to internal sensations that are perceived as dangerous or fearful. Interoceptive exposure can facilitate a decrease in catastrophic interpretation of physical sensations. This therapeutic technique, in which patients are exposed to somatic cues, breaches the association between physical sensations and fear by demonstrating that the somatic sensations do not arise because of impending danger and do not result in predicted negative consequences. Indeed, patients with panic disorder will often notice and report more problematic cardiac functioning than those without panic disorder.[166] Second, many NCCP patients exhibit high levels of worry and reassurance-seeking behavior (eg, requests for medical examinations, bodily checking, pulse checking, verbal complaints, seeking reassurance). The function of these behaviors is to reduce anxiety; however, safety seeking typically provides only temporary benefits as the patient comes to doubt the veracity of the testing and may worry that further disease has progressed since the last testing. CBT targets identify and alter cognitive misappraisals (eg, selectively attending to and misinterpreting physician reassurances). Another advantage is that the syndrome of NCCP is characterized by a psychiatrically heterogeneous sample of anxiety disorders, with frequent depression comorbidity.[45] Transdiagnostic CBT targets have been shown to improve comorbid depressive disorders and somatoform disorders. Some of the author's recent work has shown that CBT for anxiety is associated with significant improvements in comorbid depressive disorders.[167] Moreover, because some transdiagnostic CBT approaches are typically delivered in a modular format,[162] the approach affords the clinician the flexibility that may be most practical to tailored delivery with NCCP patients presenting in medical settings.

Possible Impact of CBT on Traditional CAD Risk Factors

Although still exploratory with NCCP patients, transdiagnostic CBT may indirectly reduce specific cardiovascular risk factors in anxious patients with NCCP. There are several reasons to believe that CBT treatment response might indirectly influence specific cardiovascular risk factors. First, research has shown that traditional cardiovascular risk factors are present among patients with NCCP, and this risk is associated with elevated anxiety and chest pain.[65] Second, anxiety is associated with established cardiovascular risk factors, including smoking,[168] hypertension,[169] and physical inactivity.[170] Thirty-two percent to 64% of patients with chest pain and normal coronary angiograms use nicotine.[169] The exact nature and directionality of the anxiety-smoking relationship is unclear. For example, although 19% of patients with panic disorder report that they increased their smoking due to anxiety,[171] panic attacks are not believed to induce smoking.[172] Also, the presence of an anxiety disorder is negatively associated with regular physical inactivity (ie, sedentary behavior).[170] NCCP patients have lower cardiac outputs on exercise tolerance tests,[173] and preliminary findings suggest that NCCP patients with high interoceptive sensitivity (ie, fearful of and vigilant to internal somatic sensations) produce lower outputs on exercise tolerance tests.[174] Third, low heart rate variability (HRV) predicts poor cardiac outcomes[175–177] and is associated with anxiety disorder diagnosis.[178,179] HRV is a recognized method to noninvasively study the activity and patterns of the autonomic nervous system.[180] Derived from an ambulatory electrocardiogram, HRV provides a measurement of sympathetic acceleration and parasympathetic response. High HRV suggests normal autonomic nervous system responsiveness. Further, the unique predictive ability of anxious symptoms to reduced vagal control has been documented,[181,182] even after controlling for depressive symptoms.[183] In sum, there is reason to speculate that CBT may indirectly reduce some traditional cardiovascular risk factors (ie, smoking, increased physical activity, and increased HRV) in patients treated with CBT.

Summary

Evidence-based psychological treatments customized to the chest pain patient's target problems and safety precautions are apt to be optimal. Motivational approaches may be useful to elicit behavior change among individuals less keen on change. The safety and efficacy of some pharmacotherapy and psychotherapies (CBT, IPT) have been supported in patients with CAD and comorbid depression. Pharmacotherapy and psychotherapy (CBT) are promising for patients with NCCP in reducing symptoms of emotional distress. Transdiagnostic treatments for emotional disorders have advantages for the patient with chest pain, and may lead to improved outcomes. Improving our understanding of how psychological problems manifest and are treated will likely lead us to design better ways to help each individual chest pain patient.

ACKNOWLEDGMENTS

The author thanks Cassandra J. McDonnell, MA and Adnan Smajic, BA for their assistance in manuscript preparation.

REFERENCES

1. Burt CW. Summary statistics for acute cardiac ischemia and chest pain visits to United States EDs. 1995-1999. Am J Emerg Med 1999;17:552–9.

2. American Heart Association. Heart and stroke statistical update. Dallas (TX): American Heart Association; 2009.

3. Zevallos JC, Chiriboga D, Herbert JR. An international perspective on coronary heart disease and related risk factors. In: Ockene IS, Ockene JK, editors. Prevention of coronary heart disease. Boston: Little, Brown; 1992. p. 147–70.

4. Mannheimer C, Camici P, Chester MR, et al. The problem of chronic refractory angina. Eur Heart J 2002;23:355–70.

5. Bass CM, Mayou RA. Chest pain and palpitations. In: Mayou RA, Bass CM, Sharpe M, editors. Treatment of functional somatic syndromes. Oxford: Oxford University Press; 1995. p. 328–52.

6. Sheps DS, Creed F, Clouse RE. Chest pain in patients with cardiac and noncardiac disease. Psychosom Med 2004;66:861–7.

7. Roberts R, Kleinman N. Earlier diagnosis and treatment of acute myocardial infarction necessitates the need for a "new diagnostic mind-set". Circulation 1994;89:872–81.

8. Newby LK, LaPointe NM, Chen AY, et al. Long-term adherence to evidence-based secondary prevention therapies in coronary artery disease. Circulation 2006;113:203–12.

9. Bellg AJ. Clinical cardiac psychology. In: Camic PM, Knight SJ, editors. Clinical handbook of health psychology. 2nd edition. Cambridge: Hogrefe & Huber; 2004. p. 29–57.

10. Rybarczyk BD. Diversity among American men: the impact of aging, ethnicity, and race. In: Kilmartin C, editor. The masculine self. New York: MacMillan; 1994. p. 113–31.

11. Carney RM, Freedland KE. Depression in patients with coronary heart disease. Am J Med 2008;121:S20–7.

12. Barefoot JC, Helms MJ, Mark DB, et al. Depression and long-term mortality risk in patients with coronary artery disease. Am J Cardiol 1996;78:613–7.

13. Carney RM, Rich MW, Freedland KE, et al. Major depressive disorder predicts cardiac events in patients with coronary artery disease. Psychosom Med 1988;50:627–33.

14. White KS. Cardiovascular disease and anxiety disorders. In: Zvolensky MJ, Smits JAS, editors. Health behaviors and physical illness in anxiety and its disorders: contemporary theory and research. New York: Springer; 2007. p. 279–315.

15. Lampert R, Shusterman V, Burg MM, et al. Effects of psychologic stress on repolarization and relationship to autonomic and hemodynamic factors. J Cardiovasc Electrophysiol 2005;16:372–7.

16. Kawachi I, Colditz GA, Ascherio A, et al. Prospective study of phobic anxiety and risk of coronary heart disease in men. Circulation 1994;89:1992–7.

17. Kawachi I, Sparrow D, Vokonas PS, et al. Symptoms of anxiety and risk of coronary heart disease. The Normative Aging Study. Circulation 1994;90:2225–9.

18. Haines AP, Imeson JD, Meade TW. Phobic anxiety and ischaemic heart disease. Br Med J 1987;295:297–9.

19. Eaker ED, Pinsky J, Castelli WP. Myocardial infarction and coronary death among women in the Framingham Study. Am J Epidemiol 1992;135:854–64.

20. Zaubler TS, Katon W. Panic disorder and medical comorbidity: a review of the medical and psychiatric literature. Bull Menninger Clin 1996;60:A12–38.

21. First MB, Spitzer RL, Gibbon M, et al. Structured clinical interview for DSM-IV axis I disorders. New York: New York State Psychiatric Institute, Biometrics Research Department; 1997.

22. DiNardo PA, Brown TA, Barlow DH. Anxiety disorders interview schedule for DSM-IV: lifetime version (ADIS-IV-L). San Antonio (TX): Psychological Corporation; 1994.
23. American Psychiatric Association. Diagnostic and statistical manual of mental disorders. Text revision. 4th edition. Washington, DC: American Psychiatric Association; 2000.
24. Skala JA, Freedland KE, Carney RM. Heart disease. Cambridge (MA): Hogrefe & Huber; 2005.
25. Ninomiya JK, L'Italien G, Criqui MH, et al. Association of the metabolic syndrome with history of myocardial infarction and stroke in the Third National Health and Nutrition Examination Survey. Circulation 2004;109:42–6.
26. Boudreaux ED, Baumann BM, Perry J, et al. Emergency department initiated treatments for tobacco (EDITT): a pilot study. Ann Behav Med 2008;36: 314–25.
27. Bock B, Becker B, Partridge R, et al. Smoking cessation among patients in the chest pain observation unit. Ann Behav Med 2005;61:29S.
28. Norell M, Lythall D, Coghlan G, et al. Limited value of the resting electrocardiogram in assessing patients with recent onset chest pain: lessons from a chest pain clinic. Br Heart J 1992;67:53–6.
29. White KS, Craft JM, Gervino EV. Anxiety and hypervigilance to cardiopulmonary sensations in non-cardiac chest pain patients with and without psychiatric disorders. Behav Res Ther 2010. [Epub ahead of print].
30. Goodacre S, Mason S, Arnold J, et al. Psychologic morbidity and health related quality of life in patients assessed in a chest pain observation unit. Ann Emerg Med 2001;38:369–76.
31. MacDonald IG, Daly J, Jelinek VM, et al. Opening Pandora's box: the unpredictability of reassurance by a normal test result. Br Med J 1996;313: 329–32.
32. Donkin L, Ellis CJ, Powell R, et al. Illness perceptions predict reassurance following a negative stress testing result. Psychol Health 2006;21:421–30.
33. Nijher G, Weinman J, Bass CM, et al. Chest pain in people with normal coronary arteries. Br Med J 2001;323:1319–20.
34. Sanders D, Bass C, Mayou RA, et al. Non-cardiac chest pain: why was a brief intervention apparently ineffective? Psychol Med 1997;27:1033–40.
35. Petrie KJ, Muller JT, Schirmbeck F, et al. Effect of providing information about normal test results on patients' reassurance: randomised controlled trial. Br Med J 2007;334:353–4.
36. Biggs AM, Aziz Q, Tomenson B, et al. Effect of childhood adversity on health related quality of life in patients with upper abdominal or chest pain. Gut 2004;53:180–6.
37. Eslick GD, Jones MP, Talley NJ. Non-cardiac chest pain: prevalence, risk factors, impact and consulting—a population-based study. Aliment Pharmacol Ther 2003;17:1115–24.
38. Wong WM, Lai KC, Lau CP, et al. Upper gastrointestinal evaluation of Chinese patients with non-cardiac chest pain. Aliment Pharmacol Ther 2002;16: 465–71.
39. Cheung TK, Hou X, Lam KF, et al. Quality of life and psychological impact in patients with noncardiac chest pain. J Clin Gastroenterol 2009;43:13–8.
40. Eifert GH, Hodson SE, Tracey DR, et al. Heart-focused anxiety, illness beliefs, and behavioral impairment: comparing healthy heart-anxious patients with cardiac and surgical inpatients. J Behav Med 1996;19:385–99.

41. Nezu AM, Nezu CM, Jain D, et al. Social problem solving and noncardiac chest pain. Psychosom Med 2007;69:944–51.

42. Lavey EB, Winkel RA. Continuing disability of patients with chest pain and normal coronary arteriograms. J Chronic Dis 1979;32:191–6.

43. Jerlock M, Gaston-Johansson F, Danielson E. Living with unexplained chest pain. J Clin Nurs 2005;14:956–64.

44. Beitman BD, Kushner MG, Basha I, et al. Follow-up status of patients with angiographically normal coronary arteries and panic disorder. JAMA 1991;265:1545–9.

45. White KS, Raffa SD, Jakle KR, et al. Morbidity of DSM-IV axis I disorders in noncardiac chest pain: psychiatric morbidity linked with increased pain and health care utilization. J Consult Clin Psychol 2008;76:422–30.

46. Tew R, Guthrie EA, Creed FH, et al. A long-term follow-up study of patients with ischemic heart disease versus patients with nonspecific chest pain. J Psychosom Res 1995;39:977–85.

47. Papanicolaou MN, Califf RM, Hlatky MA, et al. Prognostic implications of angiographically normal and insignificantly narrowed coronary arteries. Am J Cardiol 1986;58:1181–7.

48. Aikens JE, Michael E, Levin T, et al. The role of cardioprotective avoidance beliefs in noncardiac chest pain and associated emergency department utilization. J Clin Psychol Med Settings 1999;6:317–32.

49. Richter JE. Approach to the patient with noncardiac chest pain. In: Yamada T, editor. Textbook of gastroenterology. Philadelphia: Lippincott; 1995. p. 648–70.

50. Galmiche JP, Clouse RE, Balint A, et al. Functional esophageal disorders. Gastroenterology 2006;130:1459–65.

51. Beedassy A, Katz PO, Gruber A, et al. Prior sensitization of esophageal mucosa by acid reflux predisposes to reflux-induced chest pain. J Clin Gastroenterol 2000;31:121–4.

52. Cooke RA, Anggiansah A, Smeeton NC, et al. Gastroesophageal reflux in patients with angiographically normal coronary arteries: an uncommon cause of exertional chest pain. Br Heart J 1994;72:231–6.

53. Fass R, Naliboff B, Higa L, et al. Differential effect of long-term esophageal acid exposure on mechanosensitivity and chemosensitivity in humans. Gastroenterology 1998;115:1363–73.

54. Bass C. Unexplained chest pain and breathlessness. Med Clin North Am 1991;75:1157–73.

55. Eslick GD, Talley NJ. Natural history and predictors of outcome for non-cardiac chest pain: a prospective 4-year cohort study. Neurogastroenterol Motil 2008;20:989–97.

56. Bugiardini R, Bairey Merz CN. Angina with "normal" coronary arteries: a changing philosophy. J Am Med Assoc 2005;293:477–84.

57. Johnson BD, Shaw LJ, Pepine CJ, et al. Persistent chest pain predicts cardiovascular events in women without obstructive coronary artery disease: results from the NIH-NHLBI-sponsored women's ischaemia syndrome evaluation (WISE) study. Eur Heart J 2006;27:1408–15.

58. Robinson JG, Wallace R, Limacher M, et al. Cardiovascular risk in women with non-specific chest pain (from the Women's Health Initiative Hormone Trials). Am J Cardiol 2008;102:693–9.

59. Kemp HG, Kronmal RA, Vlietstra RE, et al. Seven year survival of patients with normal or near normal coronary arteriograms: a CASS registry study. J Am Coll Cardiol 1986;7:479–83.

60. Lichtlen PR, Bargheer K, Wenzlaff P. Long-term prognosis of patients with anginalike chest pain and normal coronary angiographic findings. J Am Coll Cardiol 1995;25:1013–8.

61. Robinson JG, Wallace R, Limacher M, et al. Elderly women diagnosed with nonspecific chest pain may be at increased cardiovascular risk. J Womens Health 2006;15:1151–60.

62. Bodegard J, Erikssen G, Bjornholt JV, et al. Possible angina detected by the WHO angina questionnaire in apparently healthy men with a normal exercise ECG: coronary heart disease or not? A 26 year follow up study. Heart 2004; 90:627–32.

63. Fraker TD, Fihn SD, Gibbons RJ. Chronic stable angina. In: Fuster V, editor. The AHA guidelines and scientific statements handbook. Hoboken (NJ): Wiley-Blackwell; 2009. p. 1–24.

64. Topol EJ, Nissen SE. Our preoccupation with coronary luminology: the dissociation between clinical and angiographic findings in ischemic heart disease. Circulation 1995;92:2333–42.

65. White KS, Gervino EV. Traditional cardiovascular risk factors in patients with non-cardiac chest pain: risk and its association with anxiety and chest pain, in press.

66. Dammen T, Ekeberg O, Arnesen H, et al. Personality profiles in patients referred for chest pain: Investigation with emphasis on panic disorder patients. Psychosomatics 2000;41:269–76.

67. Wielgosz AT, Fletcher RH, McCants CB, et al. Unimproved chest pain in patients with minimal or no coronary disease: a behavioral phenomenon. Am Heart J 1984;108:67–72.

68. Ockene IS, Shay MJ, Alpert JS, et al. Unexplained chest pain in patients with normal coronary arteriograms: a follow-up study of functional status. N Engl J Med 1980;303:1249–52.

69. Potts SG, Bass CM. Psychosocial outcome and use of medical resources in patients with chest pain and normal or near normal coronary arteries: a long-term follow-up study. Q J Med 1993;86:583–93.

70. Eslick GD. Epidemiology of non-cardiac chest pain. Germany: VDM Verlag; 2008.

71. Raczynski JM, Taylor H, Cutter G, et al. Diagnosis, symptoms, and attribution of symptoms among black and white inpatients admitted for coronary artery heart disease. Am J Public Health 1994;84:951–6.

72. Husser D, Bollmann A, Kühne C, et al. Evaluation of noncardiac chest pain: diagnostic approach, coping strategies and quality of life. Eur J Pain 2006;10: 51–5.

73. Wulsin LR, Arnold LM, Hillard JR. Axis I disorders in ER patients with atypical chest pain. Int J Psychiatry Med 1991;21:37–46.

74. Mayou RA. Chest pain, palpitations and panic. J Psychosom Res 1998;44: 53–70.

75. White KS, Raffa SD. Anxiety and other emotional factors in noncardiac chest pain. Mental Fitness 2004;3:60–7.

76. Eifert GH, Zvolensky MJ, Lejuez CW. Heart-focused anxiety and chest pain: a conceptual and clinical review. Clin Psychol Sci Pract 2000;7:403–17.

77. Aikens JE, Zvolensky MJ, Eifert GH. Differential fear of cardiopulmonary sensa-tions in emergency room noncardiac chest pain patients. J Behav Med 2001;24: 155–67.

78. Cheng C, Wong W, Lai K, et al. Psychosocial factors in patients with non-cardiac chest pain. Psychosom Med 2003;65:443–9.

79. Frasure-Smith N, Lesperance F, Gravel G, et al. Long-term survival differ-ences among low-anxious, high-anxious, and repressive copers enrolled in the Montreal heart attack readjustment trial. Psychosom Med 2002;64: 571–9.

80. Humes HD, DuPont HL, Harris ED, et al. Kelley's textbook of internal medicine. 4th edition. Philadelphia: Lippincott Williams & Wilkins; 2000.

81. Paffenbarger RS, Hyde RT, Wing AL, et al. The association of changes in phys-ical-activity level and other lifestyle characteristics with mortality among men. N Engl J Med 1993;328:538–45.

82. Vasan RS, Larson MG, Leip EP, et al. Impact of high-normal blood pressure on the risk of cardiovascular disease. N Engl J Med 2001;345:1291–7.

83. Multiple Risk Factor Intervention Trial Research Group. Multiple risk factor inter-vention trial: risk factor changes and mortality results. J Am Med Assoc 1982; 248:1465–77.

84. Haapanen N, Miilunpalo S, Vuori I, et al. Association of leisure time physical activity with the risk of coronary heart disease, hypertension and diabetes in middle-aged men. Int J Epidemiol 1997;26:739–47.

85. MacMahon S, Peto R, Cutler J, et al. Blood pressure, stroke and coronary heart disease. Lancet 1990;335:765–74.

86. Durrington P. Dyslipidaemia. Lancet 2003;362:717–31.

87. Shepherd J. The West of Scotland Coronary Prevention Study (WOSCOPS): benefits of pravastatin therapy in compliant subjects. Circulation 1996; 94(Suppl):539–43.

88. U.S. Department of Health and Human Services (USDHHS). Physical activity and health: a report of the Surgeon General. Pittsburgh: President's Council on Physical Fitness and Sports; 2000.

89. Botelho RJ, Skinner H. Motivating change in health behavior: Implications for health promotion and disease prevention. Prim Care 1995;22:565–89.

90. Bellg AJ. Maintenance of health behavior change in preventive cardiology: internalization and self-regulation of new behaviors. Behav Modif 2003;27: 103–31.

91. Miller WR, Rollnick S. Motivational interviewing: preparing people to change. 2nd edition. New York: Guilford Press; 2002.

92. Soria R, Legido A, Escolano C, et al. A randomised controlled trial of motiva-tional interviewing for smoking cessation. Br J Gen Pract 2006;56:768–74.

93. West DS, DiLillo V, Bursac Z, et al. Motivational interviewing improves weight loss in women with type 2 diabetes. Diabetes Care 2007;30:1081–7.

94. Swanson AJ, Pantalon MV, Cohen KR. Motivational interviewing and treatment adherence among psychiatric and dually diagnosed patients. J Nerv Ment Dis 1999;187:630–5.

95. Rubak S, Sandboek A, Lauritzen T, et al. Motivational interviewing: a systematic review and meta-analysis. Br J Gen Pract 2005;55:305–12.

96. Beck AT, Rush AJ, Shaw BF, et al. Cognitive therapy of depression. New York: Guilford Press; 1979.

97. Klerman GL. Interpersonal psychotherapy for depression. New York: Basic Books; 1984.

98. Murphy GE, Carney RM, Knesevich MA, et al. Cognitive behavior therapy, relaxation training, and tricyclic antidepressant medication in the treatment of depression. Psychol Rep 1995;77:403–20.

99. Lustman PJ, Griffith LS, Freedland KE, et al. Cognitive behavior therapy for depression in type 2 diabetes mellitus. Ann Intern Med 1998;129:613–21.

100. Elkin I, Shea MT, Watkins JT, et al. National Institute of Mental Health treatment of depression collaborative research program: general effectiveness of treatments. Arch Gen Psychiatry 1989;46:971–82.

101. Markowitz JC, Klerman GL, Perry SW. Interpersonal psychotherapy of depressed HIV-positive outpatients. Hosp Community Psychiatry 1992;43: 885–90.

102. Lesperance F, Frasure-Smith N, Koszycki D, et al. Effects of citalopram and interpersonal psychotherapy on depression in patients with coronary artery disease: the Canadian cardiac randomized evaluation of antidepressant and psychotherapy efficacy (CREATE) trial. JAMA 2007;297:367–79.

103. Shores MM, Pascualy M, Veith RC. Major depression and heart disease: treatment trials. Semin Clin Neuropsychiatry 1998;3:87–101.

104. Tabrizi K, Littman A, Williams RB Jr, et al. Psychopharmacology and cardiac disease. In: Allan R, Scheidt S, editors. Heart and mind: the practice of cardiac psychology. Washington DC: American Psychological Association; 1996. p. 397–420.

105. Sheline YI, Freedland KE, Carney RM. How safe are serotonin reuptake inhibitors for depression in patients with coronary artery disease? Am J Med 1997; 102:54–9.

106. Glassman AH, O'Connor CM, Califf RM, et al. Sertraline treatment of major depression in patients with acute MI or unstable angina. JAMA 2002;288:701–9.

107. Honig A, Kuyper AM, Schene AH, et al. Treatment of post-myocardial infarction depressive disorder: a randomized, placebo-controlled trial with mirtazapine. Psychosom Med 2007;69:606–13.

108. Rigotti N, Thorndike A, Regan S, et al. Bupropion for smokers hospitalized with acute cardiovascular disease. Am J Med 2006;119:1080–7.

109. Sorock GS, Quigley P, Rutledge M, et al. Psychotropic medication changes and the short-term risk of falls in nursing home residents: a case-crossover study. Annual meeting of the American Public Health Association Meeting. Washington, DC, November 3–7, 2007.

110. Cannon RO, Quyyumi AA, Mincemoyer R, et al. Imipramine in patients with chest pain despite normal coronary angiograms. N Engl J Med 1994;330:1411–7.

111. Varia I, Logue E, O'Connor C, et al. Randomized trial of sertraline in patients with unexplained chest pain of non-cardiac origin. Am Heart J 2000;140:367–72.

112. Mayou RA, Bass CM, Bryant BM. Management of non-cardiac chest pain: from research to clinical practice. Heart 1999;81:387–92.

113. Mayou RA, Bryant BM, Sanders D, et al. A controlled trial of cognitive behavioural therapy for non-cardiac chest pain. Psychol Med 1997;27:1021–31.

114. Klimes I, Mayou RA, Pearce MJ, et al. Psychological treatment for atypical non-cardiac chest pain: a controlled evaluation. Psychol Med 1990;20:605–11.

115. Van Peski-Oosterbaan AS, Spinhoven P, Van der Does AJ, et al. Cognitive change following cognitive behavioural therapy for non-cardiac chest pain. Psychother Psychosom 1999;68:214–20.

116. Van Peski-Oosterbaan AS, Spinhoven P, van Rood Y, et al. Cognitive behavioral therapy for noncardiac chest pain: a randomized trial. Am J Med 1999;106: 424–9.

117. Esler JL, Barlow DH, Woolard RH, et al. A brief cognitive-behavioral intervention for patients with noncardiac chest pain. Behav Ther 2003;34:129–48.

118. Lahmann C, Loew TH, Tritt K, et al. Efficacy of functional relaxation and patient education in the treatment of functional somatoform heart disorders: a randomized, controlled clinical investigation. Psychosomatics 2008;49:378–85.

119. Ryan M, Gevirtz R. Biofeedback-based psychophysiological treatment in a primary care setting: an initial feasibility study. Appl Psychophysiol Biofeedback 2004;29:79–93.

120. Miller V, Jones H, Whorwell PJ. Hypnotherapy for non-cardiac chest pain: long-term follow-up. Gut 2007;56:1643.

121. Esler JL, Bock BC. Psychological treatments for noncardiac chest pain: recommendations for a new approach. J Psychosom Res 2004;56:263–9.

122. Katon W, Hall ML, Russo J, et al. Chest pain: relationship of psychiatric illness to coronary arteriographic results. Am J Med 1988;84:1–9.

123. Dammen T, Ekeberg O, Arnesen H, et al. The detection of panic disorder in chest pain patients. Gen Hosp Psychiatry 1999;21:323–32.

124. Bass C, Wade C, Hand D, et al. Patients with angina with normal and near normal coronary arteries: clinical and psychosocial state 12 months after angiography. Br Med J 1983;287:1505–8.

125. Serlie AW, Erdman RA, Passchier J, et al. Psychological aspects of non-cardiac chest pain. Psychother Psychosom 1995;64:62–73.

126. Kessler RC, Chiu WT, Demler O, et al. Prevalence, severity, and comorbidity of twelve-month DSM-IV disorders in the national comorbidity survey replication (NCS-R). Arch Gen Psychiatry 2005;62:617–27.

127. Bass CM, Wade C. Chest pain with normal coronary arteries: a comparative study of psychiatric and social morbidity. Psychol Med 1984;14:51–61.

128. Lydiard RB, Brawman Mintzer O, Ballenger JC. Recent developments in the psychopharmacology of anxiety disorders. J Consult Clin Psychol 1996;64:660–8.

129. Pollack MH, Smoller JW. Pharmacologic approaches to treatment-resistant panic disorder. In: Pollack MH, Otto MW, editors. Challenges in clinical practice: pharmacologic and psychosocial strategies. New York: Guilford Press; 1996. p. 89–112.

130. Noyes R, Garvey MJ, Cook BL, et al. Problems with tricyclic antidepressant use in patients with panic disorder or agoraphobia: results of a naturalistic follow-up study. J Clin Psychiatry 1989;50:163–9.

131. Noyes R, Garvey MJ, Cook B, et al. Controlled discontinuation of benzodiazepine treatment for patients with panic disorder. Am J Psychiatry 1991;148:517–23.

132. Barlow DH, Gorman JM, Shear MK, et al. Cognitive-behavioral therapy, imipramine, or their combination for panic disorder: a randomized controlled trial. JAMA 2000;283:2529–36.

133. Dammen T, Arnesen H, Ekeberg O, et al. Psychological factors, pain attribution and medical morbidity in chest-pain patients with and without coronary artery disease. Gen Hosp Psychiatry 2004;26:463–9.

134. Norton PJ, Price EC. A meta-analytic review of adult cognitive-behavioral treatment outcome across the anxiety disorders. J Nerv Ment Dis 2007;195:521–31.

135. Deacon BJ, Abramowitz JS. Cognitive and behavioral treatments for anxiety disorders: a review of meta-analytic findings. J Clin Psychol 2004;60:429–41.

136. Stewart RE, Chambless DL. Cognitive-behavioral therapy for adult anxiety disorders in clinical practice: a meta-analysis of effectiveness studies. J Consult Clin Psychol 2009;77:595–606.
137. Andrews G. Comorbidity of the neurotic disorders: the similarities are more important than the differences. In: Rapee RM, editor. Current controversies in the anxiety disorders. New York: Guilford; 1996. p. 3–20.
138. Andrews G. Classification of neurotic disorders. J R Soc Med 1990;83: 606–7.
139. Brown TA. Validity of the DSM-III-R and DSM-IV classification systems for anxiety disorders. In: Rapee RM, editor. Current controversies in the anxiety disorders. New York: Guilford; 1996. p. 21–45.
140. Brown TA, Campbell LA, Lehman CL, et al. Current and lifetime comorbidity of the DSM-IV anxiety and mood disorders in a large clinical sample. J Abnorm Psychol 2001;110:585–99.
141. Brown TA, Barlow DH. A proposal for a dimensional classification system based on the shared features of the DSM-IV anxiety and mood disorders: implications for assessment and treatment. Psychol Assess 2009;21:256–71.
142. Gershuny BS, Sher KJ. The relation between personality and anxiety: findings from a 3-year prospective study. J Abnorm Psychol 1998;107:252–62.
143. Watson D, Clark LA, Carey G. Positive and negative affectivity and their relation to the anxiety and depressive disorders. J Abnorm Psychol 1988;97: 346–53.
144. Mineka S, Watson D, Clark LA. Comorbidity of anxiety and unipolar mood disorders. Annu Rev Psychol 1998;49:377–412.
145. Brown TA, Chorpita BF, Barlow DH. Structural relationships among dimensions of DSM-IV anxiety and mood disorders and dimensions of negative affect, positive affect, and autonomic arousal. J Abnorm Psychol 1998;107:179–92.
146. Etkin A, Wager TD. Functional neuroimaging of anxiety: a meta-analysis of emotional processing in PTSD, social anxiety disorder, and specific phobia. Am J Psychiatry 2007;164:1476–88.
147. Phan KL, Fitzgerald DA, Nathan PJ, et al. Association between amygdala hyperactivity to harsh faces and severity of social anxiety in generalized social phobia. Biol Psychiatry 2006;59:424–9.
148. Straube T, Glauer M, Dilger S, et al. Effects of cognitive-behavioral therapy on brain activation in specific phobia. Neuroimage 2006;29:125–35.
149. Tillfors M, Furmark T, Marteinsdottir I, et al. Cerebral blood flow during anticipation of public speaking in social phobia: a PET study. Biol Psychiatry 2002;52: 1113–9.
150. Mayberg HS, Liotti M, Brannan SK, et al. Reciprocal limbic cortical function and negative mood: converging PET findings in depression and normal sadness. Am J Psychiatry 1999;156:675–82.
151. Barlow DH, Allen LB, Choate ML. Toward a unified treatment for emotional disorders. Behav Ther 2004;35:205–30.
152. Otto MW, Smits JA, Reese HE. Cognitive-behavioral therapy for the treatment of anxiety disorders. J Clin Psychiatry 2004;65(Suppl 5):34–43.
153. Norton PJ, Hope DA. Preliminary evaluation of a broad-spectrum cognitive-behavioral group therapy for anxiety. J Behav Ther Exp Psychiatry 2005;36: 79–97.
154. Erickson DH, Janeck AS, Tallman K. A cognitive-behavioral group for patients with various anxiety disorders. Psychiatr Serv 2007;58:1205–11.

155. McEvoy PM, Nathan P. Effectiveness of cognitive behavior therapy for diagnostically heterogeneous groups: a benchmarking study. J Consult Clin Psychol 2007;75:344–50.

156. Norton PJ, Philipp LM. Transdiagnostic approaches to the treatment of anxiety disorders: a quantitative review. Psychother Theor Res Pract Train 2008;45: 214–26.

157. Ellard KK, Fairholme CP, Boisseau CL, et al. Unified protocol for the transdiagnostic treatment of emotional disorders: protocol development and initial outcome findings. Cogn Behav Pract 2010;17:102–13.

158. Kring AM, Sloan DM, editors. Emotion regulation and psychopathology: a transdiagnostic approach to etiology and treatment. New York: Guilford Press; 2009. p. 461.

159. Norton PJ, Hayes SA, Hope DA. Effects of transdiagnostic group treatment for anxiety on secondary depression. Depress Anxiety 2004;20:198–202.

160. Barlow DH. Clinical handbook of psychological disorders. New York: Guilford; 2008.

161. Barlow DH. Anxiety and its disorders: the nature and treatment of anxiety and panic. 2nd edition. New York: Guilford Press; 2002.

162. Allen LB, McHugh K, Barlow DH. Emotional disorders: a unified approach. In: Barlow DH, editor. Clinical handbook of psychological disorders. 4th edition. New York: Guilford; 2008. p. 216–49.

163. Barlow DH. Anxiety and its disorders: the nature and treatment of anxiety and panic. New York: Guilford Press; 1988.

164. Barlow DH, Craske MG, Cerny JA, et al. Behavioral treatment of panic disorder. Behav Ther 1989;20:261–82.

165. Craske MG. Models and treatment of panic: behavioral therapy of panic. J Cogn Psychother 1991;5:199–214.

166. Barlow DH, Brown TA, Craske MG. Definitions of panic attacks and panic disorder in the DSM-IV: implications for research. J Abnorm Psychol 1994; 103:553–64.

167. Allen LB, White KS, Barlow DH, et al. Cognitive-behavioral therapy (CBT) for panic disorder: relationship of anxiety and depression comorbidity with treatment outcome. Psychopathol Behav Assess 2010. [Epub ahead of print].

168. Goodwin RD, Lewinson PM, Seeley JR. Cigarette smoking and panic attacks among young adults in the community. Biol Psychiatry 2005;58:686–93.

169. Chambers J, Bass C. Chest pain and normal coronary anatomy: review of natural history and possible aetiological factors. Prog Cardiovasc Dis 1990; 33:161–84.

170. Goodwin RD. Association between physical activity and mental disorders among adults in the United States. Prev Med 2003;36:698–703.

171. Amering M, Bankier B, Berger P, et al. Panic disorder and cigarette smoking behavior. Compr Psychiatry 1999;40:35–8.

172. Breslau N, Klein DF. Smoking and panic attacks. Arch Gen Psychiatry 1999;56: 1141–7.

173. Bradley LA, Richter JE, Scarinci IC, et al. Psychosocial and psychophysical assessments of patients with unexplained chest pain. Am J Med 1992;92: 65–73.

174. Stein DS, White KS, Berman S, et al. Psychological and sociodemographic factors in non-cardiac chest pain patients impacting performance on the cardiac exercise tolerance test, in press.

175. Liao D, Cai J, Rosamond WD, et al. Cardiac autonomic function and incident coronary heart disease: a population-based case-cohort study: the ARIC study. Atherosclerosis risk in communities study. Am J Epidemiol 1997;145: 696–706.
176. Bigger JT Jr, Fleiss JL, Steinman RC, et al. Frequency domain measures of heart period variability and mortality after myocardial infarction. Circulation 1992;85: 164–71.
177. Dekker JM, Crow RS, Folsom AR, et al. Low heart rate variability in a 2-minute rhythm strip predicts risk of coronary heart disease and mortality from several causes: the ARIC Study. Circulation 2000;102:1239–44.
178. Kawachi I, Sparrow D, Vokonas P, et al. Decreased heart rate variability in men with phobic anxiety (data from the Normative Aging Study). Am J Cardiol 1995; 75:882–5.
179. Yeragani VK, Sobolewski E, Igel G, et al. Decreased heart-period variability in patients with panic disorder: a study of Holter ECG records. Psychiatry Res 1998;78:89–99.
180. Heart rate variability: standards of measurement, physiological interpretation, and clinical use. Task Force of the European Society of Cardiology and the North American Society of Pacing and Electrophysiology. Circulation 1996;93: 1043–65.
181. Melzig CA, Weike AI, Hamm AO, et al. Individual differences in fear-potentiated startle as a function of resting heart rate variability: implications for panic disorder. Int J Psychophysiol 2009;71:109–17.
182. Martens EJ, Nyklicek I, Szabo BM, et al. Depression and anxiety as predic-tors of heart rate variability after myocardial infarction. Psychol Med 2008;38: 375–83.
183. Watkins LL, Blumenthal JA, Carney RM. Association of anxiety with reduced baroreflex cardiac control in acute post-MI patients. Am Heart J 2002;143: 460–6.
184. Derogatis LR, Fitzpatrick M. The SCL-90, the brief symptom inventory (BSI), and the BSI-18. In: Maruish ME, editor. The use of psychological testing for treatment planning and outcome assessment. 3rd edition. New York: Erlbaum; 2000. p. 1–42.
185. Derogatis LR, Melisaratos N. The brief symptom inventory: an introductory report. Psychol Med 1983;13:595–605.
186. Zigmond AS, Snaith RP. The hospital anxiety and depression scale. Acta Psychiatr Scand 1983;67:361–70.
187. Ware JE, Sherbourne CD. The MOS 36-item short-form health survey (SF-36): I. Conceptual framework and item selection. Med Care 1992;30:473–83.
188. Hafkenscheid A. Reliability of a standardized and expanded brief psychiatric rating scale: a replication study. Acta Psychiatr Scand 1993;88:305–10.
189. Teng EL, Chui HC. The modified mini-mental state (3MS) examination. J Clin Psychiatry 1987;48:314–8.
190. Kiernan RJ, Mueller J, Langston JW, et al. The neurobehavioral cognitive status examination: a brief but quantitative approach to cognitive assessment. Ann Intern Med 1987;107:481–5.
191. Beck AT, Steer RA. Beck anxiety inventory. San Antonio (TX): The Psychological Corporation; 1993.
192. Beck AT, Steer RA, Ball R, et al. Comparison of beck depression inventories-IA and -II in psychiatric outpatients. J Pers Assess 1996;67:588–97.

193. Spitzer RL, Kroenke K, Williams JB. Validation and utility of a self-report version of PRIME-MD: the PHQ primary care study. JAMA 1999;282:1737–44.
194. Spitzer RL, Williams JB, Kroenke K, et al. Utility of a new procedure for diagnosing mental disorders in primary care. The PRIME-MD 1000 study. JAMA 1994;272:1749–56.
195. Brown TA, DiNardo P, Barlow DH. Anxiety disorder interview schedule for DSM-IV: current version (ADIS-IV). Cary (NC): Oxford University Press; 1994.
196. First MB, Spitzer RL, Gibbon M, et al. Structured clinical interview for DSM-IV axis I disorders-patient edition. New York: New York Biometrics Research Department; 1995.

Skin and Breast Disease in the Differential Diagnosis of Chest Pain

Jim Muir, MBBS, FACD, FACRRM (Hon)[a,*],

Michael Yelland, MBBS, PhD, FRACGP, FAFMM, Grad Dip Musculoskeletal Medicine[b]

KEYWORDS
- Chest pain • Skin diseases • Herpes zoster
- Breast • Neoplasm

Pain is not a symptom commonly associated with skin disease. This is especially so when considering the known skin problems that have a presenting symptom of chest pain that could potentially be confused with chest pain from other causes.

PAINFUL SKIN CONDITIONS

Several extremely painful and tender skin conditions present with dramatic clinical signs. Inflammatory disorders such as pyoderma gangrenosum, skin malignancies, both primary and secondary, acute bacterial infections such as erysipelas or cellulitis, and multiple other infections are commonly extremely painful and tender. As these conditions manifest with obvious skin signs such as swelling, erythema, localized tenderness, fever, lymphangitis, and lymphadenopathy, there is little chance of misdiagnosis of symptoms as caused by anything other than a cutaneous pathology.

Several skin tumors can be painful or tender. These include blue rubber bleb nevus, eccrine spiradenoma, neuromas, neurilemmomas, glomus tumors, angiolipomas, leiomyomas, dermatofibromas, squamous cell carcinomas and other skin malignancies especially when perineural infiltration is present, endometriomas, and granular cell tumors. Once again in almost all cases of pain related to a skin tumor a lesion can be readily identified, often by the patient. For a painful skin condition to be

[a] Department of Dermatology, Mater Misericordiae Hospital, Raymond Terrace, South Brisbane, QSD 4101, Australia
[b] School of Medicine, Logan Campus, Griffith University, University Drive, Meadowbrook, QSD 4131, Australia
* Corresponding author.
E-mail address: arnoldmuir@optusnet.com.au

Med Clin N Am 94 (2010) 319–325
doi:10.1016/j.mcna.2010.01.006
0025-7125/10/$ – see front matter © 2010 Elsevier Inc. All rights reserved.

medical.theclinics.com

misdiagnosed as cardiac, pulmonary, or other forms of chest pain, the pain must arise in the absence of readily identifiable skin disease.

HERPES ZOSTER

The classic condition to cause significant pain without obvious skin changes is herpes zoster. Although herpes zoster affects 20% to 30% of people in their lifetime, up to 50% of those more than 80 years old will be affected.[1] Herpes zoster is the reactivation of varicella zoster (chicken pox) virus that has lain dormant in the spinal dorsal root ganglion since initial infection. This produces the well-known, dermatomally distributed eruption commonly known as shingles. Most often unilateral and confined to a single dermatome, herpes zoster can involve multiple dermatomes and be bilateral. In severe cases, scarring and depigmentation may follow the healing of the acute lesions. There is often significant associated pain preceding, accompanying, and following resolution of the skin eruption. Pain persisting more than a month after the typical skin eruption is termed postherpetic neuralgia.

The pain is variable in intensity but can be severe. It may be localized or more diffuse. The onset of pain is usually around 4 days before any skin lesions appear.[2] This prodromal pain has been labeled as "preherpetic neuralgia."[3] There may be associated fever, malaise, and often tenderness or hyperesthesia in the affected area. Obviously in the prodromal phase before the onset of the skin lesions, the source of this pain can be obscure and erroneously attributed to other causes. For example, involvement of abdominal dermatomes can lead to the diagnosis of intraabdominal pathology such as biliary colic,[4] duodenal ulcer, appendicitis, or renal colic. A rare presentation is where there is no skin eruption following the prodromal pain. This is termed "zoster sine eruption" or "zoster sine herpete." The diagnosis may be supported by demonstrating an increase in IgM and eventually IgG varicella antibody titers.[5,6]

Of particular interest are reports of 6 zoster patients in whom pain preceded any skin eruption for between 7 and more than 100 days. The distribution of the pain did not always occur in the same dermatomes where the rash eventually developed.[3] Clearly it would be extremely difficult to diagnose the cause of such a pain before the onset of skin signs. Pain from such an atypical presentation of zoster would be even more likely to be attributed to other causes.

During this phase of pain without skin lesions, there is the likelihood that diagnoses other than herpes zoster will be considered.[7] Of especial pertinence to chest pain is the fact that zoster-related pain is more likely in older patients and will more often be severe. As older patients are also more at risk of chest pain from cardiac and pulmonary causes, the increasing incidence of zoster with increasing age also adds to the likelihood of diagnostic confusion.

Thoracic dermatomes are commonly affected. These features enhance the risk of confusion with cardiac pain[8,9] or pleurisy. Herpes zoster can be complicated by pleuropericarditis and even complete heart block.[10] Temporary electrocardiographic abnormalities can be seen.[11]

Diagnosing herpes zoster during this prodromal phase is clearly difficult. Clues to the diagnosis include a history of varicella or herpes zoster, the presence of localized skin tenderness or hyperesthesia in the painful area, and the localization of pain to a dermatome. Obviously all efforts would need to be made to exclude other serious or indeed life-threatening causes of chest pain. Often the diagnosis is only made with the onset of the typical skin lesions of grouped vesicles and pustules on an erythematous base in a dermatomal distribution. Then the diagnosis can usually be made on clinical grounds alone. Swabs from a blister base reveal varicella zoster virus

DNA when submitted for confirmatory polymerase chain reaction. Only rarely is biopsy necessary.

Treatment is with pain relief and a variety of systemic antiviral agents (acyclovir, famciclovir, valacyclovir). Treatment should be instituted within 72 hours of the appearance of the rash and continued for 7 days.[12] There is evidence that valacyclovir is superior to acyclovir.[13] The former agent has the advantages of better bioavailability and less frequent dosing.

An episode of herpes zoster usually resolves completely within 4 weeks. Scarring and depigmentation may occur. There should be no confusion as to the cause of pain once the typical skin lesions have developed. It should be noted that there are case reports of herpes zoster being temporally associated with and perhaps triggered by thoracic surgery with zoster arising in the surgical scars.[14]

Pain that persists or recurs more than a month after the onset of herpes zoster is termed postherpetic neuralgia. It is more common in older female patients especially if there was significant prodromal pain, a more severe rash, and more severe acute pain.[15] Again there is little risk of misdiagnosis of this pain as a history of acute herpes zoster will be found.

Once established postherpetic neuralgia is notoriously difficult to treat. Treatments used include gabapentin,[16] pregabalin,[17] topical capsaicin cream,[18] tricyclic antidepressants,[19] and in selected cases epidural injections of local anesthetic and steroid.[20]

A condition little known outside of dermatologic circles is notalgia paresthetica. It is characterized by itch and less commonly pain in the interscapular region of the back. This is the area innervated by the posterior primary rami of the thoracic nerves T2 to T6. Entrapment of these nerves is speculated to be causal.[21] Typically the condition occurs in older patients and there is a long history of discomfort, itch, or even hyperesthesia in the region. Skin changes can be minimal or related to chronic rubbing and scratching with thickening and darkening of the skin in the affected area. Sensory disturbances may be detectable on pin-prick testing. Biopsy of the affected skin can reveal necrotic epidermal keratinocytes and melanophages in the dermis.[22] Amyloid deposition, which is probably reactive, is also documented. Treatment is difficult and the condition tends to run a prolonged course. Agents such as topical capsaicin, topical local anesthetics, and oral amitryptiline have been used in treatment. Unfortunately there is little published evidence to support any intervention.

SKIN NEOPLASMS

As outlined earlier, several skin neoplasms can be painful. It would be uncommon for any of these lesions to present diagnostic confusion as to the source of the pain. Histology is characteristic in each case.

Glomus tumors are benign vascular skin tumors that resemble the gloumus apparatus. They are essentially vascular lesions.[23] Typically these lesions are solitary, pink to purple, domed dermal nodules. They vary in size from 1 to 20 mm diameter. Classically they are found on the distal extremities and are very painful. Symptoms can be spontaneous or triggered by pressure and temperature change. Glomangiomas, which have more prominent vessels and less prominent glomus cells, are reported on the trunk. These present as larger hemangioma-like lesions that may be congenital, are not restricted to the extremities, and although less likely to be painful, they can be.[24] Treatment is usually by surgical excision.

Eccrine spiradenomas are tumors derived from sweat glands and present as single, gray to pink, dermal nodules. They arise on the head, neck, and trunk but less often the extremities. Several variants are described (multiple, giant, linear, congenital). Malignant transformation can occur. They can be tender and painful. Histology is distinctive. Treatment and often diagnosis is by excision.[25]

Leiomyomas in the skin are benign smooth muscle lesions that can be vascular (angileiomyoma) in origin or derived from arrector pili muscle (piloleiomyomas). Both forms can be painful but angioleiomyomas are more likely to cause symptoms. Piloleiomyomas are often multiple and occur on the face, back, and limbs. They are firm red-brown nodules. Trauma and cold can trigger pain. Angioleiomyomas, on the other hand, are usually solitary nodules on the extremities. Pain and tenderness are seen in most cases. Many treatments are described including excision, analgesics, nifedipine, phenoxybenzamine hydrochloride, gabapentin, and doxazosin. More recently botulinum toxin has been used with success.[26]

Angiolipomas, as the name suggests, arise in the subcutis and are far more vascular than lipomas. They are believed to be hamartomas of blood vessels and fat. Onset soon after puberty is common and they present as soft sometimes bluish nodules on the trunk or limbs and are often multiple. They are often easier felt than seen. Unlike simple lipomas, mild pain and tenderness with pressure or movement is common. There is a noninfiltrating and a more rare but aggressive infiltrating type. The latter can mimic malignancy and is likely to recur after surgery. Treatment is usually surgical for single lesions. If multiple, β blockers can be useful in relieving pain.[27]

The blue rubber bleb nevus syndrome is an extremely rare disorder characterized by multiple venous malformations affecting primarily the skin and gastrointestinal tract. Multiple other organs can be affected. The skin lesions are dark blue nodules up to several centimeters in diameter. As expected with vascular lesions, they are compressible. They can be widespread and disfiguring. Pain and tenderness may be seen. In most cases, onset occurs in childhood.[27]

Traumatic neuromas are a result of nerve injury. They thus complicate trauma, surgery, and scars. Lying in the subcutaneous tissue, these firm, oval, pea-sized lesions are more easily felt than seen. Spontaneous pain and tenderness can occur. Traumatic neuromas are a well-known complication of amputation stumps and are also found on the foot; they have been related to wearing high-heeled shoes. Intercostal nerve injury is felt to be a major factor in postthoracotomy pain. It has been reported that injury to these nerves occurs routinely with rib retraction.[28] Another painful lesion derived from nerve tissue is the neurilemmoma or schwannoma. These slow-growing benign tumors, derived from Schwann cells, usually arise in association with a major nerve. Bilateral acoustic schwannomas are typical of neurofibromatosis type 2. The other common sites are the head and neck and near the limb joints. Up to one-third are associated with pain, tenderness, and parasthesia. Rounded and well defined, they are usually solitary and up to 5 cm in diameter. Other sites include deep soft tissues, retroperitoneum, mediastinum, and tongue. Scwannomas can involve the intercostal nerves and cause pain.[29] They may be palpable.[30] Retroperitoneal schwannomas are a rarely reported cause of chest pain. Treatment is by local resection and recurrence is rare.[31]

BREAST LESIONS AND CHEST PAIN

Chest pain may also result from breast lesions. In a survey of presenting symptoms in patients with breast cancer in 2 health service districts in Wales, pain or soreness was the initial symptom in 12% of women, only second to a painless lump at 68%.[32] Similar figures of 10% for pain and 76% for painless lump as presenting symptoms of breast cancer were reported by an Australian breast unit.[33]

Not all painful breast lesions are malignant. Women with fibrocystic disease of the breast typically complain of pain and tenderness, most marked in the premenstrual period, with some continuing throughout the cycle.[34] The incidence of fibrocystic disease is 90 per 100,000 woman-years; the incidence increases up to the age of 45 years and then declines sharply.[35] In contrast, the incidence of breast cancer increase with age, being 50 per 100,000 woman-years in women less than 50 and 300 per 100,000 woman-years in women more than 50 years.[36]

Given these rates, breast lesions are still be a relatively uncommon source of chest pain, but breast examination and investigations, including mammography, ultrasound, and magnetic resonance imaging, may be indicated when other causes of chest pain are not found or if the pain is of a cyclical nature.

SUMMARY

There are several skin and breast lesions that can cause pain or tenderness. In most cases the presence of a skin lesion, if not its definitive diagnosis, will be clinically evident. In most instances treatment of these painful skin lesions is by simple excision, which will also provide histologic confirmation of the diagnosis. It would be rare for a cutaneous cause of skin pain to be mistaken for another cause. The prodromal pain of herpes zoster is most likely to cause diagnostic confusion. The painful skin lesions are usually identified by the patient as being the source of their discomfort. The specific diagnosis may not be apparent without submission of lesional tissue for histology. Chest pain is an uncommon presenting symptom of benign and malignant breast lesions. Breast examination and investigation may be appropriate when other causes of chest pain are not evident.

REFERENCES

1. Johnson RW. Herpes zoster and postherpetic neuralgia: a review of the effects of vaccination. Aging Clin Exp Res 2009;21(3):236–43.
2. Johnson RW. Zoster associated pain: what is known, who is at risk and how can it be managed? Herpes 2007;14(Suppl 2):30–4.
3. Gilden DH, Dueland AN, Cohrs R, et al. Preherpetic neuralgia. Neurology 1991; 41:1215–8.
4. Hassan I, Donohue JH. Herpes zoster mistaken for biliary colic and treated by laparoscopic cholecystectomy; a cautionary case report. Surg Endosc 1996; 10(8):848–9.
5. Barrett AP, Katelaris CH, Morris JG, et al. Zoster sine herpete of the trigeminal nerve. Oral Surg Oral Med Oral Pathol 1993;75(2):173–5.
6. Schuchmann JA, McAllister RK, Armstrong CS, et al. Zoster sine herpete with thoracic motor paralysis temporally associated with thoracic epidural steroid injection. Am J Phys Med Rehabil 2008;87(10):853–8.
7. Morgan R, King D. Characteristics of patients with shingles admitted to a district general hospital. Postgrad Med J 1998;74(868):101–3.
8. Goh CL, Khoo L. A retrospective study of the clinical presentation and outcome of herpes zoster in a tertiary dermatology outpatient referral clinic. Int J Dermatol 1997;36(9):667–72.
9. Franken RA, Franken M. Pseudo-myocardial infarction during an episode of herpes zoster. Arq Bras Cardiol 2000;75(6):523–30.
10. Ma TS, Collins TC, Habib G, et al. Herpes zoster and its cardiovascular complications in the elderly–another look at a dormant virus. Cardiology 2007;107(1): 63–7.

11. Pastinszky I, Kenedi I. Electrocardiographic changes associated with herpes zoster. Acta Med Acad Sci Hung 1963;19:23–30.

12. Dworkin RH, Johnson RW, Breuer J, et al. Recommendations for the management of herpes zoster. Clin Infect Dis 2007;44(Suppl 1):S1–26.

13. Beutner KR, Friedman DJ, Forszpaniak C, et al. Valaciclovir compared with acyclovir for improved therapy for herpes zoster in immunocompetent adults. Antimicrob Agents Chemother 1995;39(7):1546–53.

14. Godfrey EK, Brown C, Stambough JL. Herpes zoster–varicella complicating anterior thoracic surgery: 2 case reports. J Spinal Disord Tech 2006;19(4): 299–301.

15. Jung BF, Johnson RW, Griffin DR, et al. Risk factors for postherpetic neuralgia in patients with herpes zoster. Neurology 2004;62(9):1545–51.

16. Irving G, Jensen M, Cramer M, et al. Efficacy and tolerability of gastric-retentive gabapentin for the treatment of postherpetic neuralgia: results of a double-blind, randomized, placebo-controlled clinical trial. Clin J Pain 2009;25(3):185–92.

17. Zareba G. Pregabalin: a new agent for the treatment of neuropathic pain. Drugs Today (Barc) 2005;41(8):509–16.

18. Peikert A, Hentrich M, Ochs G. Topical 0.025% capsaicin in chronic post-herpetic neuralgia: efficacy, predictors of response and long-term course. J Neurol 1991; 238(8):452–6.

19. Saarto T, Wiffen PJ. Antidepressants for neuropathic pain. Cochrane Database Syst Rev 2005;(4):CD005454. DOI: 10.1002/14651858.CD005454.pub2.

20. van Wijck AJ, Opstelten W, Moons KG, et al. The PINE study of epidural steroids and local anaesthetics to prevent postherpetic neuralgia: a randomised controlled trial. Lancet 2006;367(9506):219–24.

21. Savk O, Savk E. Investigation of spinal pathology in notalgia paresthetica. J Am Acad Dermatol 2005;52(6):1085–7.

22. Layton AM, Cotterill JA. Notalgia Paraaesthetica – a report of three cases and their treatment. Clin Exp Dermatol 1991;16:197–8.

23. Weedon D. Weedons skin pathology. 3rd edition. Amsterdam: Elsevier; 2009. p. 907.

24. Carvalho VO, Taniguchi K, Giraldi S, et al. Congenital plaquelike glomus tumor in a child. Pediatr Dermatol 2001;18(3):223–6.

25. Weedon D. Weedon's skin pathology. 3rd edition. Amsterdam: Elsevier; 2009. p. 786.

26. Onder M, Adişen E. A new indication of botulinum toxin: leiomyoma-related pain. J Am Acad Dermatol 2009;60(2):325–8.

27. Burns DA, Breathnach SM, Cox N, et al. editors. Rook's textbook of dermatology. 7th edition. Oxford (UK): Blackwell Publishing Ltd; 2006. p. 15.83–15.85, 55.34–55.35.

28. Rogers ML, Henderson L, Mahajan RP, et al. Preliminary findings in the neuro-physiological assessment of intercostal nerve injury during thoracotomy. Eur J Cardiothorac Surg 2002;21(2):298–301.

29. Yang J, Guo QN, Zhang R, et al. Intraosseous schwannoma of rib. J Clin Pathol 2009;62(2):185–6.

30. Sakurai H, Hada M, Mitsui T. Extrathoracic neurilemoma of the lateral chest wall mimicking a subcutaneous tumor: report of a case. Ann Thorac Cardiovasc Surg 2006;12(2):133–6.

31. Choudry HA, Nikfarjam M, Liang JJ, et al. Diagnosis and management of retro-peritoneal ancient schwannomas. World J Surg Oncol 2009;7:12.

32. MacArthur C, Smith A. The symptom presentation of breast cancer: is pain a symptom? Community Med 1983;5(3):220–3.

33. National Breast Cancer Centre. The investigation of a new breast symptom: a guide for general practitioners. February 2006. Available at: http://nbocc.org. au/view-document-details/ibs-the-investigation-of-a-new-breast-symptom-guide-for-gps. Accessed December 29, 2009.

34. Greenblatt RB, Samaras C, Vasquez JM, et al. Fibrocystic disease of the breast. Clin Obstet Gynecol 1982;25(2):365–71.

35. Cole P, Mark Elwood J, Kaplan SD. Incidence rates and risk factors of benign breast neoplasms. Am J Epidemiol 1978;108(2):112–20.

36. Ravdin PM, Cronin KA, Howlader N, et al. The decrease in breast-cancer incidence in 2003 in the United States. N Engl J Med 2007;356(16):1670–4.

Evaluation of Chest Pain in the Pediatric Patient

Jennifer Thull-Freedman, MD, MSc[a,b]

KEYWORDS

- Cardiac • Electrocardiogram • Pediatric chest pain
- Pulmonary embolism

Many causes of chest pain in children are benign and self-limited. Nonetheless, serious and life-threatening etiologies exist, and the challenge to the practitioner is to be able to identify the few patients who have a serious cause for their pain. Furthermore, chest pain is a worrisome symptom for families who often fear a cardiac cause, and the symptom may lead to school absence and limitation of activities. The differential diagnosis for pediatric chest pain is extensive (**Box 1**), and physicians caring for children must be familiar with the possible causes for chest pain and attempt to identify an etiology. In many cases a thorough history and physical examination are sufficient to identify the source of the pain, and diagnostic testing can be performed on a selective basis to address concerns identified. Only after a serious cause has been excluded should reassurance and symptomatic care be offered.

EPIDEMIOLOGY

Chest pain accounts for approximately 0.3% to 0.6% of pediatric emergency department (ED) visits.[1–3] The frequency of visits is fairly constant throughout the year,[4] with a slight excess in summer months reported in one study.[1]

In EDs treating children up to 18 years of age, the median age for presentation with chest pain was 12 to 13 years.[1,5,6] The reported male to female ratio is fairly even, ranging from 1:1 to 1.6:1.[1,5,6] In adolescents, relatively more girls present with chest pain.[5] Many ED studies report that most children present with acute pain of less than 1 day in duration.[2,6] In contrast, a study done in Turkey reported that 59% of patients described pain greater than 1 month in duration.[7]

[a] Department of Paediatrics, Division of Paediatric Emergency Medicine, University of Toronto, Toronto, ON, Canada
[b] Department of Paediatrics, Division of Paediatric Emergency Medicine, The Hospital for Sick Children, 555 University Avenue, Toronto, ON M5G 1X8, Canada
E-mail address: jennifer.thull-freedman@sickkids.ca

Med Clin N Am 94 (2010) 327–347
doi:10.1016/j.mcna.2010.01.004
0025-7125/10/$ – see front matter © 2010 Elsevier Inc. All rights reserved.

medical.theclinics.com

Box 1
Differential diagnosis of pediatric chest pain

Cardiovascular

- Arrhythmia
- Coronary artery disease (anomalous coronary arteries, acute Kawasaki disease [coronary arteritis], premature atherosclerosis [eg, dyslipidemia])
- Coronary artery vasospasm (toxicologic ingestion [cocaine, marijuana])
- Structural (hypertrophic cardiomyopathy, valvular stenosis [pulmonary, aortic], mitral valve prolapse)
- Myocarditis
- Pericarditis
- Endocarditis
- Congenital absence of pericardium
- Aortic aneurysm or dissection (Marfan, Turner, and Noonan syndromes)

Respiratory

- Asthma
- Pneumonia
- Pneumothorax/pneumomediastinum
- Pulmonary embolism
- Pleuritis/pleural effusion (eg, systemic lupus erythematosus)
- Pleurodynia (coxsackievirus)
- Chronic cough
- Airway foreign body

Abdominal and gastrointestinal

- Esophagitis (gastroesophageal reflux disease, eosinophilic esophagitis, bulimia, pill esophagitis)
- Esophageal foreign body
- Esophageal spasm/dysmotility
- Gastritis
- Hiatal hernia
- Referred pain from abdominal trauma (Kehr sign)
- Cholecystitis

Musculoskeletal and chest wall

- Chest wall strain (exercise, overuse injury, forceful coughing)
- Skeletal (chest wall or thoracic spine) anomaly
- Trauma (contusion/rib fracture)
- Costochondritis/Tietze syndrome
- Slipping rib
- Precordial catch (Texidor twinge)
- Breast tenderness
- Cutaneous (eg, herpes zoster)

Psychiatric

- Anxiety
- Panic
- Somatoform disorder (eg, conversion)
- Depression
- Emotional distress

Hematologic and oncologic

- Sickle cell disease
- Chest wall, thoracic, or mediastinal tumor

Neurologic

- Migraine
- Spinal nerve root compression

CAUSES OF CHEST PAIN IN CHILDREN

Most of what is known about frequency of various causes of pediatric chest pain comes from studies performed in pediatric EDs and cardiology clinics. **Table 1** provides a list of frequencies of causes according to organ system. In general, the most frequent cause reported is musculoskeletal pain, including costochondritis. These conditions represent between 7% and 69% of cases presenting to an ED, with the reported frequency dependent somewhat on how strictly musculoskeletal pain is defined and whether it is used as a diagnosis of exclusion or reported in combination with idiopathic causes. Respiratory causes including asthma are the second most common organic etiology identified, representing 13% to 24% of cases. Gastrointestinal and psychogenic causes are identified in less than 10% of cases, and a cardiac cause is found infrequently, representing not more than 5% of cases. An idiopathic etiology was frequently assigned in several studies, accounting for 20% to 61% of diagnoses made.[5,6,8,9] Children who were given a diagnosis of nonorganic chest pain were more likely to have pain greater than 6 months in duration and more likely to have a family history of chest pain or heart disease.[5] Children who were given a diagnosis of organic disease were more likely to have pain of acute origin, pain awakening them from sleep, fever, or abnormal examination findings. Children less

Cause	Emergency Department or Pediatric Clinic (%)[1,4–6,8,9]	Cardiology Clinic (%)[4,10–12]
Idiopathic/cause unknown	12–61	37–54
Musculoskeletal/costochondritis	7–69	1–89
Respiratory/asthma	13–24	1–12
Gastrointestinal/gastroesophageal reflux disease	3–7	3–12
Psychogenic	5–9	4–19
Cardiac	2–5	3–7

Table 1
Frequency of causes in children complaining of chest pain

than 12 years of age were two times more likely to have a cardiac or respiratory cause for their pain, whereas adolescents were 2.5 times more likely to have a psychogenic cause.[5] Rowe and colleagues[1] demonstrated an increased frequency of traumatic causes in boys.

Chest Wall

Direct trauma has been reported as the cause for chest pain in approximately 5% of cases.[4,5] Frequent or severe cough can cause chest wall pain because of muscle strain. Children who engage in a new or intense physical activity may experience delayed-onset muscle soreness of the pectoralis or shoulder muscles. Delayed-onset muscle soreness typically peaks within 2 days following activity. Because of the lag in development of soreness, children and parents may not recognize the association of the pain with the preceding activity before seeking medical attention. The pain of delayed-onset muscle soreness can generally be reproduced by palpation or engagement of the involved muscle group. Treatment is with nonsteroidal anti-inflammatory agents and rest.

Chest wall deformities, such as pectus excavatum or pectus carinatum (**Fig. 1**), can be associated with musculoskeletal chest pain. Patients with chest wall deformities should be examined carefully for findings consistent with Marfan syndrome, which is associated with an increased risk of aortic root dilation and dissection and spontaneous pneumothorax (**Fig. 2**). Pectus excavatum in isolation may also be associated with aortic root dilation, even when other stigmata of Marfan syndrome are absent.[13]

Costochondritis is defined as a pain localized to a costal cartilage that is reproducible on palpation. Many patients complaining of chest pain are found to have areas of tenderness at the costochondral or costosternal junctions (26%–41%).[1,2] A diagnosis of costochondritis is assigned when pain reproducible by palpation is not attributed to

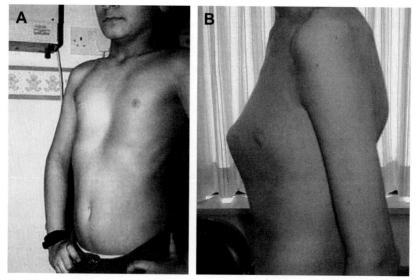

Fig. 1. (*A*) Pectus excavatum. (*From* Chaudhry B, Harvey D. Mosby's color atlas and text of pediatrics and child health. Edinburgh: Mosby; 2001. p. 186; with permission.) (*B*) Pectus carinatum. (*From* Warner BW. Pediatric surgery. In: Townsend CM, editor. Sabiston textbook of surgery. 18th edition. Philadelphia: WB Saunders; 2008. p. 2074; with permission.)

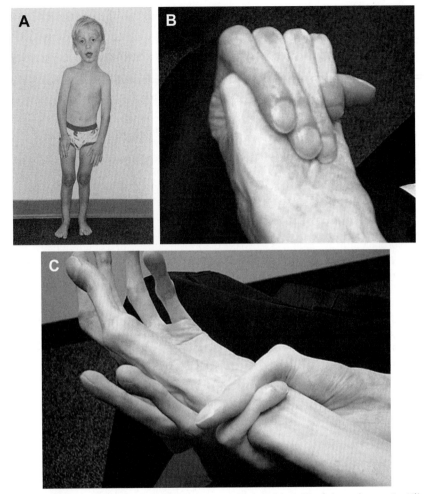

Fig. 2. (*A*) Marfan syndrome. (*From* Robinson LK, Fitzpatrick E. Marfan syndrome. In: Kliegman RM, editor. Nelson textbook of pediatrics. 18th edition. Philadelphia: Saunders/Elsevier; 2007. p. 2891; with permission.) (*B*) Thumb sign. When the hand is clenched without assistance, the entire thumbnail projects beyond the border of the hand. (*From* Zitelli BJ. Picture of the month. Arch Pediatr Adolesc Med 2005;159:721–3; with permission.) (*C*) Wrist sign. When the wrist is grasped by the contralateral hand, the thumb overlaps the terminal phalanx of the fifth digit. (*From* Zitelli BJ. Picture of the month. Arch Pediatr Adolesc Med 2005;159:721–3; with permission.)

another specific diagnosis. The causes and natural history of this condition are not well understood. Postulated etiologies include minor trauma, cough, and postviral reaction. In adults, costochondritis can be associated with fibromyalgia and other rheumatologic conditions in a minority of individuals[14]; however, in children this association has not been described. In a study that was limited by a large loss to follow-up, 62% of adolescents (15% of the original population) who had been diagnosed with costochondritis still reported pain after 1 year.[15]

Tietze syndrome is a specific form of costochondritis characterized by localized, painful, nonsuppurative costochondral swelling. Mukamel and colleagues[16] described a series of eight Israeli children between 10 months and 12 years of age with a clinical diagnosis of Tietze syndrome. Masses were usually tender; varied in size from 1 to 4 cm; and were located in lower, middle, and upper costochondral junctions. None had fever or systemic symptoms, although elevated erythrocyte sedimentation rate was reported in some. All cases resolved within 2 months. The etiology of this condition is unknown.

Slipping rib syndrome is an unusual cause of lower chest pain that results when the medial fibrous attachments of the 8th, 9th, or 10th ribs are inadequate or ruptured, allowing the costal cartilage tips to sublux and possibly impinge on intercostals nerves. In some cases there may be a preceding trauma. Patients may be aware of a popping sensation at the onset of pain. The diagnosis is supported by a positive "hooking maneuver," which consists of hooking the fingers under the lowest costal cartilages and drawing them anteriorly and superiorly, reproducing the symptoms. Saltzman and colleagues[17] described a case series of 12 patients diagnosed with slipping rib syndrome who experienced temporary relief of pain with intercostal nerve block (nine of nine) and complete relief of pain following excision of the offending rib tip (nine of nine).

Precordial catch syndrome is a clinical diagnosis applied to a characteristic pattern of benign chest pain. The pattern was first described in 1955 by Miller and Texidor[18] and came to be known as "Texidor twinge." The pathophysiology of the syndrome is not known, and although it has been described anecdotally as a frequent cause of pediatric cardiology referral,[19] it has not been specifically studied in the pediatric population. It is described, however, as a sharp pain of sudden onset localized to the anterior chest wall that occurs mostly at rest. It tends to last from a few seconds to 3 minutes and may be exacerbated by taking a deep breath. There are no associated symptoms, and physical examination is negative.

Breast tenderness can also be the source of chest wall pain. This can be physiologic during thelarche, or caused by infectious or inflammatory conditions, such as mastitis. Cutaneous chest wall pain may occur during an episode of herpes zoster. Pain occurs in a unilateral dermatome distribution and may precede the development of characteristic skin findings by several days.

Pulmonary

Approximately 13% to 24% of children with chest pain seen in an ED or ambulatory setting are found to have a pulmonary origin for their pain.[4,6] The most frequently implicated respiratory cause is asthma. Selbst and colleagues[5] identified asthma as the diagnosis in 7% of patients presenting to the ED with chest pain. Exercise-induced asthma may be an underrecognized cause of pediatric chest pain. A study of children with chest pain who performed exercise stress testing found significant improvement in symptoms and pulmonary function after bronchodilator use.[20] In a study of pediatric patients with chest pain referred to a cardiac stress laboratory, 26% had abnormal pulmonary function testing, despite only 19% having a known history of asthma.[21]

Pneumonia has been reported in 2% to 5% of ED patients with chest pain.[5,6,8] In patients with sickle cell disease, chest pain accompanied by lower respiratory tract symptoms and an infiltrate on radiograph should be managed as an acute chest crisis (**Fig. 3**). Pleurodynia (historically "devil's grip") is characterized by fever and pleuritic chest pain. It may occur in localized epidemics and is often associated with coxsackievirus B1, although other enteroviruses have also been implicated.[22] Pleuritis and pleural effusions are uncommon causes of pleuritic chest pain but can be seen in children with infections and such conditions as collagen vascular disease, malignancy, and familial Mediterranean fever.

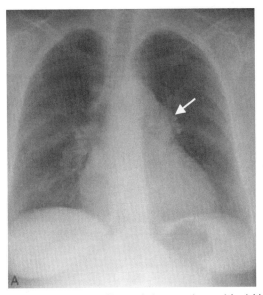

Fig. 3. Acute chest syndrome. Chest radiograph in a patient with sickle cell disease who experienced new chest pain and hypoxemia, showing new infiltrates and pulmonary hypertension as evidenced by an enlarged main pulmonary artery segment (*arrow*). (*From* Hamrick J, Claster S, Vichinsky E. Pulmonary complications of hematologic disease. In: Mason RJ, editor. Murray and Nadel's textbook of respiratory medicine. 4th edition. Philadelphia: WB Saunders; 2005. p. 2244; with permission.)

Pneumothorax and pneumomediastinum may account for up to 3% of cases of chest pain presenting to a pediatric ED (**Fig. 4**).[1,6] Chest pain is present in nearly all children with pneumothorax.[23] In a study by Lee and colleagues,[24] however, only 68% of children with pneumomediastinum had chest pain; neck pain (44%) and sore throat (33%) were also present. These entities are typically found in children with asthma; bronchiolitis; or other lower airway diseases, such as cystic fibrosis. Marfan syndrome is also a risk factor. Previously healthy children may present with a spontaneous pneumothorax from a ruptured bleb. Pneumothorax or pneumomediastinum may also occur after an episode of choking or aspiration or after inhalation of cocaine or marijuana.[25] Pneumothorax should be suspected in a child with risk factors or unexplained dyspnea, tachypnea, or decreased breath sounds. Pneumomediastinum should be suspected if subcutaneous emphysema or Hamman sign (precordial crackles that correlate with the heartbeat) are present.

Pulmonary embolism (PE) is rare in healthy children but may be seen in the presence of risk factors, such as a central venous catheter; malignancy; coagulopathy; nephrotic syndrome; major surgery (especially cardiac); trauma; or sepsis.[26,27] Nearly all children identified as having a PE are symptomatic. In a study of pediatric trauma patients with PE, 73% had dyspnea, 70% had tachypnea, 51% had rales, and 66% had pleuritic chest pain.[28] Typical electrocardiograms (ECGs) findings in PE are presented in **Table 2**.

Gastrointestinal

Gastrointestinal causes for chest pain have been identified in up to 8% of patients presenting to pediatric EDs.[9] Gastroesophageal reflux disease is the most frequently

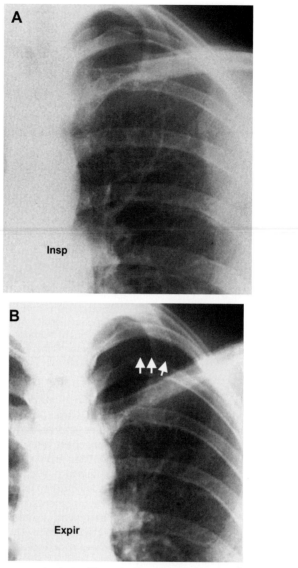

Fig. 4. Pneumothorax accentuated with expiration. (*A*) In this patient with chest pain, on a typical inspiration chest radiograph, no pneumothorax is identified. (*B*) With expiration, the superior lung margin (*arrows*) becomes smaller, but the pneumothorax stays the same size; relatively it appears bigger and can be easier to see. (*From* Mettler FA. Chest. In: Essentials of radiology. 2nd edition. Philadelphia: Saunders/Elsevier; 2005. p. 102; with permission.)

diagnosed gastrointestinal cause for chest pain in children, occurring in 3% of patients in one study.[9] Because gastroesophageal reflux disease is usually a clinical diagnosis, however, it is difficult to estimate the true contribution of gastroesophageal reflux disease in chest pain. In an uncontrolled study by Berezin and colleagues,[29] 27 children with idiopathic chest pain and no symptoms of reflux underwent endoscopy. Sixteen were found to have esophagitis, four had gastritis, and one had abnormal

Table 2 Electrocardiographic findings in conditions causing chest pain	
Condition	**ECG Finding**
Pericarditis	Sinus tachycardia
	Generalized ST-segment elevation (or depression)
	Nonspecific ST-segment/T-wave changes
	PR depression with upright P waves
	Low QRS amplitude if large effusion present
	Electrical alternans if large effusion present
Myocarditis	Sinus tachycardia
	Low QRS voltages (total <5 mm)
	ST-segment elevation
	Flattened or inverted T waves
	Incomplete atrioventricular conduction blocks
	Intraventricular conduction blocks
	Premature ventricular contractions
Pulmonary embolism	Normal in 25% of patients
	Sinus tachycardia
	Right heart strain (RBBB, T-wave inversions in anterior leads)
	Right ventricular hypertrophy
	S in I with Q and inverted T wave in III found in <25%

manometry. In another study, patients who presented to a cardiology clinic with both chest pain and epigastric tenderness had a high prevalence of esophagitis or gastritis on endoscopy (41 of 44 patients). Most of those who received treatment had resolution of symptoms.[30]

Structural abnormalities, inflammatory or motility disorders, and foreign bodies involving the esophagus or stomach may also produce chest pain in children. Eosinophilic esophagitis is an increasingly recognized disorder in children, which may cause chest pain because of esophageal inflammation, dysmotility, and reflux.[31] Bulimia nervosa is another cause of esophagitis in the pediatric population, particularly in adolescent girls. Coins and other objects lodged in the esophagus typically present with chest pain that is often accompanied by drooling and dysphagia.[32] Pill esophagitis is chemical irritation of the esophageal mucosa from certain medications, particularly iron preparations, tetracyclines, and nonsteroidal anti-inflammatory agents. The classic pediatric presentation of pill esophagitis is the adolescent patient who ingests a tetracycline antibiotic capsule with too little water, especially before going to bed.[33] Chest pain, dysphagia, and occasionally hemoptysis are present.

Esophageal rupture from nontraumatic causes (Boerhaave syndrome) has also been described as a cause of chest pain in children.[34] The perforation of the esophagus is believed to be caused by increased pressure transmitted from retching or vomiting but has also been associated with coughing, asthma, defecation, seizures, childbirth, nose-blowing, and immunosuppression. Patients may present with chest pain, vomiting, and subcutaneous emphysema (Mackler triad) and hematemesis, respiratory distress, and hemorrhagic or septic shock. Chest radiography may reveal pneumomediastinum, pneumothorax, mediastinal widening, or pleural effusion, and diagnosis is confirmed by contrast esophagram or CT scan.

Cardiac

Cardiovascular disease is identified in only 2% to 5% of patients seen in pediatric EDs for chest pain[1,4]; however, it is often the leading concern of patients and families seeking care.[8] In one study 56% of adolescents feared chest pain was cardiac.[35] The presence of fever, dyspnea, palpitations, pallor, or abnormal cardiac auscultation has been found to be statistically significantly related to a cardiac etiology.[4] Outside of North America, the frequency of cardiovascular etiologies for pediatric chest pain may by higher. A Turkish study of pediatric patients with chest pain referred for cardiology evaluation, of whom 9% had a known cardiac diagnosis, determined that 42.5% had cardiac disease, including 14% with rheumatic heart disease and 12% with evidence of dysrhythmia.[7]

In children, acute myocardial infarction (AMI) has been described in association with coronary artery anomalies; congenital heart disease; Kawasaki disease; familial hypercholesterolemia; previous heart transplant; sickle cell disease; cardiac myxoma; hypercoagulable states; substance abuse; and certain metabolic conditions, such as homocystinuria and mucopolysaccharidosis. Most information on AMI in the pediatric population comes from case reports. A population database study, however, estimated the risk in adolescents as 6.6 per 1 million patient-years.[36] Of the 123 patients between 13 and 18 years who had suffered AMI, 23% had a history of substance abuse (cocaine 41%, amphetamines 31%, cannabis 10%, multiple substances 10%). AMI was more common in males (OR = 3) and smokers (OR = 4.1) compared with patients of the same age admitted for other reasons. Pre-existing conditions (systemic lupus erythematosus and hyperlipidemia) were found in 2.5% of patients. The most common location of infarction was subendocardial, accounting for 40% of infarcts. A study of all myocardial infarction cases in a single pediatric institution in an 11-year period identified nine cases.[37] The average age was 15.5 years; eight were boys. The one female patient was 4 months postpartum. All were previously healthy except for migraine headaches in two and attention deficit disorder in one patient who was taking methylphenidate. Drug screens, hypercoagulability studies (performed in seven of nine patients), and lipid profiles were negative in all patients. All presented with chest pain and responded to nitroglycerin. Abnormal ECGs were found in eight patients, and all had elevated cardiac enzymes. Of interest, all nine patients had normal coronary angiograms, and all had normal exercise stress testing after hospitalization. The authors concluded that coronary spasm was the most likely cause for the ischemia. Intracoronary thrombus can also be a cause of AMI in children.[38] Risk factors include hypercoagulability and emboli from endocarditis or prosthetic valves.[39]

Congenital coronary artery abnormalities have also been associated with an increased risk of myocardial infarction in children. Anomalous origin of the left coronary artery from the pulmonary artery is often identified in early infancy when the pulmonary artery pressure declines, usually around 2 to 3 months of age. Patients may present with crying, poor feeding, and signs of congestive heart failure. Anomalous origin of the left coronary artery from the pulmonary artery may also present in later childhood and may present with anginal pain. The typical ECG pattern is that of an anterolateral infarction with large and wide Q waves, ST changes, and T wave inversion in leads I, aVL, V5, and V6. Other coronary artery abnormalities, including anomalous origin of the left main coronary artery or right coronary artery from the contralateral sinus of Valsalva and hypoplastic coronary arteries, may also present in childhood. Numerous case reports have been published of children, especially young athletes, who experience chest pain, myocardial ischemia, or sudden cardiac death because of the presence of coronary artery anomalies.[40,41]

Kawasaki disease has been associated with myocardial infarction both in the acute and subacute phases and as a long-term consequence. Acute cardiac complications of Kawasaki disease include coronary artery aneurysms, myocarditis, pericarditis, and arrhythmias. Aneurysms, which generally occur 10 days to 4 weeks after the onset of symptoms, are the most frequent complication and occur in 20% to 25% of untreated patients[42] and 5% of patients treated with intravenous immunoglobulin. Infarction can occur during the acute phase caused by intimal proliferative inflammation or during resolution caused by obstruction, stenosis, or irregularities of the arterial wall. Successful use of intravenous immunoglobulin to treat Kawasaki disease was first reported in 1983.[43] In a cohort of patients with acute Kawasaki disease in the preintravenous immunoglobulin era, 25% had coronary aneurysms. Forty-nine percent experienced regression of their aneurysms within 1 to 2 years after diagnosis; however, 10 to 21 years after diagnosis, 19% were found to have coronary stenosis (5% of the original cohort), and 8% had experienced myocardial infarction (2% of original cohort).[44] Presumably children with a missed diagnosis of Kawasaki disease who do not receive intravenous immunoglobulin would have a similar prognosis for stenosis or infarction.

Myocardial ischemia has also been reported in children with sickle cell disease. In a study of pediatric sickle cell patients with a history of chest pain, heart failure, abnormal ECG, left ventricular dilation, or hypokinetic left ventricle, 64% had perfusion defects on thallium-201 single-photon emission CT. Three children who were started on hydroxyurea therapy underwent repeat single-photon emission CT, and all showed improvement. No occlusion of coronary arteries was found, suggesting that pathology of the microcirculation is responsible for the defects.[45]

Myocarditis is a rare but serious cause of chest pain in children. In one study, 56% of children with myocarditis ages 10 to 17 years presented with symptoms of chest pain or palpitations, and 25% presented with lightheadedness, syncope, or seizure.[46] In children less than 10 years old respiratory presentations were more common, accounting for 47% of cases. Common physical findings include tachypnea (60%–68%); hepatomegaly (36%–50%); and tachycardia (32%–58%).[46,47] ECG abnormalities are detected in 93% to 100%, and chest radiography is abnormal in 55% to 90%. Laboratory abnormalities include elevated troponin (54%); elevated creatine kinase (73%); elevated erythrocyte sedimentation rate (38%–57%); and elevated aspartate aminotransferase (85%). Pericarditis and endocarditis can also be associated with chest pain. Typical ECG findings in myocarditis and pericarditis are presented in **Table 2**, and representative ECG examples are presented in **Figs. 5** and **6**. Partial or complete congenital absence of the pericardium is rare but may produce chest pain in children. In a series of 10 patients, the median age of presentation was 21 years (the youngest was 2 years of age). All except the youngest child presented with chest

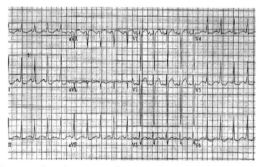

Fig. 5. Electrocardiogram showing signs of myocarditis including sinus tachycardia, T-wave changes, ST-segment changes (elevation and depression), and incomplete left bundle-branch block. (*From* Brady WJ, Ferguson JD, Ullman EA. Myocarditis: emergency department recognition and management. Emerg Med Clin North Am 2004;22:865–85; with permission.)

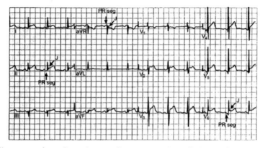

Fig. 6. Electrocardiogram showing signs of acute pericarditis, including widespread J-point and ST-segment elevation and deflection of the PR segments in the direction opposite that of the P wave, generally PR depression with upright P waves. (*From* Breitbart RE. Pericardial diseases. In: Keane JF, editor. Nadas' pediatric cardiology. 2nd edition. Philadelphia: Saunders/Elsevier; 2006. p. 460; with permission.)

pain, which was typically stabbing and nonexertional, and often could be induced or relieved by postural changes. Chest radiographs of 7 of the 10 showed displacement of the cardiac silhouette to the left with loss of the right heart border.[48]

Arrhythmias are one of the more common causes of cardiac-related chest pain in children. ED studies by Massin and coworkers[4] and Lin and coworkers[6] reported arrhythmias in approximately 2% of children presenting with chest pain. Tachyarrhythmias are associated with decrease in duration of diastole and may cause chest pain because of a reduction in myocardial blood flow. In one study, 14% of children over the age of 1 year presenting with supraventricular tachycardia reported having chest pain.[49] Structural heart disease may also cause chest pain. Left ventricular outflow obstruction caused by aortic stenosis or hypertrophic cardiomyopathy causes pain that is typically exertional and is caused by subendocardial ischemia. In hypertrophic cardiomyopathy, the physical examination is characterized by a harsh systolic ejection murmur that is heard best at the apex and lower left sternal border. An increase in the intensity of the murmur is seen when the patient assumes an upright posture from a squatting, sitting, or supine position, and with the Valsalva maneuver. A decrease in intensity is heard after going from a standing to a sitting or squatting position, or with passive elevation of the legs. The decrease in intensity occurs when increased ventricular filling increases the size of the outflow tract and decreases the gradient across the obstruction. Mitral valve prolapse has been reported in pediatric patients with chest pain. The role of mitral valve prolapse, however, in causing chest pain is unclear. In adults, the prevalence of chest pain in patients with mitral valve prolapse is similar to that in the general population.[50] It has been hypothesized, however, that severe mitral valve prolapse could cause pain because of papillary muscle dysfunction or ischemia.

Children with severe pulmonary stenosis or pulmonary hypertension are at risk for myocardial ischemia. Pain often occurs with exercise. The murmur of pulmonary stenosis is audible at the upper left sternal border and may radiate to the ipsilateral axilla and back. Pulmonary arterial hypertension is a serious and often fatal condition that may be initially difficult to diagnose and rarely may present with chest pain. It may be idiopathic or secondary to congenital heart disease; pulmonary disease; or systemic disease, such as collagen vascular disease. In a study of 63 pediatric patients with an average age at presentation of 5.8 years, the most common symptoms were exercise-induced dyspnea (98%); dyspnea at rest (25%); chest pain (3%); and syncope (13%).[51]

Aortic aneurysm and dissection have been described both in healthy pediatric patients and in those with known risk factors. Approximately 3.5% of aortic dissections occur in children under 19 years of age,[52] and aortic dissection is responsible for approximately 1 in 3000 pediatric deaths.[53] Risk factors include congenital anomalies, such as coarctation of the aorta and aortic valvular stenosis. Other causes include Marfan syndrome (see **Fig. 2**), Ehler-Danlos syndrome, Turner syndrome (**Fig. 7**), trauma, cocaine use, and weight lifting. A study of patients under 28 years of age with Marfan syndrome found a prevalence of aortic root dilation of 83%. Half of the patients studied began to develop aortic root dilation by 10 years of age.[54] Before the development of preventative medical and surgical therapy, life expectancy for Marfan patients was greatly reduced and aortic dissection and other

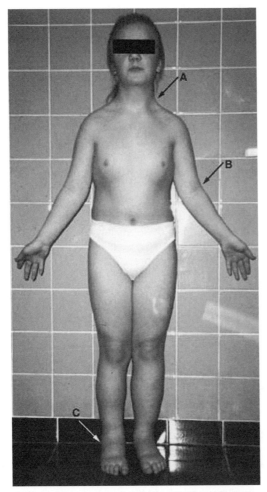

Fig. 7. A patient with Turner syndrome and typical features including webbed neck (*A*), cubitus valgus (*B*), ankle edema (*C*), and short stature and widely spaced nipples. (*From* Gawlik A, Malecka-Tendera E. Hormonal therapy in a patient with delayed diagnosis of Turner's syndrome. Nat Clin Pract Endocrinol Metab 2008;4(3):173–7; with permission.)

cardiovascular complications were responsible for over 90% of deaths.[55] Turner syndrome is another cause of aortic dissection in children. Approximately half of girls with Turner syndrome have underlying cardiac defects, most commonly bicuspid aortic valve and aortic coarctation. A study describing 85 cases of aortic dissection in Turner syndrome reported an average age of 30.7 (range, 4–64) years. Fifteen percent had underlying hypertension, 30% had congenital heart disease, and 34% had both. In 11% of the cases, however, no risk factors were identified.[56] The prevalence of aortic root dilation in Turner syndrome is approximately 6% of patients.[57] Pectus excavatum may be associated with aortic root dilation, even when other stigmata of Marfan syndrome are absent. In one study, patients with isolated pectus excavatum without a suspected connective tissue disorder were evaluated with echocardiograms. The patients with pectus excavatum had a significantly higher prevalence of aortic root dilatation than controls. Several patients underwent genetic testing and were diagnosed with Marfan syndrome despite lacking the usual phenotypic appearance.[13] The pain of aortic dissection is often described as severe and knifelike or tearing. It tends to be located in the anterior or posterior chest, neck, jaw, or shoulder. The chest radiograph is likely to show mediastinal widening, pleural effusion, abnormal aortic contour, or cardiomegaly. Diagnosis can be confirmed by echocardiography.

Psychiatric

In studies based in a pediatric ED, chest pain has been attributed to a psychiatric cause in approximately 5% to 9% of cases.[1,4] One study found adolescents to be 2.5 times as likely to have a psychogenic cause for their chest pain compared with younger children.[5] A history of a stressful event, such as death or hospitalization in the family, family separation, or school changes, has been reported in 31% of adolescents with chest pain.[35] Other reported psychiatric causes include anxiety disorders and depression. A study of 27 children referred to a cardiology clinic for chest pain found that 56% of children who did not have a cardiac etiology were given a *Diagnostic and Statistical Manual-IV* diagnosis of an anxiety disorder, including panic disorder (33%), generalized anxiety disorder (26%), social phobia (19%), and other specific phobia (19%). One child had major depression.[58] A study of 36 children diagnosed with psychogenic chest pain found that 55% had other somatic complaints and 30% had sleep disturbances.[59]

APPROACH TO THE PEDIATRIC PATIENT WITH CHEST PAIN

The primary goals in evaluation of a child with chest pain are to rule out cardiac and other serious causes and to classify the origin of the pain. A thorough history and physical examination are often sufficient to accomplish these goals. In cases in which the cause remains unclear or if concerning features are identified, further evaluation and sometimes referral are warranted.

History

A complete history is perhaps the most important part of the assessment of a child with chest pain. The history should begin with the onset of pain, with the knowledge that acute pain is more likely to be caused by an identifiable organic cause. One study reported that 31% of children stated that the pain had awakened them from sleep; this was shown to be associated with a higher likelihood of an organic cause.[5] The family should be asked about events that may have precipitated the pain, such as exercise, trauma, eating, potential foreign body ingestion, or psychologic stressors. In many cases the child's description of the pain does not help in identifying the etiology, with most children indicating an anterior location to their pain, and 90% of children characterizing their pain as moderate to severe.[1] Descriptions of pain being sharp, constant, or radiating can be nonspecific and have not been found to be significantly associated with cardiorespiratory causes.[5] Most studies of pediatric chest pain are small, however, and include few patients with serious organic causes, so the studies may not be powered to demonstrate such an association. Characteristic pain patterns have been described with certain conditions. Chest wall pain is often localized and sharp, and exacerbated by moving or taking a deep breath. Pleural or pulmonary pain may also be accentuated with inspiration or cough, although pain is less likely to be well-localized than musculoskeletal pain, and less likely to be reproduced with palpation. Pleuritic pain is often sharp and superficial, whereas pulmonary pain, such as that associated with asthma, is more likely to be diffuse and deep. A description of midsternal or precordial pain that worsens after eating or when lying down may be esophageal. The classic description of cardiac pain is that of pressure, crushing, or a squeezing sensation that may radiate to the neck or arm. There is little information on whether this classic description is typical in pediatric cases. Pain that is mitigated by sitting up and leaning forward may be caused by pericarditis. The presence of blood or other irritants in the peritoneal cavity may cause referred chest or shoulder pain (Kehr sign). Psychogenic pain is expected to be vague, poorly localized, varying in location, and possibly associated with other somatic complaints.

Pain associated with palpitations or syncope should be considered a possible indicator of cardiac disease, and pain associated with exertion could be either cardiac or related to a respiratory cause, such as exercise-induced asthma. A history of fever is likely to be reported with pneumonia, but may also be present with myocarditis, pericarditis, or pleural effusion. A history of drooling or reluctance to swallow may be present in a child with an esophageal foreign body. The presence of joint pain or rash may suggest collagen vascular disease. The patient and family should be asked about emotional stressors or presence of anxiety or depression. Adolescents should be asked about use of medications, especially oral contraceptives and pills that have been associated with esophagitis, such as tetracycline. They should also be interviewed privately and asked about use of illicit substances, such as cocaine or marijuana. A complete review of systems is beneficial in identifying relevant information that may not be volunteered by the patient.

In taking the past medical history, certain illnesses should be asked about directly, such as Kawasaki disease, asthma, sickle cell disease, diabetes, or connective tissue disorders, such as Marfan syndrome. The family history should focus on history of unexplained or sudden death, serious underlying conditions, and whether family members have a history of chest pain or heart disease. Although a family history of heart disease may help to identify a child at risk of the same, it has actually been demonstrated that a family history of heart disease or chest pain is associated with a higher likelihood of nonorganic disease.[5]

It should be recognized that the symptom of chest pain is often very worrisome for children and their families. In a study of adolescents seen in a pediatric chest pain, 61% reported that they did not know what was causing their pain, but 56% were afraid of heart disease or a heart attack, and 12% were worried they had cancer.[35] It is important to recognize this fear and address patients' and families' concerns during the assessment. Children who present to EDs with chest pain are likely to have missed school, with estimates ranging from 30% to 41%.[2,5,35] Families should be specifically asked about school absenteeism so that recommendations for returning to school can be given.

Physical Examination

Physical examination abnormalities have been reported in 39% to 49% of pediatric ED patients with chest pain.[2,6] The examination should include a full set of vital signs and an assessment of the general appearance, noting level of alertness, color, and presence of distress or anxiety. Fever may suggest the presence of pneumonia or another infectious or inflammatory condition, and tachycardia or tachypnea suggests the possibility of cardiac, respiratory, or other serious organic etiology. The chest wall should be inspected for signs of trauma, asymmetry, pectus carinatum or excavatum, or costosternal swelling. Tenderness of the chest wall or costochondral and costosternal junctions has been reported in 24% to 54%[2,6] of pediatric ED patients with chest pain and suggests a musculoskeletal etiology.

After chest wall tenderness, abnormal lung auscultation is the second most commonly identified abnormality in the examination of pediatric chest pain patients, occurring in approximately 13% of patient seen in an ED setting.[6] Auscultation of the lungs for crackles, wheezes, and decreased breath sounds may suggest pneumonia, asthma, or pneumothorax. Pneumomediastinum may cause subcutaneous emphysema, which can be detected by crepitus on palpation of the supraclavicular area or neck. The heart should be auscultated to identify the presence of an irregular rhythm, murmur, rub, gallop, or muffled heart sounds. The rub of pericardial effusion is best appreciated when the patient is leaning forward. If a large effusion is present, the patient may have distant heart sounds, jugular venous distention, narrow pulse pressure, and increased pulsus paradoxus. Patients with myocarditis may have tachycardia, gallop rhythm, displaced point of maximal impulse, or a murmur of mitral regurgitation. If coarctation or aortic dissection is suspected, four-limb blood pressures should be obtained.

Palpation of the abdomen may reveal epigastric tenderness in patients with a gastrointestinal cause for their pain. In a study of children referred to a pediatric cardiology clinic in Iran for evaluation of their chest pain, 33% had epigastric tenderness, and of these, 93% had positive findings on endoscopy.[30] If a history of trauma is present, the abdomen should be assessed from tenderness and peritoneal signs. Hepatomegaly may be a sign of heart failure. The skin and extremities should be examined for evidence of trauma, chronic disease, or dysmorphology. Xanthomas on the hands, elbows, knees, and buttocks are characteristic of familial dyslipidemia. Range of motion and resistance testing of the upper extremities may reveal a musculoskeletal source for pain, such as muscle strain or delayed-onset muscle soreness. Special attention should be given to identifying findings associated with Marfan syndrome or other connective tissue disorders, because these conditions carry an increased likelihood of serious pathology.

Investigations

If concern for serious etiology is raised by the history or physical examination, or if pain is severe or disruptive to usual activities, further investigation is warranted (**Table 3**). Although it may be difficult to identify a precise cause for the pain, it is important to exclude life-threatening pathology. A chest radiograph should be obtained if there is unexplained pain of acute onset, respiratory distress, abnormal pulmonary or cardiac auscultation, fever, significant cough, history of drooling or foreign body ingestion, or significant underlying medical conditions. In a study by Rowe and colleagues,[1] chest radiography was obtained in 50% of patients presenting to an ED with chest pain. Of 18 positive results, 15 were infiltrates, and there were two cases of pneumomediastinum and one pneumothorax. Lin and colleagues[6] described 103 children who visited

Table 3
Worrisome signs and symptoms to prompt further work-up in pediatric patients (partial list)

Workup	History/Symptom	Sign
Chest radiograph	Fever	Fever
	Cough	Tachypnea, rales, distress
	Shortness of breath	Ill-appearing
	History of trauma	Evidence of significant trauma
	Pain awakening from sleep	Unexplained tachycardia
	History of drug use (eg, cocaine)	Pathologic heart auscultation
	Association with exercise	Decreased breath sounds
	Acute onset of severe pain	Subcutaneous air/crepitus
	Underlying medical problems (eg, Marfan syndrome, lupus, Kawasaki disease)	Tall, thin habitus, pes excavatum or carinatum
	Foreign body ingestion	Drooling
Electrocardiogram	Shortness of breath	Pathologic heart auscultation
	Association with exercise	Unexplained tachycardia
	Association with syncope	Unexplained respiratory distress
	Palpitations	Diminished perfusion
	History of drug use	Decreased pulses
	Precordial trauma	Evidence of trauma
	Personal or family history of heart disease	Ill-appearing

Adapted from Gokhale J, Selbst SM. Chest pain and chest wall deformity. Pediatr Clin North Am 2009;56:52; with permission.

an ED in Taiwan for chest pain; chest radiographs were obtained in 98%. Abnormalities were found in 28% and were reported as pulmonary infiltrates (13%); hyperinflation (7%); pneumonia (5%); and pneumothorax (3%). A 12-lead ECG should be obtained if there is pain or syncope with exertion, abnormal cardiac auscultation, a clinical suspicion for myocarditis or pericarditis, or serious underlying medical conditions that carry an increased risk of cardiac disease. The ECG should be evaluated with age-appropriate criteria for evidence of arrhythmia, conduction delay, preexitation, hypertrophy, or ischemia. In a study by Selbst and colleagues,[5] 191 children with ill-defined or potentially cardiac-related chest pain received ECGs. Of these, 16% were abnormal. All abnormalities were minor or were previously known, however, except in four patients. Of these, three had arrhythmias identified by physical examination, and one child with systemic lupus erythematosus who was febrile had changes consistent with pericarditis. In a study by Rowe and colleagues,[1] ECG was performed in 18% of patients presenting with chest pain. Of ECGs obtained, six (10%) were positive, with four being previously known or unrelated findings, one patient with ST segment and T-wave changes found to have myocarditis, and one with a history of palpitations found to have Wolff-Parkinson-White syndrome.[1] Lin and colleagues[6] described 103 children who visited an ED in Taiwan for chest pain; ECGs were obtained in 85%. Four (4.6%) showed abnormalities, including first-degree AV block, second-degree AV block, premature ventricular contraction, and Wolff-Parkinson-White syndrome.

Laboratory investigations are rarely necessary in the evaluation of children with chest pain, but may be useful when certain conditions are suspected. A complete blood count may be obtained for suspected infectious causes or in a patient with an underlying condition, such as sickle cell disease. In a patient with suspected cardiac ischemia or myocarditis, cardiac enzymes and aspartate aminotransferase may be useful.[46,47] Troponin is elevated in 54% of pediatric patients with myocarditis[47] and may also be elevated with pericarditis. D-dimer may be obtained if PE is suspected, although there are limited data about D-dimer test performance in pediatrics. One study found that children with PE were as likely as control patients with similar risk factors to have a D-dimer value within the normal range,[60] and in another study D-dimer was normal in 40% of pediatric patients with PE.[61] Other tests that are rarely necessary but may be useful include a drug screen when there is a concern about possible substance abuse, Holter monitor if arrhythmia is suspected, exercise stress test or pulmonary function test for unexplained exertional pain, and endoscopy for possible gastrointestinal sources of pain.

Treatment and Referral

If musculoskeletal pain is identified, analgesics (ibuprofen or acetaminophen) should be offered. Patients with infectious, respiratory, or cardiac sources for their pain need treatment directed at their underlying condition. If esophagitis or gastritis is suspected, a therapeutic trial of an H_2 blocker or proton pump inhibitor can be initiated. Patients with possible exercise-induced asthma may be offered a trial of a β-agonist if more serious respiratory or cardiac disorders are not suspected. For patients with idiopathic or undiagnosed pain, analgesics and close follow-up are appropriate.

Patients being seen in a nonhospital setting should be referred to an ED if experiencing significant distress, if trauma has occurred, or if serious pathology cannot be ruled out. Consultation or referral to a cardiologist may be appropriate if there is exertional pain; history of palpitations, syncope, or presyncope; abnormal cardiac auscultation, chest radiograph, or ECG; concerning family history; or significant recurrent pain of unknown etiology. Referral to a gastroenterologist or pulmonologist may be considered for specific concerns. If significant anxiety, depression, or emotional stress is present, the patient should be referred to a psychiatrist, psychologist, or primary care provider with experience in mental health issues.

SUMMARY

Chest pain is common in children seen in EDs, ambulatory clinics, and cardiology clinics. Although most children have a benign cause for their pain, some have serious and life-threatening conditions. The symptom must be carefully evaluated before reassurance and supportive care are offered. Because serious causes of chest pain are uncommon and not many prospective studies are available, it is difficult to develop evidence-based guidelines for evaluation. The clinician evaluating a child with chest pain should keep in mind the broad differential diagnosis and pursue further investigation when the history and physical examination suggest the possibility of serious causes.

REFERENCES

1. Rowe BH, Dulberg CS, Peterson RG, et al. Characteristics of children presenting with chest pain to a pediatric emergency department. CMAJ 1990;143(5):388–94.
2. Gastesi Larrañaga M, Fernandez Landaluce A, Mintegi Raso S, et al. Chest pain in pediatric emergency departments: a usually benign process. An Pediatr (Barc) 2003;59(3):234–8.
3. Massin MM, Montesanti J, Gerard P, et al. Spectrum and frequency of illness presenting to a pediatric emergency department. Acta Clin Belg 2006;61:161–5.

4. Massin MM, Bourguignont A, Coremans C, et al. Chest pain in pediatric patients presenting to an emergency department or to a cardiac clinic. Clin Pediatr (Phila) 2004;43(3):231–8.
5. Selbst SM, Ruddy RM, Clark BJ, et al. Pediatric chest pain: a prospective study. Pediatrics 1988;82(3):319–23.
6. Lin CH, Lin WC, Ho YJ, et al. Children with chest pain visiting the emergency department. Pediatr Neonatol 2008;49(2):26–9.
7. Cagdas DN, Pac FA. Cardiac chest pain in children. Anadolu Kardiyol Derg 2009; 9:401–6.
8. Driscoll DJ, Glicklich LB, Callen WJ. Chest pain in children: a prospective study. Pediatrics 1976;57(5):648–51.
9. Zavaras-Angelidou KA, Weinhouse E, Nelson DB. Review of 180 episodes of chest pain in 134 children. Pediatr Emerg Care 1992;8(4):189–93.
10. Evangelista JA, Parsons M, Renneburg AK. Chest pain in children: diagnosis through history and physical examination. J Pediatr Health Care 2000;14(1): 3–8.
11. Lam JC, Tobias JD. Follow-up survey of children and adolescents with chest pain. South Med J 2001;94(9):921–4.
12. Yildirim A, Karakurt C, Karademir S, et al. Chest pain in children. Int Pediatr 2004; 19(3):175–9.
13. Rhee D, Solowiejczyk D, Altmann K, et al. Incidence of aortic root dilatation in pectus excavatum and its association with Marfan syndrome. Arch Pediatr Adolesc Med 2008;162(9):882–5.
14. Disla E, Rhim HR, Reddy A, et al. Costochondritis: a prospective analysis in the emergency department setting. Arch Intern Med 1994;154(21):2466–9.
15. Brown RT, Jamil K. Costochondritis in adolescents: a follow-up study. Clin Pediatr 1993;32(8):499–500.
16. Mukamel M, Kornreich L, Horev G, et al. Tietze's syndrome in children and infants. J Pediatr 1997;131:774–5.
17. Saltzman DA, Schmitz ML, Smith SD, et al. The slipping rib syndrome in children. Pediatr Anesth 2001;11:740–3.
18. Miller AJ, Texidor TA. Precordial catch, a neglected syndrome of precordial pain. JAMA 1955;159:1364–5.
19. Gumbiner CH. Precordial catch syndrome. South Med J 2003;96(1):38–41.
20. Weins L, Sabath R, Ewing L. Chest pain in otherwise healthy children and adolescents is frequently caused by exercise-induced asthma. Pediatrics 1992;90: 350–3.
21. Danduran MJ, Earing MG, Sheridan DC, et al. Chest pain: characteristics of children/adolescents. Pediatr Cardiol 2008;29:775–81.
22. Ikeda RM, Kondracki SF, Drabkin PD, et al. Pleurodynia among football players at a high school. JAMA 1993;270:2205–6.
23. Wilcox DT, Glick PL, Karamanoukian HL, et al. Spontaneous pneumothorax: a single-institution, 12-year experience in patients under 16 years of age. J Pediatr Surg 1995;30(10):1452–4.
24. Lee CH, Wu CC, Lin CY. Etiologies of spontaneous pneumomediastinum in children of different ages. Pediatr Neonatol 2009;50(5):190–5.
25. Damore DT, Dayan PS. Medical causes of pneumomediastinum in children. Clin Pediatr 2001;40:87–91.
26. Van Ommen CH, Heijboer H, Buller HR, et al. Venous thromboembolism in childhood: a prospective two-year registry in the Netherlands. J Pediatr 2001;139(5): 676–81.

27. Monagle P, Adams M, Mahoney M, et al. Outcome of pediatric thromboembolic disease: a report from the Canadian childhood thrombophilia registry. Pediatr Res 2000;47(6):763–6.

28. Vavilala MS, Nathens AB, Jurkovich GJ, et al. Risk factors for venous thromboembolism in pediatric trauma. J Trauma 2002;52(5):922–7.

29. Berezin S, Medow MS, Glassman MS, et al. Chest pain of gastrointestinal origin. Arch Dis Child 1988;63:1457–60.

30. Sabri MR, Ghavanini AA, Haghigat M, et al. Chest pain in children and adolescents: epigastric tenderness as a guide to reduce unnecessary work-up. Pediatr Cardiol 2003;24:3–5.

31. Ferreira CT, Vieira MC, Vieira SM, et al. [Eosinophilic esophagitis in 29 pediatric patients]. Arq Gastroenterol 2008;45(2):141–6 [in Portuguese].

32. Nijhawan S, Shimpi L, Mathur A, et al. Management of ingested foreign bodies in upper gastrointestinal tract: report on 170 patients. Indian J Gastroenterol 2003; 22(2):46–8.

33. Biller JA, Flores AF, Buie T, et al. Tetracycline-induced esophagitis in adolescent patients. J Pediatr 1992;120:144–5.

34. Kundra M, Yousaf S, Maqbool, et al. Boerhaave syndrome: unusual cause of chest pain. Pediatr Emerg Care 2007;23(7):489–91.

35. Pantell RH, Goodman BW. Adolescent chest pain: a prospective study. Pediatrics 1983;71:881–7.

36. Mahle WT, Campbell RM, Favaloro-Sabatier J. Myocardial infarction in adolescents. J Pediatr 2007;151:150–4.

37. Lane JR, Ben-Shachar G. Myocardial infarction in healthy adolescents. Pediatrics 2007;120(4):e938–43.

38. Duvernoy CS, Bates ER, Fay WP, et al. Acute myocardial infarction in 2 adolescent males. Clin Cardiol 1998;21:687–90.

39. Aragon J. A rare noncardiac cause for acute myocardial infarction in a 13-year-old patient. Cardiol Rev 2004;12:31–6.

40. Bria S, Chessa M, Abella R. Aborted sudden death in a young football player due to anomalous origin of the left coronary artery: successful surgical correction. J Cardiovasc Med 2008;9:834–8.

41. Amabile N, Fraisse A, Quilici J. Hypoplastic coronary artery disease: report of one case. Heart 2005;91:e12.

42. Newburger JW, Takahashi M, Burns JC, et al. The treatment of Kawasaki syndrome with intravenous gamma globulin. N Engl J Med 1986;315:341–7.

43. Furusho K, Sato K, Soeda T, et al. High-dose intravenous gammaglobulin for Kawasaki disease. Lancet 1983;2(8363):1359.

44. Kato H, Sugimura T, Akagi T. Long-term consequences of Kawasaki disease: a 10- to 21-year follow-up study of 594 patients. Circulation 1996;94:1379–85.

45. Montalambert M, Maunoury C, Acar P. Myocardial ischaemia in children with sickle cell disease. Arch Dis Child 2004;89:359–62.

46. Freedman SB, Haladyn JK, Floh A, et al. Pediatric myocarditis: emergency department clinical findings and diagnostic evaluation. Pediatrics 2007;120:1278–85.

47. Durani Y, Egan M, Baffa J, et al. Pediatric myocarditis: presenting clinical characteristics. Am J Emerg Med 2009;27:942–7.

48. Gatzoulis MA, Munk MD, Merchant N, et al. Isolated congenital absence of the pericardium: clinical presentation, diagnosis, and management. Ann Thorac Surg 2000;69:1209–15.

49. Vos P, Pulles-Heintzberger CF, Delhaas T. Supraventricular tachycardia: an incidental diagnosis in infants and difficult to prove in children. Acta Paediatr 2003;92:1058–61.

50. Freed LA, Levy D, Levine RA, et al. Prevalence and clinical outcome of mitral-valve prolapse. N Engl J Med 1999;341:1.

51. van Loon RL, Roofthooft MT, van Osch-Gevers M, et al. Clinical characterization of pediatric pulmonary hypertension: complex presentation and diagnosis. J Pediatr 2009;155:176–82.

52. Fikar CR, Amrhein JA, Harris P. Dissecting aortic aneurysm in childhood and adolescence. Clin Pediatr 1981;20:78–83.

53. Fikar CR, Koch W. Etiologic factors of acute aortic dissection in children and young adults. Clin Pediatr 2000;39:71–80.

54. Van Karnebeek CD, Naeff MS, Mulder BJ, et al. Natural history of cardiovascular manifestations in Marfan syndrome. Arch Dis Child 2001;84(2):129–37.

55. Murdoch JL, Walker BA, Halpern BL, et al. Life expectancy and causes of death in the Marfan syndrome. N Engl J Med 1972;286:804–8.

56. Carlson M, Silberbach M. Dissection of the aorta in Turner syndrome: two cases and review of 85 cases in the literature. J Med Genet 2007;44:745–9.

57. Lin AE, Lippe B, Rosenfeld RG. Further delineation of aortic dilation, dissection, and rupture in patients with Turner syndrome. Pediatrics 1998;102(1):e12.

58. Lipsitz JD, Masia C, Apfel H, et al. Noncardiac chest pain and psychopathology in children and adolescents. J Psychosom Res 2005;59:185–8.

59. Asnes RS, Santulli R, Bemporad JR. Psychogenic chest pain in children. Clin Pediatr (Phila) 1981;20(12):788–91.

60. Biss TT, Brandão LR, Kahr WH, et al. Clinical probability score and D-dimer estimation lack utility in the diagnosis of childhood pulmonary embolism. J Thromb Haemost 2009;7(10):1633–8.

61. Rajpurkar M, Warrier I, Chitiur M, et al. Pulmonary embolism: experience at a single children's hospital. Thromb Res 2007;119(6):699–703.

An Algorithm for the Diagnosis and Management of Chest Pain in Primary Care

Michael Yelland, MBBS, PhD, FRACGP, FAFMM, Grad Dip Musculoskeletal Medicine[a],*, William E. Cayley Jr, MD, MDiv[b], Werner Vach, Dip Stats, PhD[c]

KEYWORDS

- Chest pain • Algorithm • Diagnosis • Evidence

BACKGROUND AND SIGNIFICANCE

In response to the demands that chest pain assessment has placed on the health system, chest pain assessment protocols and services have been established in several countries to provide more effective and cost-efficient methods of dealing with the assessment and management of chest pain. Many of them are focused on risk stratification for life-threatening causes of chest pain, for example the Rouan decision rule for myocardial infarction (MI)[1] or the Wells score for pulmonary embolism (PE).[2] These protocols are mostly oriented toward use in the emergency department setting. They need some adaptation to make them relevant to the primary care setting, in which the spectrum of causes of chest pain is different to that in the emergency setting.[3] The emergency department protocols generally do not venture into the diagnosis of other causes of chest pain that are not life threatening, commonly referred to as noncardiac chest pain (NCCP).[4]

The diagnosis of NCCP is challenging as it is a condition with many causes; individuals may have more than 1 cause of NCCP or have chest pain from cardiac and noncardiac causes simultaneously. History, examination, and investigations all have limited sensitivity and specificity and a definitive pathology often difficult or impossible to define. The noncardiac causes of chest pain have been classified broadly as

[a] School of Medicine, Logan Campus, Griffith University, University Drive, Meadowbrook, Queensland 4131, Australia
[b] University of Wisconsin Department of Family Medicine, UW Health Eau Claire Family Medicine Residency, 617 West Clairemont, Eau Claire, WI 54701, USA
[c] Institute of Medical Biometry and Medical Informatics, University Medical Center Freiburg, Stefan Meier Straße 26, Freiburg 79104, Germany
* Corresponding author.
E-mail address: m.yelland@griffith.edu.au

Med Clin N Am 94 (2010) 349–374
doi:10.1016/j.mcna.2010.01.011
0025-7125/10/$ – see front matter © 2010 Elsevier Inc. All rights reserved.

gastroenterologic, soft-tissue, musculoskeletal, pulmonary, and psychiatric.[5] The morbidity in this group with NCCP is considerable.[4,5] There has been a debate in the literature about how to deal with these patients once coronary artery disease (CAD) has been excluded. Some propose that providing a definitive diagnosis may be less important than addressing the patients' fears by providing an explanation and reassurance.[6] They call for the development of better, noninvasive algorithms for use by general practitioners to avoid unnecessary referrals to hospital. Others strongly endorse the importance of a definitive diagnosis and argue that the inability to provide a definitive diagnosis may relate to the psychological and psychiatric complications of chest pain.[7] They claim that it is possible to achieve this in up to 85% of cases. If this is indeed possible, there may be opportunities to develop better algorithms for positive diagnosis coupled with good-quality explanation, reassurance, and medical management of chest pain to reduce the physical and psychological morbidity of NCCP and the associated costs to the individual and the health system.

Few algorithms are designed to guide practitioners on all major causes of chest pain, particularly in the outpatient primary care setting. Cayley[8] has devised an algorithm derived from the best available evidence, incorporating the Rouan rule for MI,[1] the Wells score for PE,[2] a 2-question screen for panic disorder,[9] and selective symptoms and signs with the best, albeit limited, diagnostic usefulness. However, it does not fully address diagnosis of gastroenterologic, musculoskeletal, soft-tissue, and psychological causes of chest pain. This article updates and expands this algorithm to provide the primary care practitioner with a flexible, efficient, and evidence-based approach to the primary care patient with chest pain. The algorithm covers the common causes and the rare but life-threatening causes and is based on several principles that translate evidence into practice and that also recognize the realities of working in primary care.

PRINCIPLES UNDERPINNING THE CHEST PAIN ALGORITHM

Given the large number of potential causes of chest pain in primary care and multiple clinical features and investigations used for the diagnosis or exclusion of each cause, the authors have devised an algorithm that guides the diagnostic processes for chest pain in primary care. This algorithm combines problem-solving and decision-making approaches.[10] In the problem-solving approach, clinical features lead to a limited number of hypotheses based on pattern recognition, spot diagnosis, and clinical experience. These hypotheses inform subsequent information gathering. In the decision-making process, the diagnosis is refined using probabilistic reasoning.[11] Probabilistic reasoning is based on knowledge of the pretest probability or prevalence of a condition and how this translates to the posttest probability based on knowledge of the diagnostic accuracy of the clinical feature or test. This principle is often not applied explicitly by exact computation of posttest probabilities, but in a more informal, implicit manner following 2 basic rules in deciding between 2 possible causes with a positive diagnostic test result:

1. If the 2 possible causes have equal prevalence, but the diagnostic tests differ in their accuracy, prioritize the cause with the better test.
2. If the 2 diagnostic tests have equal accuracy, prioritize the cause with the higher prevalence.

The algorithm presented in **Fig. 1** describes a logical order to diagnosis that is safe, efficient, and comprehensive. A key consideration for safety in diagnosis is to start by assessing conditions that have the potential to threaten life. Similar to the assessment

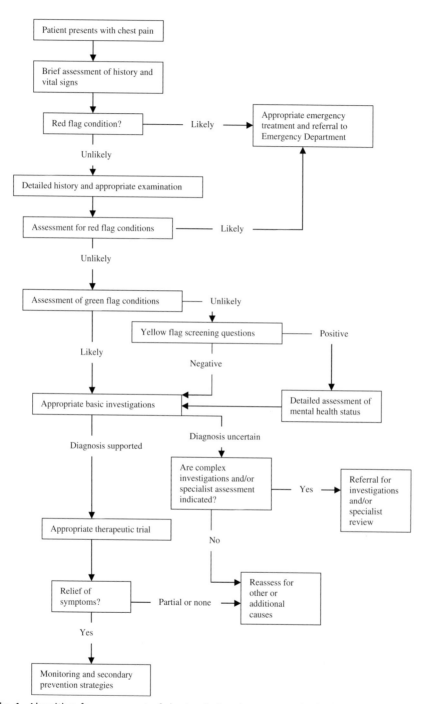

Fig. 1. Algorithm for assessment of chest pain in primary care. The key elements for use in the algorithm are summarized in **Tables 6, 7** and **8**. The algorithm proposed here, although based on available evidence, does not constitute a validated decision rule.

of low back pain, indicators of life-threatening physical causes are labeled as red flags, indicators of non–life-threatening physical causes as green flags, and psychosocial indicators as yellow flags.[12] The assessment of red flags takes priority over green and yellow flags. The assessment of green flags comes next, and it is the step in which the principle of probabilistic reasoning is most prominent. As all potential green flag conditions are of equal medical importance (in the sense of their need to be treated), and as the diagnostic elements of the green flags can be easily performed, it is reasonable to consider these potential causes simultaneously and to select the most likely causes for further consideration. Although assessment of yellow flags may occur throughout the consultation, decisions about their contribution to the sensation of chest pain are left until after the green flags have been adequately assessed, with the intention of increasing the diagnostic confidence about psychogenic causes or factors.

The key diagnostic elements used in the processes of the algorithm are described and tabulated later in this article. Here, the term "element" includes various symptoms, signs, and investigations or diagnostic rules or scores based on pieces of diagnostic information. A diagnostic element may also include a pragmatic trial of treatment, in which the response may support or refute a provisional diagnosis.

In choosing the elements for use in the algorithm, several properties of the elements in the primary care setting have been considered. These elements include their diagnostic performance, risks, benefits, cost, and usefulness.

Diagnostic Performance

Single history, examination, and investigation elements

The diagnostic performance of single elements with positive or negative results is variously described by the properties of sensitivity and specificity, positive and negative likelihood ratios (LRs), positive and negative predictive values, and odds ratios. Definitions of these terms can be viewed at http://www.cebm.utoronto.ca/glossary/index.htm#s. Positive predictive value expresses the probability that the disease is present when the test is positive. A high positive predictive value is desirable in the early phase of the algorithm to make quick and accurate decisions about treatment; however, a lower positive predictive value is acceptable later in the algorithm when making decisions about therapeutic trials for low-risk conditions. The negative predictive value expresses the probability that the disease is absent when the test is negative. This factor is most important for ruling out red flag causes confidently early in the algorithm but also later to rule out additional diagnoses.

Clinical prediction rules

Clinical prediction rules (CPRs), also called diagnostic rules or diagnostic scores, aim to quantify the contribution of history, physical examination and diagnostic tests and stratify patients into levels of probability of having a condition.[13] A validated CPR offers more diagnostic confidence than an unvalidated rule.

Accessibility

The following considerations affect the accessibility of elements to primary care physicians.

Cost

Lower cost elements, such as clinical assessment and simple surgery tests, are preferred but when an expensive investigation has a high diagnostic accuracy that leads to definitive diagnosis, this may be incorporated.

Time

Because of the time constraints in primary care, elements that are simpler and more rapidly administered are favored. With respect to tests or treatments, elements with a more rapid response time are more useful diagnostically.

Resources

Equipment, if needed for the element, should be available in primary care. If it is not widely available, such as bedside troponin testing, an alternative, such as laboratory testing, should be considered.

Level of training required

The element should be able to be performed in primary care. If the level of training is higher than that generally present in the primary care setting, the element should be included only as an option with an alternative.

Risks Versus Benefits

Risks

The risk of adverse events is balanced against the potential benefits of diagnostic and treatment elements of the algorithm. Higher risks are more acceptable for red flag causes than for green or yellow flag causes. The risk of missing a red flag cause by not including an element is also a consideration.

Benefits

Benefits include reassurance as well as relief of symptoms and reduction of risk of future events. With therapeutic trials, the size of the treatment effect and the predictive value of a response to treatment, if available, will influence their inclusion in the algorithm.

Diagnostic Confidence

In the process of applying the algorithm, there will be branching points with decisions about the use of an expensive or high-risk test or therapeutic trial that will be affected by the diagnostic confidence at that point. For example, patients who are categorized as at high risk of acute coronary syndrome (ACS) will have a strong indication for referral for coronary angiography.

Quality of Evidence

This article uses the strength of recommendation taxonomy (SORT) for clinical review articles based on the quality and consistency of available evidence (http://www.aafp.org/online/en/home/publications/journals/afp/afpsort.html).[14]

- A = consistent, good-quality patient-oriented evidence
- B = inconsistent or limited-quality patient-oriented evidence
- C = consensus, disease-oriented evidence, usual practice, expert opinion, or case series for studies of diagnosis, treatment, prevention, or screening.

In the interests of efficiency, we have limited the choice of elements to those with the best evidence or at least some evidence supporting them. Despite this the level of evidence for many elements, particularly those related to NCCP, is still only at level C.

The Epidemiology of Chest Pain in Primary Care

Patients with chest pain place a considerable burden on the health systems of many countries. The proportion of general practice consultations for chest pain varies from at least 1% in the United Kingdom[15] to 1.5% in Sweden[16] and 2.7% in Switzerland.[17]

In the British general practice setting the rate of new diagnoses of chest pain has been estimated at 15.5 per 1000 person-years.[18]

The diagnostic probabilities across the spectrum of causes depend on the setting. The prevalences of diagnostic categories for chest pain in primary care have been defined for at least 3 countries, based on studies of often unvalidated medical diagnoses from medical records and patient questionnaires (**Table 1**). In Belgium they have been compared with the spectrum of chest pain diagnoses in a hospital emergency department setting, highlighting some major differences. Cardiac diagnoses accounted for 54% in hospital compared with 13% in primary care.[3] Of the noncardiac causes, musculoskeletal chest pain comprised 6% of hospital diagnoses compared with 21% in primary care. Pulmonary diagnoses accounted for 12% in hospital compared with 20% in primary care but only 20% of the latter were serious diagnoses (ie, pneumonia, pleuritis, pneumothorax, and lung cancer) and the remainder were for tracheitis or bronchitis. Over the 3 countries, musculoskeletal diagnoses comprised 21% to 51% of totals, making them the most common amongst the noncardiac categories.[3,17,19] The prevalence of gastroenterologic diagnoses was 8% to 19% and of psychogenic diagnoses was 8% to 17%.

The key diagnostic elements for specific causes of chest pain are outlined in the following section. In the spirit of probabilistic reasoning we have addressed them in order of decreasing prevalence within each diagnostic category. However, as we were unable to find comparative data on the prevalence of many of these specific causes, the estimates of prevalence for some causes are based on our clinical experience.

DIAGNOSTIC ELEMENTS FOR COMMON CAUSES OF CHEST PAIN IN PRIMARY CARE
Cardiovascular Causes

ACS
Three key clinical features of chest pain can help predict the risk of CAD: (1) location (is it substernal chest pain?), (2) aggravating factors (is it exertional?), and (3) alleviating factors (is it relieved by rest or nitroglycerin?). Chest pain with all 3 characteristics is considered angina chest pain, and is high risk for CAD in all age groups. If only 2 of

Table 1
The prevalence of diagnostic categories for chest pain in patients with chest pain in the primary care setting versus the emergency department setting

Diagnosis	Primary Care (USA)[18] (%)	Primary Care (Switzerland)[16] (%)	Primary Care (Belgium)[3] (%)	Emergency Department (Belgium)[3] (%)
Cardiovascular[a]	16	16	13	54
Musculoskeletal	36	51	21	6
Pulmonary	5	10	20	12
Gastroenterologic	19	8	10	3
Psychogenic	8	11	17	9
Total noncardiac	68	80	68	30
Other			10	10
Uncertain/not specified	16	4	1	5

[a] Including pulmonary embolism.

the 3 characteristics are present, chest pain is considered atypical angina, which carries intermediate risk for CAD in women older than 50 years and in all men. Nonanginal chest pain, with only 1 of the 3 characteristics present, carries intermediate risk for CAD in women older than 60 years and men older than 40 years.[20]

Patients whose chest pain puts them at moderate to high risk of CAD deserve prompt assessment for the risk of ACS. ACS includes acute myocardial infarction (AMI) and unstable angina. However, studies in emergency department settings show that only a few features of angina chest pain have adequate usefulness to meaningfully increase or decrease the diagnostic likelihood of AMI. Exertional chest pain (LR 2.35) and pain radiating to the shoulder or both arms (LR 4.07) increase the likelihood of AMI. Similarly, exertional chest pain (LR 2.06), and pain radiating to the shoulder, the left arm, or both arms (LR 1.62) are the features most predictive of any ACS.[21] Symptoms that are not predictive for either ACS or AMI include the site or nature of the pain and the presence of nausea, vomiting, or diaphoresis.[22] The only physical finding that is helpful in diagnosis of ACS or MI is chest wall tenderness. Presence of chest wall tenderness (LR 0.3) or reproduction of chest pain with palpation (LR 0.23) both significantly decrease the likelihood that chest pain is caused by ACS or AMI.[22,23]

The most important initial test for the patient at risk of ACS or AMI is an electrocardiogram (ECG). Electrocardiographic findings that most strongly suggest ACS or AMI are new ST segment increase (LR 16), new Q waves (LR range, 8.7), and a new conduction defect (LR 6.3). Although a normal ECG result markedly decreases the likelihood of an MI (LR range, 0.1–0.3), no ECG abnormality is sensitive enough for AMI or ACS that its absence completely excludes the diagnosis.[24]

The Rouan decision rule can help predict which patients with chest pain and a normal or nonspecific ECG are at higher risk for MI (**Table 2**).[1] However, emergency department data indicate that up to 3% of patients initially diagnosed with a noncardiac cause of chest pain suffer death or MI within 30 days of presentation; thus patients with cardiac risk factors such as male sex, greater age, diabetes, hyperlipidemia, previous CAD, or heart failure warrant close follow-up.[25]

The most common markers of myocardial damage are creatine kinase (CK), its MB subform (CKMB), troponin T (TnT), and troponin I (TnI). A CKMB level greater than 6.0 ng/mL within 9 hours of presentation for emergency care modestly increases the likelihood of MI or death in the next 30 days.[26]

Increased levels of either troponin (TnT > 2 ng/mL or TnI > 1 ng/mL) support the diagnosis of MI or ACS and increase the likelihood of death or recurrent MI within 30 days. Increase of troponin takes 4 to 6 hours and may remain increased for 5 to 14 days.[27]

Table 2
Rouan decision rule: clinical characteristics and risk of MI

Clinical Characteristics	No. of Factors Present	Risk of MI (%)
Age > 60 years	0	Up to 0.6
Male gender	1	Up to 3.4
Pain described as pressure	2	Up to 4.8
Pain radiates to arm, shoulder, neck or jaw	3	Up to 12
Diaphoresis	4	Up to 26
History of previous MI or angina		

Data from Rouan GW, Lee TH, Cook EF, et al. Clinical characteristics and outcome of acute myocardial infarction in patients with initially normal or nonspecific electrocardiograms (a report from the Multicenter Chest Pain Study). Am J Cardiol 1989;64:1087–92.

A survey of New Zealand general practitioners found that the majority ordered troponins at least once monthly and would be more likely to use this test if the likelihood of AMI was less than 5%, or the pain was more than 12 hours ago.[28] One study of 773 patients presenting to an emergency department with chest pain and an essentially normal ECG found that for detection of AMI, the sensitivity of TnT was 94% and of TnI was 100%. The specificity of the 2 assays was 99.7% and 98.9%, respectively (ie, only 0.3% with a normal TnI and 1.1% with a normal TnT at 6 hours died or had acute MI in the next 30 days).[29]

In the detection of MI in the emergency department without ST segment increase on presentation, a normal level of TnT and of TnI between 6 and 72 hours after the onset of chest pain is strong evidence against MI or ACS, particularly if the ECG is normal or near normal.[30,31] Thus, individuals with chest pain and a low-risk history, a normal or near-normal ECG, and normal troponins can safely be evaluated as outpatients.

Potential hazards of using troponin in the primary care setting include possible delays in appropriate referral of patients with ACS to an emergency department setting,[28] and a false-negative result if the test is performed too early.[27]

Several studies in the emergency department setting have found that the response of chest pain to administration of nitroglycerin does not reliably predict the presence or absence of cardiac chest pain, CAD, or myocardial ischemia.[32–35]

PE

No individual signs or symptoms can reliably diagnose PE, but a validated clinical prediction rule can help determine which patients have low, moderate, or high likelihood of PE, which then guides further evaluation. The Wells clinical prediction rule (**Table 3**) has been subjected to more than 10 years of testing and development, and validated in numerous settings.[36–39] Other clinical prediction rules have been developed and validated, but to date the Wells rule is the most widely tested.

Table 3
Simplified Wells scoring system for PE

Clinical Finding	Score
Symptoms of DVT (objectively measured leg swelling or pain with palpation of leg veins)	3.0
No alternate diagnosis more likely than PE	3.0
Heart rate >100 beats per minute	1.5
Immobilization (bed rest, except for access to bathroom, for 3 or more consecutive days) or surgery in past 4 weeks	1.5
Previous objectively diagnosed DVT or PE	1.5
Hemoptysis	1.0
Malignancy (patients receiving treatment of cancer, those with cancer and cessation of treatment in past 6 months, those with cancer receiving palliative care)	1.0

Interpretation		
<2 points = low probability of PE	(1%–28%)	(LR 0.13)
2–6 points = moderate probability of PE	(28%–40%)	(LR 1.82)
>6 = high probability of PE	(38%–91%)	(LR 6.75)

Data from Wells PS, Anderson DR, Rodger M, et al. Derivation of a simple clinical model to categorize patients probability of pulmonary embolism: increasing the models utility with the SimpliRED D-dimer. Thromb Haemost 2000;83:416–20.

D-dimer testing has also become an important part of the evaluation for PE and deep vein thrombosis (DVT), but not all assays are the same; quantitative enzyme-linked immunosorbent assay (ELISA) D-dimer assays are more sensitive, and have been more thoroughly tested in clinical settings, than whole-blood agglutination assays.[40] A low clinical suspicion for PE (eg, a Wells score <2) plus a normal quantitative ELISA D-dimer assay safely rules out PE with a negative predictive value greater than 99.5%. Helical computed tomography (CT) can be combined with clinical suspicion and other testing such as lower extremity ultrasound to rule in or rule out PE if further testing is needed.[36,40–43]

Several different sequential testing protocols have been proposed that all involve essentially the same elements:

1. For patients with low clinical suspicion for PE (Wells score <2) and a normal D-dimer, no further evaluation or treatment;
2. For patients with moderate or high clinical suspicion for PE (Wells score 2 or greater), and abnormal CT or venous ultrasound, treat for PE or DVT regardless of D-dimer
3. For patients with an abnormal D-dimer, plus a normal CT and venous ultrasound, consider serial ultrasound if clinical suspicion is low to moderate and pulmonary angiography if clinical suspicion is high.

Patients who are initially diagnosed as free of PE by such an approach, and are not treated, have a less than 1% chance of PE in the subsequent 3 months.[42,44,45]

Heart failure

Heart failure by itself is unlikely to cause chest pain, but it may accompany ACS, valvular disease, MI, or other critical cardiac conditions. A displaced apical impulse and a previous history of MI support this diagnosis. Because virtually all patients with heart failure have exertional dyspnea, its absence is helpful at ruling out this diagnosis.[46] An abnormal ECG and cardiomegaly on chest radiograph can increase the likelihood of heart failure among patients with chest pain, and increased b-type natriuretic peptide (BNP) levels have been found reliable for detecting heart failure in patients presenting with acute dyspnea.[47–49] For any patient suspected of having heart failure based on clinical examination or laboratory testing, echocardiography is crucial to making the final diagnosis.[50,51]

Aortic dissection

Dissection of the thoracic aorta is a rare, red flag condition that occurs at a rate of only 6 to 10/100,000 patient years.[52] Left untreated, it has a mortality of 50% at 48 hours. The acute/sudden severe onset of pain is the cardinal feature of aortic dissection, with a sensitivity of 84%. The description of the pain as ripping or tearing has an LR for aortic dissection from 1.2 to 10.8.[52] Hypertension is the most common predisposing factor, being present in 78% of patients.[53]

Pulmonary Causes of Chest Pain

Acute bronchitis and pneumonia

It is important to differentiate bronchitis from pneumonia, as the latter is a more severe infection that may require more aggressive treatment, including hospitalization.[54] Chest radiograph is considered the reference standard test for patients suspected to have pneumonia, and is the standard against which clinical evaluations for pneumonia are compared.[55] When deciding whether to proceed to chest radiograph, the presence of fever or focal chest signs such as increased vocal resonance or dullness to percussion are the most useful clinical tools in differentiating these 2 conditions.[55] In 1 sample of patients with acute cough and a 5% to 10% prevalence of pneumonia, in whom focal auscultatory signs were present, the chance of pneumonia increased to 39%, and reduced to only 2% when the signs were absent.[56] The absence of focal chest findings does not completely rule out pneumonia in the patient with chest pain and cough.[55] A large study in 1984 developed a decision rule (**Table 4**) using 7 clinical findings to predict the likelihood of pneumonia.[57]

A Cochrane review has shown modest benefits for treating acute bronchitis with antibiotics, including reduction in cough, days feeling unwell, and days of limited activity.[58] There is a stronger indication for treating those subgroups at high risk of complications including those aged more than 75 years, and those with insulin-dependent diabetes, preexisting chronic obstructive pulmonary disease, cardiac failure, and serious neurologic disorders.[58]

Lung cancer

Chest pain is a presenting symptom in 53% of patients with lung cancer.[59] Respiratory symptoms with a higher frequency at presentation include dyspnea (86%), cough (81%), hoarseness (54%), and hemoptysis (26%). None of these symptoms are diagnostic of lung cancer, but other common symptoms, such as tiredness (86%) and lack of appetite (76%), are too general to indicate lung cancer, let alone a respiratory cause of any kind.

Smoking is the major risk factor for lung cancer, with hazard ratios (compared with those who have never smoked) ranging from 2 for former smokers to 55 for heavy smokers.[60] One review has summarized that the relative risk of developing lung cancer in ever-smokers is 24.2 for men and 12.5 for women.[61]

Sputum cytology, a test that can readily be arranged in primary care, has a specificity of 99% and a sensitivity of 66% in the detection of lung cancer.[62] Further investigation requires referral for bronchoscopy, cytobrushing, transbronchial biopsy, or transthoracic needle aspirate.

Pneumothorax

Pneumothorax is a rare, red flag cause of chest pain, with an incidence of 14 per 100,000 person-years in men and 3 per 100,000 years in women.[63,64] Spontaneous

Table 4
Diehr diagnostic rule for pneumonia in adults with acute cough

Finding	Points	Score	LR (+)	LR (−)	Probability of Pneumonia (%)
Rhinorrhea	−2				
Sore throat	−1				
Night sweats	1	−3	1.1	0	5
Myalgia	1	−1	2.5	0.37	12
Sputum all day	1	0	4.9	0.47	21
Respiratory rate >25 breaths per minute	2	1	8.3	0.70	30
Temperature >100°F	2	3	11	0.90	37

The LR (+) and LR (−) columns are grouped under the header "Interpretation" → "LR". The Probability of Pneumonia (%) column is separate.

Data from Diehr P, Wood RW, Bushyhead J, et al. Prediction of pneumonia in outpatients with acute cough—a statistical approach. J Chronic Dis 1984;37:215–25.

pneumothorax may be primary (usually in the 20- to 40-year age-group) or secondary to underlying pulmonary disease (usually in the 60 years and older age-group). Other causes of pneumothorax are chest trauma and medical procedures. Acute, pleuritic chest pain and dyspnoea occur together in 64% to 85% of patients.[64] Signs of tachycardia are most common followed by tachypnea and hypoxia. Diagnosis is by chest radiograph, ultrasound, or CT scan.

Musculoskeletal Chest Wall Pain

Most musculoskeletal chest wall pain is labeled by an umbrella term chest wall syndrome, which encompasses a range of diagnostic labels including anterior chest wall syndrome, atypical chest pain, musculoskeletal chest pain syndrome, cervico-thoracic angina (CTA), and costochondritis.[17] All of these diagnoses are clinically based and lack a true reference standard for diagnosis, such as a radiological or pathologic test. The cause of chest wall syndrome is poorly understood. Musculoskeletal chest pain caused by trauma is discussed separately to the chest wall syndrome, as is that associated with the generalized pain syndrome labeled fibromyalgia.

Chest wall syndrome

In a Swiss primary care cohort study of 672 patients with chest pain,[17] using a standardized history and examination protocol, 45% were diagnosed with conditions that fell within the broad category of chest wall syndrome. The clinical characteristics that best discriminated this syndrome from other causes of chest pain were chest wall pain reproducible by palpation, chest pain that was neither squeezing nor oppressive, pain localized to left chest wall, nonexercise-induced chest pain, pain influenced by mechanical factors or simply well localized on the chest wall (**Table 5**). Diagnoses were not validated by other clinicians or investigations.

In an Australian study of musculoskeletal signs comparing patients from primary care with pain in the chest or abdomen with pain-free controls, the prevalence of pain with cervical and thoracic spinal movements was 60% to 70% versus 20% to 35% and thoracic spinal tenderness was 65% versus 25%.[65]

Further useful information on clinical features of musculoskeletal pain comes from hospital studies of patients with chest pain undergoing coronary angiography. In an early study of patients with chest pain and negative coronary angiography, chest wall tenderness was found in 69% of patients compared with none of a control group without chest pain.[66] However, there was a correlation between the sites of tenderness and pain in only 23% of the case group. Christensen and colleagues[67] have

Table 5	
The 6 most discriminative clinical characteristics of chest wall syndrome versus the other conditions causing chest pain	
Clinical Characteristic	**Odds Ratio (95% CI)**
Pain is	
• Not squeezing or oppressive	2.53 (1.21–5.28)
• Localized on the left or median-left part of the chest wall	2.28 (1.58–3.28)
• Well localized on the chest wall	2.10 (1.37–3.22)
• Nonexercise-induced chest pain	1.58 (1.00–2.49)
• Influenced by movement or posture	1.54 (1.06–2.24)
• Reproducible by palpation	5.72 (1.20–5.28)

Data from Verdon F, Burnand B, Herzig L, et al. Chest wall syndrome among primary care patients: a cohort study. BMC Fam Pract 2007;851.

made a diagnosis of musculoskeletal chest pain labeled as CTA in 18% of a cohort of patients with known or suspected stable angina referred to a hospital for coronary angiography. This diagnosis was based on a detailed history and spinal/chest wall palpation findings and produced a group in which 80% had negative myocardial perfusion scintigraphy compared with 50% in the remaining non-CTA group. They found that combining several clinical features may be more accurate in making a musculoskeletal diagnosis than using 1 feature alone. The diagnosis of CTA is most closely associated with:

- The grading of angina by a physician as noncardiac or atypical angina (Canadian Cardiovascular Society [CCS] guidelines)
- The presence of neck pain
- Reduced motion palpation of the T3 to T5 vertebrae
- The presence of spinal tenderness.

Indirect support for the diagnosis of musculoskeletal chest pain in the CTA group came from improvements in pain and general health with a trial of manual therapy compared with no change in these parameters in those without CTA treated by other means.[68] The same research team is about to publish a similar analysis of a cohort of patients with acute chest pain but with a more rigorous assessment of manual therapy using randomized clinical trial design.[69]

Costochondritis

Costochondritis, also called costosternal syndrome, is a condition characterized by pain and tenderness at the costochondral or chondrosternal articulations without a notable swelling as in the less common condition of Tietze syndrome.[70] Usually multiple levels are affected and they lack swelling or induration. Pain is reproduced by palpation of the affected cartilage segments and may radiate on the chest wall.

Corticosteroid injections have been used as a treatment of costochondritis with sulfasalazine added for recurrent cases. This approach has been shown in a retrospective case series to reduce investigation and hospitalizations for chest pain.[71] Otherwise there is little research in this area. Trial of analgesics or antiinflammatory medication, rest, and reassurance has been recommended, but there are no data about their efficacy.[72]

Trauma

Chest pain may arise from ribs and muscles that have suffered direct or indirect trauma.[70] This trauma is usually clear from the history. Less obvious may be rib fractures resulting from repetitive strain of coughing and also as stress fractures in sports such as golf, rowing, pitching, and bodybuilding.[71] Clinical features include pain on inspiration and chest or upper limb movements and localized tenderness at the site of the strain or fracture. Not all fractures may be detected by plain radiographs, so if a clinical suspicion of fracture remains, bone scintigraphy, CT scanning,[73] or ultrasonography[74] may be necessary.

Fibromyalgia

Fibromyalgia is a syndrome characterized by widespread chronic muscle pain and tenderness in multiple discrete points.[70] The pain must be present on both sides of the body and above and below the waist, including part of the spine or anterior chest.[75] Fatigue, insomnia, and joint pains further help to characterize fibromyalgia, as they are present in more than 70% of patients. Common muscle tender points in the chest are in the pectorals, the rotator cuff, rhomboids, and trapezius. There are no serologic or histologic markers of inflammation or other pathology in this condition. Coexisting anxiety and depression may add to the pain and suffering. The key to screening for fibromyalgia as the cause of chest pain is to check if pain is present outside the chest and then assess if its distribution and an examination of the designated points for tenderness fit the pattern for fibromyalgia. Other rheumatologic causes of widespread pain should be excluded before diagnosing fibromyalgia.

Gastroenterologic Causes of Chest Pain

In assessing possible gastroenterologic causes of chest pain, attention should first be paid to several important symptoms that may herald serious conditions: the so-called alarm symptoms. These symptoms include repeated vomiting, decreased appetite, weight loss, dysphagia, odynophagia (pain on swallowing), hematemesis, anemia, and melena (**Box 1**).[76]

Differentiating cardiac pain from esophageal pain is difficult, but features that are more indicative of esophageal pain in the emergency department setting are an atypical response to exercise, pain that continued as a background ache, retrosternal pain without lateral radiation, pain that disturbed sleep, and the presence of certain esophageal symptoms.[77] These esophageal symptoms include dysphagia and odynophagia, heartburn, and regurgitation, Of these symptoms, the only 3 significantly more common in patients with NCCP with gastroesophageal reflux disease (GERD) versus those without GERD are heartburn (57% vs 21%) and regurgitation (49% vs 16%) and pain relieved by antacid (43% vs 16%).[77] These translate to sensitivities of 40% to 49% and specificities of 81% to 84%.

Although upper gastrointestinal (GI) endoscopy or 24-hour esophageal pH monitoring have been used as reference standards for the diagnosis of GERD,[78,79] neither shows a perfect correlation with symptoms. The cheaper and more accessible alternative in primary care is an empiric trial of high-dose acid suppression using a proton pump inhibitor (PPI). The range for the sensitivity of this test is 65% to 90% and for the specificity, 75% to 88%, using upper GI endoscopy or 24-hour esophageal pH monitoring as a reference standard.[78,80] Treatment success at 12 months is also higher than for endoscopy or monitoring (84% vs 74%).[81] Several schedules of therapeutic trials of PPIs ranging from 1 day to 4 weeks have been tested but the one with the best balance between accuracy and usefulness is a 7-day trial of lansoprazole (60 mg in the morning and 30 mg in the evening).[76] At the threshold of 50% reduction in symptoms, this test has a sensitivity of 78% and specificity of 82% in

---

Box 1
Alarm symptoms requiring endoscopic investigation for gastroenterologic conditions in patients with NCCP

Repeated vomiting

Decreased appetite

Weight loss

Dysphagia

Odynophagia (pain on swallowing)

Hematemesis

Anemia

Melena

Data from Faybush EM, Fass R. Diagnosis of noncardiac chest pain: In: Fass R, Eslick GD, editors. Noncardiac chest pain: a growing medical problem. San Diego: Plural Publishing; 2007.

the diagnosis of GERD and is able to diagnose most of the responders within the first 48 hours. Others recommend a longer PPI trial period of 1 to 2 months before investigating for other causes of chest pain (see the article by Oranu and Vaezi elsewhere in this issue for further explanation of this topic).

Failing a clear response to the PPI test, if the primary care practitioner still suspects an esophageal cause for the pain, referral is needed to a gastroenterologist for investigation of esophageal motility with esophageal manometry or visceral hyperalgesia with an intraesophageal balloon distension test.[76] Alternatively, the practitioner should revisit the history and examination to check for causes other than gastroesophageal disorders.

Skin and Soft-Tissue Causes

In assessment of skin and soft tissue as a cause of chest pain, the detection of a tender skin lesion at the site of pain may uncover an obvious cause of the pain. Skin lesions such as glomus tumors, eccrine spiradenomas, leiomyomas, angiolipomas, and traumatic neuromas are unlikely to cause diagnostic uncertainty (see the article by Muir and Yelland elsewhere in this issue for further explanation of this topic). Painful breast lesions including cancer and fibrocystic disease are somewhat more difficult to detect and require deeper palpation and special tests for diagnosis.[82,83] The main difficulty is in the exclusion of herpes zoster as a cause in the prodromal period of about 4 days before the emergence of skin lesions in a dermatomal distribution. The commonest symptoms in this period are dermatomal pain (41%), itching (27%), and paresthesia (12%).[84] Antiviral therapies given before the emergence of the rash may reduce pain during treatment and for a month after this, but have no effect on pain at 3 months and beyond.[85]

Psychogenic Chest Pain

The proportion with a primary diagnosis of psychogenic chest pain is difficult to estimate with any accuracy. The precise contribution of the psychiatric disorder to the chest pain is difficult to define. In an article elsewhere in this issue on psychological causes of chest pain, White avoids labeling certain types of chest pain as purely psychogenic; rather she discusses the increased likelihood of psychiatric problems in patients with NCCP, showing nearly twice the prevalence of psychiatric impairment compared with in patients with CAD[86] and 2 to 3 times the prevalence of anxiety compared with patients with cardiac disease and with the general population. The situation is made more complex by the association between stress and myocardial ischemia. In patients without documented CAD, mental stress can induce myocardial ischemia in 16% to 21%.[87] Furthermore, in patients with documented CAD, mental stress-induced transient myocardial ischemia has been found in 34% to 74%.[87] Therefore it is prudent to view psychological disorders as contributors to the sensation of chest pain rather than the cause per se. It is also prudent to remember that psychological and physical conditions commonly coexist.

An assessment of the contribution of psychological factors to chest pain commences with a thorough assessment of the physical causes of chest pain outlined in this article followed by an assessment for panic, anxiety, and depression. Panic disorder has a reported prevalence of 8% in primary care patients with NCCP.[88]

Given the time constraints of primary care, the use of 2 questions as a brief diagnostic screen for panic disorder in primary care[9] has been suggested to screen for underlying panic disorder. These are:

- "In the past 6 months, have you ever had a spell or an attack when all of a sudden you felt frightened, anxious, or very uneasy?"

- "In the past 6 months, have you ever had a spell or an attack when for no reason your heart suddenly began to race, you felt faint, or you couldn't catch your breath?"

A positive response to either item is a positive screen. In a primary care setting, this brief questionnaire has good sensitivity (94%–100%) and negative predictive value (94%–100%) so it is useful for excluding panic disorder. However, its low specificity (25%–59%) and positive predictive value (range 18%–40%) mean that a positive result requires more thorough assessment.

Similarly, there is a rapid screen for depression using the following 2 questions[89]:

- "During the past month have you often been bothered by feeling down, depressed, or hopeless?"
- "During the past month have you often been bothered by little interest or pleasure in doing things?"

As with the screen for panic disorder, a positive response to 1 or both questions is regarded as positive screen. In the primary care setting this screen has a sensitivity of 97% (95% confidence interval [CI], 83%–99%) and a specificity of 67% (95% CI, 62%–72%). The associated positive LR of 2.9 (2.5–3.4) and negative LR of 0.05 (0.01–0.35)[89] make it a useful screening tool for depression.

A therapeutic trial of treatment of anxiety or depression is not only desirable to reduce the episodes of chest pain, but may act as a diagnostic tool. Several psychological interventions for NCCP are discussed elsewhere in this issue in the article by White on psychological causes of chest pain. These include cognitive behavioral therapy (CBT), hypnotherapy, relaxation training, and biofeedback. Of these, the best evidence for effectiveness in the short- and long-term is for CBT.[90]

Other evidence from therapeutic trials for psychological disorders is not specific to patients with chest pain, but may give some guide to treatment. For panic disorder, combined psychotherapy and antidepressant therapy is more effective than either therapy alone.[91] When appropriate psychological interventions are not available or have been unsuccessful, there is a role for a trial of selective serotonin reuptake inhibitors for depression. These drugs have evidence for effectiveness compared with placebo in the primary care setting.[92] They may be preferred to tricyclic antidepressants in patients with chest pain because of their lower cardiotoxicity in overdose.[93]

Applying the Algorithm in Practice

The chest pain algorithm shown in **Fig. 1** acts as a guiding framework for the clinical application of the diagnostic elements described in the body of this article. The diagnostic elements relating to history, examination, and investigation are summarized in **Tables 6** and **7** and those relating to therapeutic trials in **Table 8**.

Early in the red flag algorithm it is important to take a brief history and check the vital signs to assess if emergency treatment and referral to an emergency department are necessary. If the patient seems stable, a more detailed assessment for red flag conditions can be performed, with urgent treatment and referral if red flags are found.

Not all cardiac and pulmonary causes are red flags. Certain cardiac and pulmonary causes can be safely managed in the community and may depend on the availability of community-based treatments and the ability to refer for complex investigations and specialist review if indicated. For example, a patient with stable angina can be managed with medication and referral to a cardiologist for coronary angiography.

Table 6
Cardiac and pulmonary causes of chest pain, their flag status, and associated diagnostic elements derived from history, examination, and investigation (the evidence for each element is classified according to SORT)

Condition	Flag Status	Element	Evidence Rating	References[a]
Cardiovascular				
ACS	Red	Classification of chest pain as anginal, atypical anginal, or nonanginal helps determine cardiac risk	C	20
		Exertional chest pain and pain radiating to the shoulder or both arms increases the risk of ACS	B	21
		The Rouan decision rule aids risk stratification for MI	C	1
		ECG findings of new ST segment increase, Q waves, and conduction defects strongly suggest ACS or AMI	C	22
		Serum troponin is an accurate predictor of AMI of death or recurrent MI within 30 days	C	29
		Patients with chest pain and a negative initial cardiac evaluation should have further testing with stress ECG, perfusion scanning, or angiography depending on their level of risk	C	20
Heart failure	Red or green	The absence of exertional dyspnea makes heart failure unlikely	C	46
		An abnormal ECG and cardiomegaly on chest radiograph suggest heart failure in patients with chest pain	C	47
		Increased BNP levels suggest heart failure in patients with acute dyspnea	C	47–49

PE	Red	A Wells score of less than 2 plus a normal D-dimer assay should rule out PE	A	2,9,42
		In patients with an abnormal D-dimer assay or a Wells score indicating moderate to high risk, helical CT and lower extremity venous ultrasound examination should be used to rule in or rule out PE	A	42,45
Dissecting aortic aneurysm	Red	Sudden severe onset of pain	C	52
		Pain described as ripping or tearing	C	52
Pulmonary				
Pneumonia	Red or green	Focal chest signs in lower respiratory tract infections increase the likelihood of pneumonia	B	56
		The Diehr diagnostic rule predicts the likelihood of pneumonia based on clinical findings	A	56
Lung cancer	Red	The most common respiratory symptoms in patients presenting with lung cancer are dyspnea, cough, hoarseness, and hemoptysis	B	59
		Smoking is a risk factor for lung cancer	A	59,60
		Sputum cytology has a specificity of 99% and a sensitivity of 66% in the detection of lung cancer	A	62
Pneumothorax	Red	Acute, pleuritic chest pain with dyspnea, tachycardia, tachypnea, and hypoxia are suggestive of pneumothorax	C	63,64

[a] The evidence for each element is classified according to SORT.
Data from Ebell MH, Siwek J, Weiss BD, et al. Strength of recommendation taxonomy (SORT): a patient-centered approach to grading evidence in the medical literature. Am Fam Physician 2004;69(3):548–56.

Table 7
Noncardiac causes of chest pain, their flag status, and associated diagnostic elements derived from history, examination, and investigation (the evidence for each element is classified according to SORT)

Condition	Flag Status	Element	Evidence Rating	References
Musculoskeletal				
Chest wall syndrome	Green	Pain is not squeezing or oppressive	B	17
		Pain is well localized	B	17
		Musculoskeletal chest pain is more likely in patients with chest wall tenderness	B	65,66
		Presence of paraspinal tenderness	B	65,67
		CTA most closely predicted by	B	67
		• The grading of angina by a physician as noncardiac or atypical angina (CCS guidelines)		
		• The presence of neck pain		
		• Reduced motion palpation of T3–T5		
		• The presence of spinal tenderness		
Costochondritis	Green	Tenderness to palpation of costochondral junctions; reproduces patient's pain; usually multiple sites on same side of chest	C	72,95
Chest trauma	Green	History of direct trauma or repetitive trauma Localized pain and tenderness	C	73,95
Fibromyalgia	Green	Widespread pain and tenderness	C	75
Gastrointestinal				
Life-threatening GI conditions	Red	Alarm symptoms for investigation	C	76
		• Repeated vomiting		
		• Decreased appetite		
		• Weight loss		
		• Dysphagia		
		• Odynophagia (pain on swallowing)		
		• Hematemesis		
		• Anemia		
		• Melena		

GERD	Green	Patients with heartburn and regurgitation are more likely to have abnormal esophageal pH results than those without these symptoms	C	77
		Symptoms significantly more common in patients with NCCP who have GERD are heartburn, regurgitation, and pain relieved by antacid	B	96
Skin and soft tissue				
Herpes zoster	Green	Dermatomal pain, itching, or paresthesia	C	84
Skin tumor	Red or green	Skin or soft-tissue lump	C	
Breast lesion	Red or green	Anterior chest pain ± breast lump	C	82,83
Psychogenic chest pain				
Panic disorder	Yellow	A 2-question screen can accurately exclude panic disorder if negative but requires further evaluation if positive	B	9
Depression	Yellow	A 2-question screen for depression is a valid screening tool	B	89

Data from Ebell MH, Siwek J, Weiss BD, et al. Strength of recommendation taxonomy (SORT): a patient-centered approach to grading evidence in the medical literature. Am Fam Physician 2004;69(3):548–56.

Table 8
Conditions causing chest pain and associated diagnostic elements derived from therapeutic trials (the evidence for each element is classified according to SORT)

Condition	Element	Evidence Rating	References
Cardiovascular			
ACS	Administration of nitroglycerin does not reliably predict the presence or absence of cardiac chest pain, CAD, or myocardial ischemia	B	[32–35]
Pulmonary			
Acute bronchitis	Antibiotics have modest benefits	A	[58]
	Stronger indication for antibiotics in groups with a high risk of complications from infection	C	[54]
Musculoskeletal			
Chest wall syndrome	Manual therapy in patients with clinical features of musculoskeletal chest pain	C	[67]
Costochondritis	Local anesthetic injections Analgesics or antiinflammatory medication, rest, and reassurance	B	[71,72]
Gastrointestinal			
GERD	PPI for reflux esophagitis	B	[76]
Skin and soft tissue			
Herpes zoster	Antiviral agents for herpes zoster (not specific to chest pain patients)	B	[85]
Skin tumor or breast lesion	Excision of tumors (not specific to chest pain patients)	C	
Psychogenic			
Panic disorder	CBT	A	[90]
	Combined behavioral therapy and antidepressants in panic disorder (not specific to chest pain patients)	A	[91]
Depression	SSRIs for depression (not specific to chest pain patients)	A	[92]

Data from Ebell MH, Siwek J, Weiss BD, et al. Strength of recommendation taxonomy (SORT): a patient-centered approach to grading evidence in the medical literature. Am Fam Physician 2004;69(3):548–56.

Once red flags have been assessed as unlikely, the assessment can switch to green flags. If a green flag is found, basic investigations that can be performed quickly and locally may be performed, often to deal with any remaining uncertainty about red flags. If green flags are unlikely, the brief screening questionnaires for panic disorder and depression can be used to screen for these conditions, and a more detailed assessment of the mental health status performed if they are positive. If this screening process is negative, further investigation, at least at a basic level, may be indicated to exclude green flags with more certainty.

These assessments should lead to a provisional diagnosis and an appropriate therapeutic trial. This trial may require referral, depending on the skills of the practitioner. The response to the trial is used as a weak form of evidence to confirm or refute the provisional diagnosis. If the trial is successful, but the underlying condition is likely to continue, then follow-up should be arranged for monitoring and secondary prevention. If the trial is unsuccessful or only partly successful, the options are to search for a different cause or a second cause or to refer for further investigation and/or specialist review.

A Word of Caution

Trials of treatment are incorporated within this algorithm not only to provide treatment per se but also for their diagnostic benefit. However, throughout this process the practitioner should be mindful of investigating any symptoms suggestive of serious causes. Patients may have more than 1 cause of chest pain. Discovery of a noncardiac cause is no reason to be complacent about cardiovascular risk factors. In the emergency department setting, predictors of adverse cardiac events after an initial diagnosis of NCCP include hypercholesterolemia, diabetes, history of CAD, and history of congestive heart failure.[25] These features can act as a guide to primary care practitioners for patients, and further testing to exclude cardiac causes of chest pain is warranted when these predictors are present.

The algorithm proposed here, although based on available evidence, does not constitute a validated decision rule. It warrants testing in a clinical trial in primary care, where it could be compared with usual care for chest pain.

SUMMARY

It is apt to conclude with a quote from Anthony Komaroff, who, in 1982, wrote about the concern that algorithms would threaten the art of clinical medicine, leading to regimentation and mediocrity in decision making.[94] In their defense, he wrote:

In our view, algorithms can help us to articulate how we make decisions, to clarify our knowledge and to recognize our ignorance. They can help us to demystify the practice of medicine, and to demonstrate that much of what we call the "art" of medicine is really a scientific process, a science which is waiting to be articulated.

Although the science behind the assessment of chest pain into an algorithm has progressed considerably since 1982, this article illustrates that there is still a lot left to be validated about many of the diagnostic elements used in this assessment process. Nonetheless, there is now a lot of science that can inform the art of dealing with patients presenting with chest pain. The algorithm and its diagnostic elements presented should be used with discretion to guide, rather than replace, clinical decision making.

REFERENCES

1. Rouan GW, Lee TH, Cook EF, et al. Clinical characteristics and outcome of acute myocardial infarction in patients with initially normal or nonspecific electrocardiograms (a report from the multicenter chest pain study). Am J Cardiol 1989;64:1087–92.
2. Wells PS, Anderson DR, Rodger M, et al. Derivation of a simple clinical model to categorize patients probability of pulmonary embolism: increasing the models utility with the SimpliRED D-dimer. Thromb Haemost 2000;83:416–20.
3. Buntinx F, Knockaert D, Bruyninckx R, et al. Chest pain in general practice or in the hospital emergency department: is it the same? Fam Pract 2001;18(6):586–9.

4. Eslick GD, Talley NJ. Non-cardiac chest pain: squeezing the life out of the Australian healthcare system? Med J Aust 2000;173:233–4.

5. Eslick G, Fass R. Noncardiac chest pain: evaluation and treatment. Gastroenterol Clin North Am 2003;32:531–52.

6. Nihjer G, Weinman J, Bass C, et al. Chest pain in people with normal coronary anatomy. BMJ 2001;323:1320–1.

7. Coulshed DS, Eslick GD, Talley NJ. Non-cardiac chest pain[letter to the editor]. BMJ 2002;324:915.

8. Cayley WE Jr. Diagnosing the cause of chest pain. Am Fam Physician 2005; 72(10):2012–21.

9. Stein MB, Roy-Byrne PP, McQuaid JR, et al. Development of a brief diagnostic screen for panic disorder in primary care. Psychosom Med 1999;61:359–64.

10. Elstein AS, Schwartz A. Clinical problem solving and diagnostic decision making: selective review of the cognitive literature. BMJ 2002;324(7339):729–32.

11. Doust J. Diagnosis in general practice. Using probabilistic reasoning. BMJ 2009; 339:b3823.

12. Bogduk N, McGuirk B. Medical management of acute and chronic low back pain. An evidence-based approach. Sydney (Australia): Elsevier; 2002.

13. Van de Laar FA, Kenealy T, Fahey T, et al. Elaboration of clinical prediction rules work. Available at: http://www.cochraneprimarycare.org/en/index.html/. Accessed January 10, 2010.

14. Ebell MH, Siwek J, Weiss BD, et al. Strength of recommendation taxonomy (SORT): a patient-centered approach to grading evidence in the medical literature. Am Fam Physician 2004;69(3):548–56.

15. McCormick A, Fleming DM, Charlton J. Morbidity statistics from general practice: fourth national study 1991–1992. Available at: http://www.statistics.gov.uk/downloads/theme_health/MB5No3.pdf. Accessed February 14, 2010.

16. Nilsson S, Scheike M, Engblom D, et al. Chest pain and ischaemic heart disease in primary care. Br J Gen Pract 2003;53(490):378–82.

17. Verdon F, Burnand B, Herzig L, et al. Chest wall syndrome among primary care patients: a cohort study. BMC Fam Pract 2007;8:51.

18. Ruigomez A, Rodriguez LA, Wallander MA, et al. Chest pain in general practice: incidence, comorbidity and mortality. Fam Pract 2006;23(2):167–74.

19. Klinkman MS, Stevens D, Gorenflo DW. Episodes of care for chest pain: a preliminary report from MIRNET. J Fam Pract 1994;38:345–52.

20. Gibbons RJ, Balady GJ, Bricker JT, et al. ACC/AHA 2002 guideline update for exercise testing: summary article: a report of the American College of Cardiology/American Heart Association Task Force on Practice Guidelines (Committee to Update the 1997 Exercise Testing Guidelines). Circulation 2002;106:1883–92.

21. Berger JP, Buclin R, Haller E, et al. Right arm involvement and pain extension can help to differentiate coronary diseases from chest pain of other origin: a prospective emergency ward study of 278 consecutive patients admitted for chest pain. J Intern Med 1990;227:165–72.

22. Goodacre S, Locker T, Morris F, et al. How useful are clinical features in the diagnosis of acute, undifferentiated chest pain? Acad Emerg Med 2002;9(3):203–8.

23. Bruyninckx R, Aertgeerts B, Bruyninckx P, et al. Signs and symptoms in diagnosing acute myocardial infarction and acute coronary syndrome: a diagnostic meta-analysis. Br J Gen Pract 2008;58(547):105–11.

24. Panju AA, Hemmelgarn BR, Guyatt GH, et al. The rational clinical examination. Is this patient having a myocardial infarction? JAMA 1998;280(14):1256–63.

25. Miller CD, Lindsell CJ, Khandelwal S, et al. Is the initial diagnostic impression of "noncardiac chest pain" adequate to exclude cardiac disease? Ann Emerg Med 2004;44(6):565–74.
26. McCord J, Nowak RM, Hudson MP, et al. The prognostic significance of serial myoglobin, troponin I, and creatine kinase-MB measurements in patients evaluated in the emergency department for acute coronary syndrome. Ann Emerg Med 2003;42(3):343–50.
27. National Heart Foundation of Australia, Cardiac Society of Australia and New Zealand. Guidelines for the management of acute coronary syndromes 2006. Med J Aust 2006;184(8):S1–30.
28. Law K, Elley R, Tietjens J, et al. Troponin testing for chest pain in primary healthcare: a survey of its use by general practitioners in New Zealand. N Z Med J 2006;119(1238):U2082.
29. Hamm CW, Goldmann BU, Heeschen C, et al. Emergency room triage of patients with acute chest pain by means of rapid testing for cardiac troponin T or troponin I. N Engl J Med 1997;337(23):1648–53.
30. Ebell MH, Flewelling D, Flynn CA. A systematic review of troponin T and I for diagnosing acute myocardial infarction. J Fam Pract 2000;49:550–6.
31. Ebell MH, White LL, Weismantel D. A systematic review of troponin T and I values as a prognostic tool for patients with chest pain. J Fam Pract 2000;49:746–53.
32. Diercks DB, Boghos E, Guzman H, et al. Changes in the numeric descriptive scale for pain after sublingual nitroglycerin do not predict cardiac etiology of chest pain. Ann Emerg Med 2005;45(6):581–5.
33. Henrikson CA, Howell EE, Bush DE, et al. Chest pain relief by nitroglycerin does not predict active coronary artery disease. Ann Intern Med 2003;139(12):979–86.
34. Steele R, McNaughton T, McConahy M, et al. Chest pain in emergency department patients: if the pain is relieved by nitroglycerin, is it more likely to be cardiac chest pain? CJEM 2006;8(3):164–9.
35. Shry EA, Dacus J, Van De Graaff E, et al. Usefulness of the response to sublingual nitroglycerin as a predictor of ischemic chest pain in the emergency department. Am J Cardiol 2002;90(11):1264–6.
36. Wells PS, Anderson DR, Rodger M, et al. Excluding pulmonary embolism at the bedside without diagnostic imaging: management of patients with suspected pulmonary embolism presenting to the emergency department by using a simple clinical model and d-dimer. Ann Intern Med 2001;135(2):98–107.
37. Chunilal SD, Eikelboom JW, Attia J, et al. Does this patient have pulmonary embolism? JAMA 2003;290:2849–58.
38. Tamariz LJ, Eng J, Segal JB, et al. Usefulness of clinical prediction rules for the diagnosis of venous thromboembolism: a systematic review. Am J Med 2004;117(9):676–84.
39. Yap KS, Kalff V, Turlakow A, et al. A prospective reassessment of the utility of the Wells score in identifying pulmonary embolism. Med J Aust 2007;187(6):333–6.
40. Stein PD, Hull RD, Patel KC, et al. D-dimer for the exclusion of acute venous thrombosis and pulmonary embolism: a systematic review. Ann Intern Med 2004;140(8):589–602.
41. Musset D, Parent F, Meyer G, et al. Diagnostic strategy for patients with suspected pulmonary embolism: a prospective multicentre outcome study. Lancet 2002;360:1914–20.
42. Perrier A, Roy PM, Aujesky D, et al. Diagnosing pulmonary embolism in outpatients with clinical assessment, D-dimer measurement, venous ultrasound, and helical computed tomography: a multicenter management study. Am J Med 2004;116(5):291–9.

43. Qaseem A, Snow V, Barry P, et al. Joint American Academy of Family Physicians/
American College of Physicians panel on deep venous thrombosis/pulmonary
embolism. Current diagnosis of venous thromboembolism in primary care: a clinical practice guideline from the American Academy of Family Physicians and the
American College of Physicians. Ann Fam Med 2007;5(1):57–62.

44. van Belle A, Büller HR, Huisman MV, et al. Christopher Study Investigators. Effectiveness of managing suspected pulmonary embolism using an algorithm
combining clinical probability, D-dimer testing, and computed tomography.
JAMA 2006;295(2):172–9.

45. Institute for Clinical Systems Improvement. Healthcare guidelines. Venous thromboembolism. Diagnosis and treatment (guideline). Available at: http://www.icsi.
org/guidelines_and_more/gl_os_prot/cardiovascular/venous_thromboembolism/
venous_thromboembolism_6.html. Accessed January 15, 2010.

46. Davie AP, Caruana FL, Sutherland GR, et al. Assessing diagnosis in heart failure:
which features are any use? QJM 1997;90:335–9.

47. Talreja D, Gruver C, Sklenar J, et al. Efficient utilization of echocardiography for
the assessment of left ventricular systolic function. Am Heart J 2000;139:394–8.

48. Cardarelli R, Lumicao TG. B-Type natriuretic peptide: a review of its diagnostic,
prognostic, and therapeutic monitoring value in heart failure for primary care
physicians. J Am Board Fam Pract 2003;16:327–33.

49. Maisel AS, Krishnaswamy P, Nowak RM, et al. Rapid measurement of B-type
natriuretic peptide in the emergency diagnosis of heart failure. N Engl J Med
2002;347(3):161–7.

50. Dickstein K, Cohen-Solal A, Filippatos G, et al. ESC Guidelines for the diagnosis
and treatment of acute and chronic heart failure 2008: the Task Force for the
Diagnosis and Treatment of Acute and Chronic Heart Failure 2008 of the European Society of Cardiology. Eur Heart J 2008;29(19):2388–442.

51. Hunt SA, Abraham WT, Chin MH, et al. 2009 focused update incorporated into the
ACC/AHA 2005 guidelines for the diagnosis and management of heart failure in
adults: a report of the American College of Cardiology Foundation/American
Heart Association Task Force on Practice Guidelines: developed in collaboration
with the International Society for Heart and Lung Transplantation. Circulation
2009;119(14):e391–479.

52. Wiesenfarth J. Dissection, aortic. eMedicine. Available at: http://emedicine.
medscape.com/article/756835-overview. Accessed January 15, 2010.

53. Spittell PC, Spittell JA Jr, Joyce JW, et al. Clinical features and differential diagnosis of aortic dissection: experience with 236 cases (1980 through 1990).
Mayo Clin Proc 1993;68(7):642–51.

54. Woodhead M, Blasi F, Ewig S, et al. Guidelines for the management of adult lower
respiratory tract infections. Eur Respir J 2005;26(6):1138–80.

55. Metlay JP, Kapoor WN, Fine MJ. Does this patient have community-acquired
pneumonia? Diagnosing pneumonia by history and physical examination.
JAMA 1997;278:1440–5.

56. Woodhead MA, Macfarlane JT, McCracken JS, et al. Prospective study of the
aetiology and outcome of pneumonia in the community. Lancet 1987;1:671–4.

57. Diehr P, Wood RW, Bushyhead J, et al. Prediction of pneumonia in outpatients
with acute cough—a statistical approach. J Chronic Dis 1984;37:215–25.

58. Smith SM, Fahey T, Smucny J, et al. Antibiotics for acute bronchitis. Cochrane Database Syst Rev 2004;(4):CD000245. DOI:10.1002/14651858.CD000245.pub2.

59. Hopwood P, Stephens RJ. Symptoms at presentation for treatment in patients
with lung cancer: implications for the evaluation of palliative treatment. The

Medical Research Council (MRC) Lung Cancer Working Party. Br J Cancer 1995; 71(3):633–6.

60. Freedman ND, Leitzmann MF, Hollenbeck AR, et al. Cigarette smoking and subsequent risk of lung cancer in men and women: analysis of a prospective cohort study. Lancet Oncol 2008;9(7):649–56.

61. Peto R, Lopez AD, Boreham J, et al. Mortality from tobacco in developed countries: indirect estimation from national vital statistics. Lancet 1992;339(8804): 1268–78.

62. Schreiber G, McCrory DC. Performance characteristics of different modalities for diagnosis of suspected lung cancer: summary of published evidence. Chest 2003;123(1 Suppl):115S–28S.

63. Butler KH, Swencki SA. Chest pain: a clinical assessment. Radiol Clin North Am 2006;44(2):165–79, vii.

64. Chang AK, Barton ED. Pneumothorax, iatrogenic, spontaneous and pneumomediastinum 2005. Available at: http://www.emedicine.com/EMERG/topic469.htm. Accessed January 15, 2010.

65. Yelland MJ. Back, chest and abdominal pain. How good are spinal signs at identifying musculoskeletal causes of back, chest or abdominal pain? Aust Fam Physician 2001;30(9):908–12.

66. Wise CM, Semble EL, Dalton CB. Musculoskeletal chest wall syndromes in patients with noncardiac chest pain: a study of 100 patients. Arch Phys Med Rehabil 1992;73(2):147–9.

67. Christensen HW, Vach W, Gichangi A, et al. Cervicothoracic angina identified by case history and palpation findings in patients with stable angina pectoris. J Manipulative Physiol Ther 2005;28(5):303–11.

68. Christensen HW, Vach W, Gichangi A, et al. Manual therapy for patients with stable angina pectoris: a nonrandomized open prospective trial. J Manipulative Physiol Ther 2005;28(9):654–61.

69. Stochkendahl MJ, Christensen HW, Vach W. Diagnosis and treatment of musculoskeletal chest pain: design of a multi-purpose trial. BMC Musculoskelet Disord 2008;9:40.

70. Fam AG, Smythe HA. Musculoskeletal chest wall pain. CMAJ 1985;133(5): 379–89.

71. Freeston J, Karim Z, Lindsay K, et al. Can early diagnosis and management of costochondritis reduce acute chest pain admissions? J Rheumatol 2004; 31(11):2269–71.

72. Proulx AM, Zryd TW. Costochondritis: diagnosis and treatment. Am Fam Physician 2009;80(6):617–20.

73. De Maeseneer M, De Mey J, Debaere C, et al. Rib fractures induced by coughing: an unusual cause of acute chest pain. Am J Emerg Med 2000;18(2):194–7.

74. Kara M, Dikmen E, Erdal HH, et al. Disclosure of unnoticed rib fractures with the use of ultrasonography in minor blunt chest trauma. Eur J Cardiothorac Surg 2003;24(4):608–13.

75. Wolfe F, Smythe HA, Yunus MB, et al. The American College of Rheumatology 1990 criteria for the classification of fibromyalgia. Report of the Multicenter Criteria Committee. Arthritis Rheum 1990;33(2):160–72.

76. Faybush EM, Fass R. Diagnosis of noncardiac chest pain. In: Fass R, Eslick GD, editors. Noncardiac chest pain: a growing medical problem. San Diego (CA): Plural Publishing; 2007.

77. Alban-Davies H, Jones DB, Rhoades J. Esophageal angina as the cause of chest pain. JAMA 1982;248:227.

78. Eslick GD, Coulshed DS, Talley NJ. Diagnosis and treatment of noncardiac chest pain. Nat Clin Pract Gastroenterol Hepatol 2005;2(10):463–72.
79. Klauser AG, Schindlbeck NE, Muller-Lissner SA. Symptoms in gastro-oesophageal reflux disease. Lancet 1990;335(8683):205–8.
80. Fang J, Bjorkman D. A critical approach to noncardiac chest pain: pathophysiology, diagnosis, and treatment. Am J Gastroenterol 2001;96(4):958–68.
81. Ofman JJ, Gralnek IM, Udani J, et al. The cost-effectiveness of the omeprazole test in patients with noncardiac chest pain. Am J Med 1999;107(3):219–27.
82. MacArthur C, Smith A. The symptom presentation of breast cancer: is pain a symptom? Community Med 1983;5(3):220–3.
83. Greenblatt RB, Samaras C, Vasquez JM, et al. Fibrocystic disease of the breast. Clin Obstet Gynecol 1982;25(2):365.
84. Goh CL, Khoo L. A retrospective study of the clinical presentation and outcome of herpes zoster in a tertiary dermatology outpatient referral clinic. Int J Dermatol 1997;36(9):667–72.
85. Li Q, Chen N, Yang J, et al. Antiviral treatment for preventing postherpetic neuralgia. Cochrane Database Syst Rev 2009;(2):CD006866. DOI:10.1002/14651858.CD006866.pub2.
86. Bass C, Wade C, Hand D, et al. Patients with angina with normal and near normal coronary arteries: clinical and psychosocial state 12 months after angiography. Br Med J (Clin Res Ed) 1983;287(6404):1505–8.
87. Strike PC, Steptoe A. Systematic review of mental stress-induced myocardial ischaemia. Eur Heart J 2003;24(8):690–703.
88. Katerndahl DA, Trammell C. Prevalence and recognition of panic state in STAR-NET patients presenting with chest pain. J Fam Pract 1997;45:54–63.
89. Arroll B, Khin N, Kerse N. Screening for depression in primary care with two verbally asked questions: cross sectional study. BMJ 2003;327(7424):1144–6.
90. Kisely S, Campbell LA, Skerritt P. Psychological interventions for symptomatic management of non-specific chest pain in patients with normal coronary anatomy. Cochrane Database Syst Rev 2005;(1):CD004101.
91. Furukawa TA, Watanabe N, Churchill R. Combined psychotherapy plus antidepressants for panic disorder with or without agoraphobia. Cochrane Database Syst Rev 2007;(1):CD004364. DOI:10.1002/14651858.CD004364.pub2.
92. Arroll B, Elley CR, Fishman T, et al. Antidepressants versus placebo for depression in primary care. Cochrane Database Syst Rev 2009;(3):CD007954. DOI:10.1002/14651858.
93. Peretti S, Judge R, Hindmarch I. Safety and tolerability considerations: tricyclic antidepressants vs. selective serotonin reuptake inhibitors. Acta Psychiatr Scand 2000;403:17.
94. Komaroff AL. Algorithms and the 'Art' of medicine. Aust J Polit Hist 1982;72(1):10–2.
95. Fam AG. Approach to musculoskeletal chest wall pain. Prim Care 1988;15(4):767–82.
96. Mousavi S, Tosi J, Eskandarian R, et al. Role of clinical presentation in diagnosing reflux-related non-cardiac chest pain. J Gastroenterol Hepatol 2007;22(2):218–21.

Future Developments in Chest Pain Diagnosis and Management

Anthony F.T. Brown, MB, ChB, FRCP, FRCSEd, FACEM, FCEM[a,b,*],
Louise Cullen, MBBS (Hons), FACEM[a,b,c],
Martin Than, MBBS, FRCSEd(A&E), FACEM, FCEM[d,e]

KEYWORDS

- Acute coronary syndrome • Pulmonary embolism
- Aortic dissection • Biomarkers

The clinician's approach to a patient with chest pain should first focus on excluding the most potentially serious causes such as acute coronary syndrome (ACS), pulmonary embolism (PE), and acute aortic dissection (AAD), all of which can present without immediately obvious clinical, laboratory, radiological, or electrocardiography (ECG) findings. Once this initial phase of care is complete there is then no consensus on who, if anyone, should assess the patient next. This situation increases the risk of recurrent pain and repeat presentations.[1]

Alternate diagnoses at this stage include gastroesophageal reflux disease (GERD), musculoskeletal conditions including fibromyalgia, and psychological disorders. These conditions are often diagnosed by the primary care physician based on

Competing interests: A.F.T.B. has received an honorarium from Elixir Healthcare Education. L.C. has received research support from Inverness Medical, Radiometer Pacific, and Abbott, and an honorarium from Inverness Medical. M.T. has received research support from Abbott, Inverness Medical, and Beckman-Coulter, and an honorarium from Inverness Medical.

[a] School of Medicine, University of Queensland, Mayne Medical School, 288 Herston Road, Herston, Brisbane, Queensland 4006, Australia

[b] Department of Emergency Medicine, Royal Brisbane and Women's Hospital, Butterfield Street, Herston, Brisbane, Queensland 4029, Australia

[c] School of Public Health, Queensland University of Technology, Victoria Park Road, Kelvin Grove, Brisbane, Queensland 4059, Australia

[d] Christchurch School of Medicine, University of Otago, Riccarton Avenue, Christchurch 8011, New Zealand

[e] Department of Emergency Medicine, Christchurch Hospital, Riccarton Avenue, Private Bag 4710, Christchurch 8011, New Zealand

* Corresponding author. Department of Emergency Medicine, Royal Brisbane and Women's Hospital, Brisbane, Butterfield Street, Herston, Brisbane, Queensland 4029, Australia.

E-mail address: af.brown@uq.edu.au

response to a carefully chosen therapeutic trial, for instance a proton-pump inhibitor (PPI) for GERD, or following specialist referral.

Much of the focus of research on patients with chest pain is directed at technological advances in the diagnosis and management of ACS, PE, and AAD, despite there being no significant difference at 4 years as regards mortality, ongoing chest pain, and quality of life between patients presenting to the emergency department with noncardiac chest pain (NCCP) and those with cardiac chest pain.[2] Moreover, NCCP patients significantly outnumber patients presenting with an underlying cardiac cause, particularly to the primary care physician.

This article examines future developments in the diagnosis and management of patients with suspected ACS, PE, AAD, gastrointestinal disease, and musculoskeletal chest pain.

FUTURE DEVELOPMENTS IN ACUTE CORONARY SYNDROME

The diagnosis of ACS is based on clinical judgment, serial 12-lead ECG analysis, and cardiac biomarkers and, if these are negative, some form of stress testing. Each of these modalities for the evaluation of a patient with potential ACS has difficulties. On the one hand any delay in the diagnosis or "rule in" of an acute myocardial infarction (AMI) precludes early pharmacologic or interventional treatment known to improve outcome by limiting infarct size.[3,4] In contrast, chest pain units aimed at ensuring significant diagnoses are not missed to "rule out" patients with a low probability for ACS[5] report a negative assessment in up to 98% of all patients tested.[6,7] Despite this dichotomy in decision-making perspective, still as many as 2% to 5% of patients with ACS, that is, with either AMI or unstable angina pectoris (UAP), are missed and sent home from the Emergency Department (ED).[8]

Future developments in the assessment and management of patients with ACS presenting to the ED with chest pain will include improved ECG analysis, novel biomarkers, newer imaging techniques, risk stratification tools, improved drugs, sonothrombolysis, and stem cell transplantation (**Box 1**).

Earlier Diagnosis

The key to improving the outcome in the diagnosis of ACS lies in the development of a coordinated approach to early detection, from the time the patient first accesses medical care.[9–11] Thus, prehospital diagnosis of ST-elevation myocardial infarction (STEMI) with 12-lead ECG analysis can facilitate the primary goal of immediate opening of the infarct-related vessel, for instance by direct transfer of the patient to a hospital operating a catheter laboratory 24 hours a day.[10–12]

Box 1
Future developments in patients with suspected ACS

Improved ECG analysis

Novel biomarkers

Newer imaging techniques

Risk stratification tools

Improved drugs

Sonothrombolysis

Stem cell transplantation

Body Surface Mapping

Standard 12-lead ECG analysis identifies STEMI and dictates the need for immediate reperfusion therapy for an optimal outcome.[13–15] However, neither the ECG nor serum biomarkers have high early sensitivity to detect AMI in general, as they may remain negative immediately after the event. One option to improve the sensitivity in detecting AMI is ECG body surface mapping (BSM), which uses up to 80 ECG leads placed on the anterior and posterior chest to enable more complete visualization of cardiac electrical activity (**Fig. 1**).

The BSM output can be displayed in a 12-lead ECG format, in an 80-lead format, or on color contour or topographic maps.[16] With recent advances in computer technology, BSM has become more user-friendly in aiding direct visualization of injury patterns, particularly in the right ventricle and posterior wall of the left ventricle associated with an inferior AMI.[17,18]

BSM may also improve the diagnostic evaluation and treatment of patients with ST depression on a standard 12-lead ECG. In particular, BSM can differentiate a group of patients who in fact have ST elevation on BSM, who theoretically might therefore benefit from early reperfusion therapy.[19,20] One BSM trial has also shown the ability to detect AMI prehospital.[21] However, early detection of AMI with BSM comes at a cost of a lower specificity and higher false-positive results compared with the standard ECG.[22]

High-Frequency QRS Analysis

Another approach to improve the detection of acute myocardial ischemia is ECG analysis of the high-frequency (HF) components of the QRS complex above 100 Hz.[23,24] Those frequencies are usually not seen as notable morphologic alterations in the QRS complex on the standard 12-lead ECG machine, as these use noise-reducing filters to eliminate this HF range. However, the HF components can provide information about the severity of ischemia and myocardial infarction (MI). Although HF QRS analysis may offer additional noninvasive information in ACSs, it is currently hampered by marked interpatient variance, and a lack of large-scale clinical outcome trials in humans.[24]

Novel ACS Biomarkers

Overview

Elevation of cardiac biomarkers is pivotal to the diagnosis of AMI.[25] However, biomarkers that could detect ACS without myocardial necrosis may allow clinicians

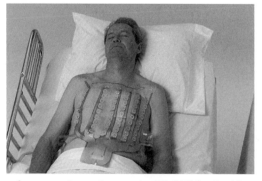

Fig. 1. ECG body surface mapping using up to 80 ECG leads. (*Courtesy of* Heartscape Technologies Inc, Columbia, MD, USA; with permission.)

to recognize biologic events happening before necrosis occurs, thereby identifying earlier patients at higher risk of an adverse event[26,27]; this could then lead to treatment targeted to limit or prevent an AMI. At present, these types of biomarker are not commercially available.

Although cardiac troponins provide important prognostic information, they do not accurately determine absolute risk for ACS.[28] Several newer cardiac biomarkers have therefore been proposed for the diagnosis and risk stratification of patients with possible ACS. These markers include copeptin, myeloperoxidase (MPO), pregnancy-associated plasma protein A (PaPP-A), placental growth factor (PlGF), CD40 ligand, ischemia modified albumin (IMA), fatty acid binding protein (h-FABP), free fatty acids, growth differentiation factor 15 (GDF-15), serum choline, glycogen phosphorylase isoenzyme BB (GPBB), and high-sensitivity C-reactive protein (hsCRP) (**Box 2**). Although many of these may provide additional short- and long-term prognostic information, at present none offer a clear diagnostic advantage over troponin alone. In addition, few are currently available in commercially approved kits.

Copeptin
Copeptin, the C-terminal part of the vasopressin prohormone, is secreted from the neurohypophysis and is activated in the endogenous stress response.[29] The measurement of copeptin in addition to a biomarker with a different pathophysiological origin such as troponin can improve the diagnostic accuracy at presentation, and possibly eliminate the need for serial sampling. One study by Reichlin and colleagues[29] found that combining copeptin and troponin T had a sensitivity of 98.8% and a specificity of 77.1% for diagnosing AMI.

Myeloperoxidase
MPO is released by neutrophils and macrophages, and so becomes elevated in coronary artery atherosclerotic lesions prone to rupture.[26,30] MPO has shown promise in risk stratification of chest pain patients with persistently normal troponin levels, and may prove useful for the disposition of patients from the ED. Of note, MPO levels

---

Box 2
Proposed new biomarkers for the diagnosis and risk stratification of patients with possible ACS

Copeptin

Myeloperoxidase

Pregnancy-associated plasma protein A

Placental growth factor

CD40 ligand

Ischemia modified albumin

Fatty acid binding protein

Free fatty acids

Growth differentiation factor 15

Serum choline

Glycogen phosphorylase isoenzyme BB

High-sensitivity C-reactive protein

have been found to be elevated at baseline in patients subsequently shown to have AMI, even when symptom onset was less than 3 hours before blood analysis.[30] However, MPO elevation is not specific to cardiac disease, as activation of neutrophils and macrophages occurs with many other disease processes.[26]

Pregnancy-associated plasma protein A
PaPP-A is a marker of neovascularization that may also play a role in detecting athero-sclerosis and plaque rupture.[26,31] Although PaPP-A appears to have little correlation with other cardiac biomarker levels, it has shown promise at predicting the need for a revascularization procedure.[31,32]

Placental growth factor
PIGF is a hormone that stimulates angiogenesis and macrophage recruitment,[32] and may thus indicate inflammation predicting early AMI.[26] However, studies to date used the higher cut-off values for the cardiac troponin reference standard that are now superseded, so new research comparing PIGF with the currently recommended levels for abnormal troponin is now necessary to reconfirm its efficacy.[31]

CD40 ligand
CD40 ligand levels reflect both inflammation and platelet/plaque interactions,[32] with encouraging results, particularly when combined with PIGF.[26,31] More studies are needed before strong conclusions can be drawn.

Ischemia modified albumin
IMA molecules are produced when the metal terminus of the albumin molecule is damaged during ischemia.[31,32] IMA should thus be useful for its strong negative predictive value for ischemia, even before necrosis. Current studies indicate good potential for IMA to rule out ACS when combined with troponin and ECG.[32] However, it is currently difficult to assess the role of IMA due to the lack of standard reference criteria for nonnecrotic ischemia.[31] IMA may also not be specific for cardiac ischemia.[26]

Fatty acid binding protein
h-FABP is released rapidly post infarction,[31] and may outperform myoglobin in the early detection of AMI. However, current studies indicate that h-FABP lacks specificity,[31] and adds little diagnostic information to the newer ultrasensitive troponin assay results.[33]

The real value of any new biomarker, including genetic and genomic markers, will be to better define ACS disease activity and to refine the risk stratification process, particularly by identifying ischemia without myocardial necrosis in ACS.

Multimarker approach
Combinations of biomarkers that complement each other in terms of their release curve improve the accuracy of the early detection of AMI, and so should reduce the delay to key interventions.[34–38] In addition, multimarkers are able to rapidly rule out AMI with a high negative predictive value.[35,37,39,40] The ability to safely and accurately exclude or "rule out" AMI improves the efficiency of a chest pain assessment unit and will allow earlier stress testing in the biomarker negative group, leading to a shorter hospital stay.

Delta troponin and ultrasensitive troponins
The use of delta troponin, the change in the troponin value over time, has improved the diagnostic accuracy for AMI.[41–43] Newer ultrasensitive troponin assays may be able to

utilize very low levels of detection, and employ a "delta approach" that measures change between initial and incremental levels at zero and from 2 to 6 hours after the onset of symptoms, or from hospital arrival.[44,45]

Unfortunately, the list of conditions other than myocardial ischemia associated with an elevated troponin continues to increase. Characteristic changes in troponin levels associated with many non-ACS related diagnoses such as PE and sepsis are not well defined. Thus, exquisitely sensitive assays may well produce their own problems in interpretation, in the light of the already long list of medical conditions associated with a raised troponin level even at currently agreed cut-off levels.[46] Particularly problematical will be if the newer ultrasensitive troponins are used indiscriminately, without careful consideration of need from the medical history and examination findings.

Newer Imaging Modalities

The choice of objective tests to identify ACS has expanded in recent times to include cardiac computed tomographic angiography (CCTA), plaque composition analysis, cardiac magnetic resonance imaging (CMRI), and positron emission tomography (PET) (**Box 3**).

Cardiac computed tomographic angiography
High-resolution CCTA offers noninvasive coronary angiography that may improve risk stratification, particularly in the intermediate-risk chest pain patient.[47] CCTA allows evaluation of global and regional left ventricular function comparable with CMRI,[48] and provides information about luminal narrowing and plaque composition. Several clinical and economic studies support the use of CCTA scanning to risk-stratify ED patients with ACS.[49–55] However, although radiation dose is an issue, CCTA when negative allows the definitive rule-out of coronary artery disease in the low- and intermediate-risk group.[51]

Plaque composition analysis
Plaque composition analysis may also prove of particular use in predicting significant ACS,[56] as these patients have more mixed and noncalcified plaques than patients with stable angina.[57,58] Outcome data on plaque analysis by CCTA are limited, but it may provide additional prognostic information for patients with possible ACS.

Alternatives to CCTA aimed at the early diagnosis of a "vulnerable" plaque include intravascular ultrasound (IVUS), palpography and virtual histology, optical coherence

---

Box 3
Newer imaging modalities to identify ACS

Cardiac computed tomographic angiography (CCTA)

"Vulnerable plaque" analysis:

    CCTA

    Intravascular ultrasound

    Palpography and virtual histology

    Optical coherence tomography

    Near-infrared spectroscopy

Cardiac magnetic resonance imaging

Positron emission tomography

tomography (OCT), and near-infrared spectroscopy[59] (see **Box 3**). However, there is at present little evidence that a local or regional therapeutic approach to asymptomatic "vulnerable" plaque reduces cardiac events compared with current optimal systemic therapy.[59]

Cardiac magnetic resonance imaging

CMRI is already established in the assessment of congenital heart disease, the great vessels, pericardial disease, and chronic coronary artery disease. CMRI also allows the assessment of a wide spectrum of causes of chest pain.[52] Although coronary anatomy imaging using coronary artery CMRI has been developed, few studies have assessed the clinical utility of CMRI for ACS in the ED setting.[60]

CMRI may be a useful alternative investigative pathway in view of its lack of radiation exposure. In addition, stress-CMRI using adenosine or dobutamine may help to predict significant coronary artery disease,[61,62] and may have a role in a select group of patients as an alternative noninvasive stress test.[63]

Positron emission tomography

As not all coronary stenoses detected by CCTA are flow limiting, additional noninvasive testing should be considered before cardiac catheterization. PET hybrid computed tomography (CT) devices allow integration of the structure and function of the heart.[64] Stress PET data may identify a hemodynamically significant stenosis, and when combined with the anatomic information from the CCTA helps guide revascularization decisions.[64,65] Again, further research is needed to define its exact role in the management of ACS in the ED setting, although access will remain limited for some time yet.

Risk Stratification Tools

Risk stratification tools are essential in determining pretest probability (PTP), as no single clinical feature or investigation result alone is diagnostic for acute coronary syndrome.[66] Accurate estimation of the PTP for ACS is fundamental to the appropriate use of resources. Several methods to determine pretest probability for ACS have been reported, including the physician's own estimate,[67] decision trees,[68] logistic regression,[69,70] attribute matching,[71,72] and computer-based artificial neural networks.[73]

Kline and colleagues[72] determined that in a population with a pretest probability of ACS of less than or equal to 2%, the risk of testing will exceed its benefits. Unnecessary investigations in this group are then averted as the person is already at a very low risk of ACS.[67]

PREtest ConsultACS

A computer-derived, quantitative pretest probability assessment derived from attribute matching has been developed for use in ACS, as well as in PE (see later discussion). PREtest ConsultACS (PREtest Consult Inc, Charlotte, NC) matches an 8-component clinical profile from any individual patient considered at risk of ACS with a prior reference database of 14,800 patients to allow an estimate of PTP probability. Those with a PTP of 2% or less, or "test negative," have a 45-day ACS outcome of just 0.3%.[74] Prospective validation in other non-US populations is in progress.

However, many models still focus on ruling in the diagnosis of AMI to facilitate the early and appropriate use of cardiology services, rather than excluding ACS by clearly identifying a rule-out population suitable for early ED discharge.[75,76] Thus the use of these tools is currently restricted by their heterogeneity and different end-point intention,[77] which emphasizes the importance of adopting a standardized data definitions set for use in ACS research. These standardized data definitions will ensure use of a common language and framework to maximize value when extrapolating research findings between different studies.[78]

Treatment Advances

Antiplatelet medication

Early diagnosis allows the earlier initiation of treatment for STEMIs and non-STEMIs, and improved outcomes. Antiplatelet medication is central to the treatment of ACS, such that aspirin is now widely used in virtually all patients with undifferentiated chest pain. This indiscriminate use of aspirin, despite significant benefit for those with ACS-related diagnoses, currently lacks validation but is assumed to be safe.

Clopidogrel is another common antiplatelet medication used with aspirin, but it shows variability in platelet inhibition.[79,80] Alternative dual antiplatelet treatment options include newer therapies such as prasugrel, which received Food and Drug Administration (FDA) approval in early 2009, and ticagrelor, both of which show improved platelet inhibition.[81–83] Ticagrelor is an oral, reversible, direct-acting inhibitor of adenosine diphosphate receptor P2Y12 that has rapid, pronounced platelet inhibition. Ticagrelor has the advantage of a survival benefit without an overall increased rate of major bleeding when compared with clopidogrel.[84]

The use of other platelet inhibitors such as the glycoprotein IIb/IIIa (GP IIb/IIIa) inhibitors in the setting of STEMI has shown variable changes in coronary artery patency.[85–87] While one small trial of prehospital treatment with a GP IIb/IIIa inhibitor has not shown clinical benefit,[88] a larger study is underway investigating the benefit of early GP IIb/IIIa inhibition prior to percutaneous coronary intervention (PCI) in the setting of non-ST elevation acute coronary syndrome (NSTEACS).[89]

Sonothrombolysis

Another emerging approach toward improving vessel patency is sonothrombolysis, using low-frequency ultrasound for thrombus dissolution. This technique may become a valuable noninvasive route to improve vessel patency with thrombolytic therapy in the large majority of patients unable to access timely percutaneous interventions.[90] Low-frequency ultrasound treatment increases tissue perfusion from coronary occlusion by thrombus dissolution.[91]

Stem cell transplantation

Finally, stem cell transplantation to improve the function of the injured myocardium is under investigation.[92] Intracoronary injection of mononuclear bone marrow cells in patients with a recent MI appears to be safe.[93] "Cellular cardiomyoplasty" trials administering intravenous allogenic human marrow stem cells (MSC) without immunosuppression to post-AMI patients are currently underway.[92]

FUTURE DEVELOPMENTS IN PULMONARY EMBOLISM

The decision whether to investigate a patient for a particular disease is a balance between the risks of harm from missing the diagnosis against the harm that might derive from the investigations themselves. Regarding PE, the threshold at which clinicians decide to commence investigating is dropping steadily,[94] and current strategies in the assessment of a patient with a suspected PE certainly have the potential to cause harm. This problem arises due to the widespread indiscriminate use of D-dimer testing, from fear of missing the diagnosis, which leads to increased diagnostic imaging by CT pulmonary angiogram (CTPA) subsequent to the high false-positive rate of the D-dimer assays. This in turn increases cost, causes delay with ED overcrowding, and exposes patients to the risks of unnecessary ionizing radiation and contrast nephropathy.

Similar to ACS, future developments in the assessment and management of patients presenting to the ED with chest pain suggestive of PE again include novel biomarkers, newer imaging techniques, risk stratification tools, and improved drugs. Additional strategies include percutaneous mechanical thrombectomy and reevaluation of the role of thrombolysis in submassive PE (**Box 4**).

Novel Pulmonary Embolism Biomarkers

Many novel biomarkers involved in inflammation, hemostasis, and vascular injury are under investigation to replace or supplement D-dimer testing in PE. Nordenholz and colleagues[95] investigated 50 potential biomarkers for their predictive value in 304 ED patients evaluated for PE, and found that only D-dimer, C-reactive protein, and MPO demonstrated sufficient diagnostic accuracy to support their use clinically, with areas under the receiver-operating characteristic (ROC) curve of greater than 0.75.

D-dimer testing using multiple rather than single cut-off levels

D-dimer testing in clinical practice is currently based on a single cut-off level for a positive and a negative result created using ROC curve analysis. Although this dichotomous approach makes the test result easy to interpret, it is oversimplistic and fails to indicate how far above or below the cut-off the test result actually lies. Linkins and colleagues[96] have suggested that the use of 3 probability-specific D-dimer cut-off points can exclude PE in a greater proportion of patients than using a single cut-off point, without sacrificing the negative predictive value.

Ischemia-modified albumin

While levels of ischemia-modified albumin are also being investigated for their diagnostic utility in ACS, a recent animal study has suggested that ischemia-modified albumin levels increase within 1 hour and up to the sixth hour post PE.[97] However, it is unclear how IMA might, if at all, usefully discriminate between different underlying causes in a patient with undifferentiated chest pain.

Growth arrest–specific gene 6

Growth arrest–specific gene 6 (Gas6) is a protein that is elevated during pulmonary or systemic infection, but not with PE. As D-dimer levels increase in all these conditions, the addition of Gas6 testing may help reduce the false-positive rate for PE, thereby increasing the specificity of the D-dimer test.[98]

Myeloperoxidase

MPO correlates with the presence of PE with an area under the ROC curve (AUC) of 0.78 compared with 0.93 for D-dimer, with a negative test helping rule out a PE.[95]

| Box 4 |
Future developments in patients with suspected PE
Novel biomarkers
Newer imaging techniques
Risk stratification tools
Improved therapeutic agents
Percutaneous mechanical thrombectomy
Reevaluation of role of thrombolysis in submassive PE

MPO may also have additional diagnostic utility again used in conjunction with D-dimer, as a combination approach reduces the high false-positive rate from using D-dimer alone.[99]

Tissue plasminogen activator and plasminogen activator inhibitor type 1

Once fibrin is formed in the thrombosis/fibrinolysis process, tissue plasminogen activator (tPA) activates plasminogen to plasmin to begin fibrin breakdown, with one of the subsequent breakdown products being D-dimer. This process is partly regulated by plasminogen activator inhibitor type 1 (PAI-1). Both tPA and PAI-1 are detectable in the circulation using an enzyme-linked immunosorbent assay once fibrinolytic system activation has occurred. Preliminary research has suggested very high sensitivity for tPA and PAI-1 in the detection of PE, but their clinical correlation is unclear.

Imaging

Various new imaging techniques are being investigated, including single photon emission computed tomography (SPECT) perfusion lung scan, magnetic resonance imaging angiography (MRA), and magnetic resonance venography of the veins of the thighs (MRV).

Single photon emission computed tomography perfusion lung scan

This nuclear medicine technique uses images in extra planes from a double- or triple-head camera, and has a better specificity than ventilation perfusion (VQ) planar scanning, with less scans reported as "indeterminate" or nondiagnostic.[100,101] At present there are relatively few published data on its clinical use.

Magnetic resonance imaging angiography

Experience with MRA is much more limited than for VQ and CTPA scanning. Therefore, MRA is usually restricted to patients with contraindications to conventional imaging. Gadolinium-enhanced angiography (Gd-MRA) has demonstrated a specificity for PE in the high ninety percent range, with a sensitivity ranging from 85% to 100%, although there is concern about the incidence of nephrogenic systemic fibrosis or nephrogenic fibrosing dermopathy (NSF/NFD) in patients given gadolinium contrast. The FDA is monitoring the situation especially in patients with moderate (glomerular filtration rate <60 mL/min) to severe renal disease. Alternative contrast techniques using contrast specifically targeting thrombus, such as iron oxide microparticles, single chain antibodies, and T1 bright methemoglobin, are under investigation.

PIOPED III

A prospective multicenter investigation known as Prospective Investigation of Pulmonary Embolism Diagnosis III (PIOPEDIII), to determine the diagnostic accuracy of Gd-MRA of the pulmonary arteries in combination with magnetic resonance venography of the veins of the thighs (MRV) in patients with clinically suspected acute PE, is currently underway.

The aim is to recruit around 1200 patients with suspected acute PE over a period of 2 years using composite reference standards to diagnose venous thromboembolism (VTE) and exclude PE. All patients with PE and a matched group without PE will undergo Gd-MRA/MRV. This combination technique could eliminate the need for iodinated contrast material and ionizing radiation in the estimated 24% of patients with suspected PE, who have relative contraindications such as renal impairment, allergy, and pregnancy.[102]

ThromboView

ThromboView (Agen Biomedical, Brisbane, Australia) consists of ^{99m}Tc-labeled deimmunized anticrosslinked fibrin (anti–D-dimer) Fab′ fragments with a high affinity and a high specificity for D-dimer given intravenously. ThromboView is under investigation as a diagnostic tool for thromboembolic events such as PE detected by SPECT. ThromboView may be superior to conventional imaging by selectively disclosing acute thrombi, as it is able to distinguish between a fresh thrombus and other filling defects within the pulmonary arteries.[103,104] A recent phase 2 study showed only comparable sensitivity and specificity to CTPA for PE. Phase 3 trials are in progress.

Decision Analysis Risk Stratification

Various new techniques are being used to provide an actual point-estimate of PTP of PE, over and above the physician's usual unstructured Gestalt estimate, assisted by validated scoring systems such as the Canadian (Wells) or Geneva scores. These methods include a back-transformed logistic regression equation, and nonlinear models such as artificial intelligence or Bayesian Network analysis.[105–107]

Probability Software Database Tools

PREtest ConsultPE (PREtest Consult Inc, Charlotte, NC) is a novel computerized method of pretest probability assessment derived from a process called attribute matching. The assessment requires the clinician to enter 10 predictor variables into a computer program (age, ± pleuritic chest pain, ± dyspnea, pulse oximetry reading, heart rate, ± prior VTE, ± recent surgery or trauma, ± estrogen use, ± hemoptysis, ± unilateral leg swelling).

Attribute matching works by a selection process whereby a computer algorithm compares the results of all 10 predictor variables obtained from the patient being evaluated to a library of 12,595 research patients previously evaluated for PE compiled from multiple hospitals. The algorithm returns only the "matched" patients who share the same profile of predictor variables as the patient under consideration. The algorithm then reports the proportion of patients with disease in this matched sample as a pretest probability, that is, the number of diseased patients divided by the total number of patients who fit the profile (**Fig. 2**).

The utility of PREtest ConsultPE includes 2 discrete steps. The clinician assesses the pretest probability of PE using a validated tool, and if the probability is low enough, no further testing is warranted. Other decision rules such as the "Charlotte Rule" were derived to allow the exclusion of a PE, but those exclusion criteria function in an "all or none" way without allowing integration into a continuum of testing available with PREtest ConsultPE.[108,109]

The "test threshold" for PE has previously been estimated at 2%,[95,104,105] which is the pretest probability that should be exceeded to justify the need for diagnostic testing. Prospectively, the summary 45-day outcome rate has been found to be 0.7% for the whole subgroup of patients with a PTP between zero and 2%. Although local standards may vary, the 1% threshold probably represents a reasonable international threshold to exclude PE.[72,108,110,111] Therefore, if the patient's pretest probability is zero to 2%, the risks inherent in further evaluation secondary to unwarranted treatment in the event of a false-positive test result outweigh the risks of the PE. Thus a patient with a quantitative PTP of 2% or less for PE does not need a D-dimer, or a CTPA, or any other pulmonary vascular imaging study, saving time, cost, and risk.

Moreover, those patients with a PTP of more than 2% may still be able to avoid exposure to unnecessary ionizing radiation by next adding biomarker testing to then

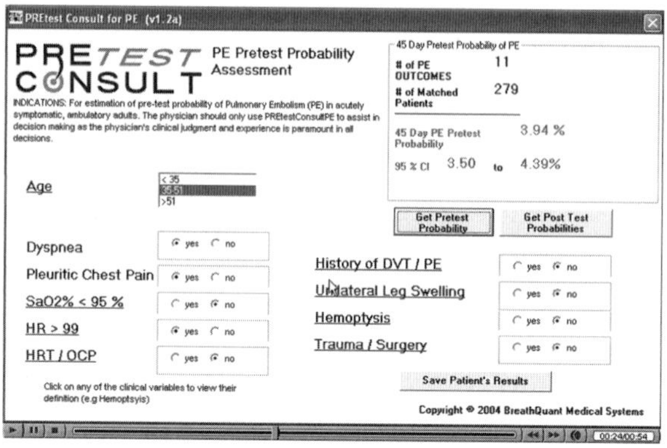

Fig. 2. Computer screen shot of the attribute matching PE computer interface. (*Courtesy of* PREtest Consult Inc, Charlotte, NC, USA; with permission.)

produce a posttest probability again below 1% (**Fig. 3**, shaded rectangle). Knowing that quantitative immunoturbidimetric or enzyme-linked colorimetric D-dimer assays demonstrate a LR(−) = 0.10 to 0.15 for the diagnosis of PE,[112–114] a pretest probability of PE less than 7.5% followed by a negative D-dimer test result of less than 500 ng/mL then produces a posttest probability less than 1%. Once again, this rules out a PE without the need for any imaging.

Improvements in Therapeutic Agents

Several new therapeutic agents, including parenteral and oral anticoagulants, have been studied.

Parenteral anticoagulants

Idraparinux is derived from fondaparinux, and binds to antithrombin with such high affinity that its half-life is comparable to that of antithrombin itself. The advantage of idraparinux is that it may be given by subcutaneous injection once weekly, and does not require coagulation monitoring. However, it must be used with caution in patients with renal insufficiency as it is excreted via the kidneys, and is contraindicated in patients with a creatinine clearance of less than 30 mL/min. Protamine sulfate, used to counteract heparin, does not reverse the anticoagulant effects of idraparinux.

SSR 126517 shares the pharmacologic features of idraparinux, but with the advantage that its anticoagulant effect is reversed by giving intravenous avidin, a tetrameric glycoprotein.

Oral anticoagulants

Warfarin Warfarin is currently the only orally available drug for long-term anticoagulation. Several problems make warfarin a difficult drug to use for physicians and patients alike; these include a narrow therapeutic margin, delayed onset of action, difficulty with reversal, many interactions with drugs and diet, a wide variation in anticoagulant effect, and the need for frequent laboratory monitoring. These problems may lead to recurrent thrombosis from undertreatment or to excessive bleeding with overtreatment. Bleeding complications with warfarin are among the most frequent adverse drug effects, with the risk of major bleeding between 1% and 5% per year. Therefore, there is an ongoing search for a replacement for warfarin for oral anticoagulation. Newer oral agents with fewer side effects than warfarin have undergone trials in VTE prevention, but treatment trials currently are limited and are usually restricted

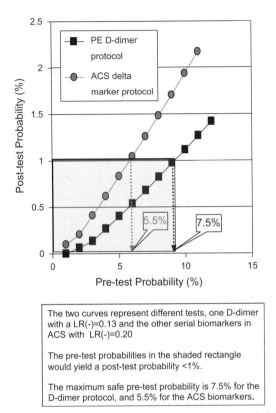

The two curves represent different tests, one D-dimer with a LR(-)=0.13 and the other serial biomarkers in ACS with LR(-)=0.20

The pre-test probabilities in the shaded rectangle would yield a post-test probability <1%.

The maximum safe pre-test probability is 7.5% for the D-dimer protocol, and 5.5% for the ACS biomarkers.

Fig. 3. Plot of pretest probability on the X-axis and the post-test probability on the Y-axis, for different tests (D-dimer and acute coronary syndrome [ACS] delta), with different odds ratios. The *shaded rectangle* represents a posttest probability of less than 1%. (*Courtesy of* PREtest Consult Inc, Charlotte, NC, USA; with permission.)

to therapy for deep venous thrombosis (DVT). These agents include dabigatran etexilate, rivaroxaban, and apixaban.

Dabigatran etexilate, rivaroxaban, and apixaban Dabigatran etexilate is an oral small molecule prodrug that acts as a thrombin inhibitor, whose absorption is pH sensitive and is reduced by around 30% by PPIs. Effective doses of dabigatran etexilate are relatively high, and it is contraindicated in patients with renal failure because it is excreted via the kidneys. Rivaroxaban selectively inhibits factor Xa and is administered orally, with 80% bioavailability. Dabigatran etexilate must also be used cautiously in patients with renal insufficiency or in patients with severe liver disease, and is monitored by Factor Xa inhibition. Finally, apixaban is an orally administered selective inhibitor of factor Xa that can be monitored using a factor Xa inhibition assay or a diluted prothrombin time.

It is hoped that these agents will provide a better therapeutic window and easier monitoring, and may be simpler to reverse in an emergency, making them more convenient and safer to use than warfarin.

Percutaneous mechanical thrombectomy

Percutaneous mechanical thrombectomy (PMT) by mechanical fragmentation and thrombus aspiration is a novel approach that may benefit patients with massive PE and right ventricular dysfunction. Patients who may particularly benefit would be those with major contraindications to thrombolysis, those at an increased bleeding risk, those who have failed thrombolysis, or when surgical thrombectomy is unavailable. Clot is fragmented via catheterization, and the fragments removed via an internal aspirator.[115]

Thrombolysis for pulmonary embolism

Although meta-analysis has shown no benefit for thrombolysis in patients with PE without shock,[116] these patients have significant morbidity at 6-month follow-up, with a 41% rate of cardiopulmonary problems, either right ventricular dysfunction on echo, heart failure (New York Heart Association score >I), or a 6-minute walk distance (6MWD) of less than 330 m.[117]

The Pulmonary Embolism Thrombolysis (PEITHO) study being conducted in Europe is seeking to demonstrate whether thrombolysis with tenecteplase plus standard anti-coagulation improves the outcome of patients presenting with high-risk submassive acute PE, when compared with standard anticoagulation alone. At present around one-third of the target of 1000 patients have been recruited.

FUTURE DEVELOPMENTS IN ACUTE AORTIC DISSECTION

AAD is one of the most common catastrophes of the aorta, classically affecting men 50 to 70 years old with hypertension, with sudden severe chest or back pain and a myriad of other possible symptoms and signs. AAD is time-critical and rapidly fatal if left untreated, particularly for ascending type A dissections.[118]

Future developments in the assessment and management of patients with AAD presenting to the ED with chest pain will once again include novel biomarkers, plus newer imaging techniques such as contrast-enhanced ultrasound, endovascular treatment, and combined interventional and surgical treatment (**Box 5**).

Novel Acute Aortic Dissection Biomarkers

Serum smooth muscle myosin heavy chain, calponin, D-dimer, and serum-soluble elastin fragments are promising tests to help rule in or rule out the diagnosis of AAD.[119,120]

Serum smooth muscle myosin heavy chain

Serum smooth muscle myosin heavy chain is specific for damage to the smooth muscle of the arterial wall, with diagnostic studies yielding a sensitivity of 90.9% and a specificity of 98% within 3 hours of symptom onset of suspected AAD, particularly with proximal lesions.[121]

Calponin

Likewise, immunoassays against basic and acidic calponin, the troponin-like protein of smooth muscle, have shown potential to detect AAD in the first 6 to 24 hours.

Box 5
Future developments in patients with suspected AAD

Novel biomarkers

Contrast-enhanced ultrasound

Endovascular treatment

Combined interventional and surgical treatment

The moderate sensitivity and specificity suggest that technical improvements in the assay are still necessary before firm recommendations on its use can be made.[122]

D-dimer

D-dimer has been used for many years when negative to rule out thromboembolic diseases such as DVT and PE. A recent Austrian study supports the routine measurement of D-dimer to exclude AAD, with 100% negative predictive value for a cut-off level of 0.1 μg/mL.[123] However, the optimal cut-off value for its clinical use is still disputed.[124]

International Registry of Acute Aortic Dissection data on D-dimer

Investigators from the International Registry of Acute Aortic Dissection (IRAD) have just published a substudy on biomarkers (IRAD-Bio) focusing on D-dimer[119] in AAD. Although small, the study was one of the largest collections of proven AAD patients within a prospectively enrolled cohort of 87 positives out of 220 patients with suspected AAD. At the widely used D-dimer cut-off level of 500 ng/mL, a negative D-dimer had a sensitivity of 95.7% within 6 hours of the onset of symptoms. In addition, the investigators also noted that D-dimer was markedly elevated in AAD and suggested that using a D-dimer of 1600 ng/mL or more was useful as a "rule-in" cut-off to identify patients with a high probability of AAD. However, the diagnostic accuracy among patients with AAD is dependent on the type, extent, and the time from presentation.

Serum-soluble elastin fragments

Although the structural protein serum-soluble elastin fragments begins to leak from the aorta during the aging process, acute aortic injury causes serum levels to elevate sharply. Testing has shown early promise with a high predictive value, but as the test takes up to 3 hours to perform it is likely to be unacceptable given the urgency of the condition.

Contrast-Enhanced Ultrasound

Contrast-enhanced ultrasound (CEUS) involves introducing gas-filled microbubbles into the circulation to provide strong contrast on ultrasonography. These microbubbles can be modified to target certain tissue types, such as inflamed blood vessels, allowing CEUS to evaluate abdominal aortic dissection, particularly in patients with contraindications to CT contrast agents such as renal failure or severe allergy. CEUS may allow a more rapid and noninvasive diagnosis, especially in critical patients from intensive care units, because of its bedside availability. As the examination is dynamic, additional information about blood flow in the true and false lumen and about renal perfusion after dissection can be obtained. Thus CEUS may provide a good alternative to multislice CTA.[125]

Endovascular Treatment

Stanford type B aortic dissections confined to the descending, distal aorta have traditionally been managed medically, but this is changing with the advent of endovascular stenting with careful patient selection. Recent generations of stent grafts are able to avoid many of the earlier stent complications such as stroke, penetration of the aorta, graft collapse, leak, migration, or aneurysm extension, although evidence of longer term durability is unclear.[124]

One remaining concern is the radiation exposure of regular CT imaging of stents needed to ensure their integrity and placement, particularly in younger patients.[126]

Combined Interventional and Surgical Treatment

The combination of surgical aortic reconstruction with endovascular stent grafting has been shown to simplify type A aortic dissection management, reduce the circulatory arrest time, reduce the risk of surgical complications, and reduce the need for subsequent surgery on the descending aorta. Again, the long-term effectiveness has not been studied.[127]

Triple Rule-Out Scan

CTA is the imaging modality of choice in the investigation of both PE and AAD. Now that CCTA is becoming established, some have suggested using a modified scanner protocol aimed at simultaneously investigating for all 3 of PE, AAD, and coronary artery disease, known as the "triple rule-out scan."

Previously, such scans were precluded as patients would have had to hold their breath for longer than 30 seconds to obtain adequate images from the lung apices to the diaphragm in older generation scanners. The advent of 64- and 128-slice CT scanners allows a faster scanning process and reduced movement artifact. Technical challenges still remain, in particular achieving consistent high levels of contrast intensity in all 3 vascular zones. Also, it is difficult to simultaneously image segmental pulmonary arteries and the distal coronary arteries supplied by the right and left ventricles, respectively.

A saline bolus to flush contrast out of the right side of the heart is used to obtain high and consistent visualization of the coronary arteries with minimal right heart enhancement in CCTA, whereas CTPA protocols are designed to achieve maximal enhancement of the pulmonary arteries and the right side of the heart. Therefore, triple rule-out scans require precise harmonization of contrast injection and imaging sequences.[128]

Radiation dosage issues

The exact radiation dose to the patient from a triple rule-out scan appears to be highly variable, depending on the scanner protocol used. For instance, the effective radiation dose can be reduced by more than 50% to 8.75 ± 2.64 mSv with ECG-based tube current modulation without loss of image quality.[129] As traditional imaging studies for ACS and PE involve a chest radiation dosage as low as 5 mSv or less, this still represents a significant step up, so poor patient selection and indiscriminate use of the triple rule-out scan would have significant radiation exposure issues.

As scanner technology and contrast protocols improve, the challenge for clinical leaders will be how to focus triple rule-out scan use to avoid spiraling costs and excessive patient radiation exposure.

FUTURE DEVELOPMENTS IN GASTROINTESTINAL DISEASE

GERD is the most common cause of esophageal chest pain, although the majority (60%) of patients have no evidence of erosive esophagitis at conventional endoscopy. Such nonerosive reflux disease (NERD) by definition should still respond to acid suppression therapy such as a PPI, albeit with a lower response rate than in erosive GERD.[130]

Novel Endoscopic Techniques

Novel alternative upper gastrointestinal endoscopy techniques are available to demonstrate subtle submucosal abnormalities such as chromoendoscopy with Lugol iodine, confocal endomicroscopy, or narrow band imaging in conjunction with zoom magnification.[130] Their exact indication is unclear, as is the role of 24-hour pH and impedance monitoring in NERD.

In addition, finding an objective marker to differentiate NERD from functional heartburn might better guide empirical therapy, as the latter is a symptom complex unrelated to the reflux of gastric contents with no correlation of symptoms with acid reflux exposure.[130]

Non-GERD–Related Esophageal Chest Pain

A large variety of therapies has been tried for non-GERD–related functional esophageal chest pain among patients with NCCP. Such treatment includes anticholinergics and muscle relaxants, botulinum toxin, psychotropic medications, cognitive-behavioral therapy, and surgery.[131]

Trials of novel visceral sensitivity modifying agents for presumed visceral hyperalgesia as a cause of NCCP, including theophylline, cilansetron (a $5\text{-}HT_3$ antagonist), tegaserod (a partial $5\text{-}HT_4$ agonist), octreotide, and fedotozine (a peripherally acting κ-opioid agonist), may demonstrate a cornerstone role, alone or in combination with a PPI.[1]

FUTURE DEVELOPMENTS IN MUSCULOSKELETAL CHEST PAIN

A careful history and examination by palpation or pressure should suggest a musculoskeletal cause for NCCP, although this does not per se rule out a more serious cardiac cause, as they may coexist.[132] Clinical predictors of musculoskeletal chest pain, including response to manual therapy, are currently under investigation for patients presenting with acute chest pain.[133]

The role of radiological examination including MRI in musculoskeletal NCCP remains unproven, and newer imaging modalities are unlikely to ever be cost effective compared with focusing on understanding better the underlying mechanisms such as spinal referred pain.[134]

SUMMARY

Future developments in the assessment and management of patients with ACS presenting to the ED with chest pain will include improved ECG analysis, novel biomarkers, newer imaging techniques, risk stratification tools, improved drugs, sonothrombolysis, and stem cell transplantation.

Similarly, developments in patients presenting to the ED with chest pain suggesting a PE will include novel biomarkers, newer imaging techniques, risk stratification tools, and safer drugs. Additional strategies may include PMT and reevaluation of the role of thrombolysis in submassive PE.

Developments for patients with suspected AAD presenting to the ED with chest pain will again include novel biomarkers, plus newer imaging techniques such as CEUS, endovascular treatment, and combined interventional and surgical treatment.

Developments in the treatment of gastrointestinal disease will include alternative endoscopic techniques, methods to differentiate non-GERD causes for pain, better recognition of functional heartburn, and validating new treatment modalities such as medication, cognitive-behavioral therapy, and surgery. Finally, developments in musculoskeletal chest pain will focus on a greater understanding of underlying mechanisms and the role, if any, of newer imaging techniques.

Most research on chest pain patients is thus focused on advances in the diagnosis and management of ACS, PE, and AAD, despite there being no significant difference at 4 years in mortality, ongoing chest pain, and quality of life between patients presenting to the ED with NCCP as opposed to cardiac chest pain. In addition, NCCP patients significantly outnumber patients presenting with an underlying cardiac cause, particularly to the primary care physician.

REFERENCES

1. Eslick GD, Coulshed DS, Talley NJ. Diagnosis and treatment of noncardiac chest pain. Nat Rev Gastroenterol Hepatol 2005;2:463–72.
2. Eslick GD, Talley NJ. Natural history and predictors of outcome for non-cardiac chest pain: a prospective 4-year cohort study. Neurogastroenterol Motil 2008; 20(9):989–97.
3. Miller TD, Christian TF, Hopfenspirger MR, et al. Infarct size after acute myocardial infarction measured by quantitative tomographic 99mTc sestamibi imaging predicts subsequent mortality. Circulation 1995;92(3):334–41.
4. Pfeffer MA, Braunwald E. Ventricular remodeling after myocardial infarction. Experimental observations and clinical implications. Circulation 1990;81(4): 1161–72.
5. Storrow AB, Gibler WB. Chest pain centers: diagnosis of acute coronary syndromes. Ann Emerg Med 2000;35(5):449–61.
6. Pilote L, Granger C, Armstrong PW, et al. Differences in the treatment of myocardial infarction between the United States and Canada. A survey of physicians in the GUSTO trial. Med Care 1995;33(6):598–610.
7. Graff LG, Dallara J, Ross MA, et al. Impact on the care of the emergency department chest pain patient from the chest pain evaluation registry (CHEPER) study. Am J Cardiol 1997;80(5):563–8.
8. Pope JH, Aufderheide TP, Ruthazer R, et al. Missed diagnoses of acute cardiac ischemia in the emergency department. N Engl J Med 2000;342(16):1163–70.
9. Terkelsen CJ, Lassen JF, Norgaard BL, et al. Reduction of treatment delay in patients with ST-elevation myocardial infarction: impact of pre-hospital diagnosis and direct referral to primary percutanous coronary intervention. Eur Heart J 2005; 26(8):770–7.
10. Ortolani P, Marzocchi A, Marrozzini C, et al. Clinical impact of direct referral to primary percutaneous coronary intervention following pre-hospital diagnosis of ST-elevation myocardial infarction. Eur Heart J 2006;27(13):1550–7.
11. Zanini R, Aroldi M, Bonatti S, et al. Impact of prehospital diagnosis in the management of ST elevation myocardial infarction in the era of primary percutaneous coronary intervention: reduction of treatment delay and mortality. J Cardiovasc Med 2008;9(6):570–5.
12. Hailer B, Naber CK, Koslowski B, et al. [STEMI network Essen—results after 1 year]. Herz 2008;33(2):153–7 [in German].
13. Indications for fibrinolytic therapy in suspected acute myocardial infarction: collaborative overview of early mortality and major morbidity results from all randomised trials of more than 1000 patients. Fibrinolytic Therapy Trialists' (FTT) Collaborative Group. Lancet 1994;343(8893):311–22.
14. Boersma E, Maas AC, Deckers JW, et al. Early thrombolytic treatment in acute myocardial infarction: reappraisal of the golden hour. Lancet 1996;348(9030): 771–5.
15. Cannon CP, Gibson CM, Lambrew CT, et al. Relationship of symptom-onset-to-balloon time and door-to-balloon time with mortality in patients undergoing angioplasty for acute myocardial infarction. JAMA 2000;283(22):2941–7.
16. Self WH, Mattu A, Martin M, et al. Body surface mapping in the ED evaluation of the patient with chest pain: use of the 80-lead electrocardiogram system. Am J Emerg Med 2006;24(1):87–112.

17. Menown IB, Allen J, Anderson JM, et al. Early diagnosis of right ventricular or posterior infarction associated with inferior wall left ventricular acute myocardial infarction. Am J Cardiol 2000;85(8):934–8.
18. Kornreich F, Montague TJ, Rautaharju PM. Body surface potential mapping of ST segment changes in acute myocardial infarction. Implications for ECG enrollment criteria for thrombolytic therapy. Circulation 1993;87(3):773–82.
19. Owens C, McClelland A, Walsh S, et al. Comparison of value of leads from body surface maps to 12-lead electrocardiogram for diagnosis of acute myocardial infarction. Am J Cardiol 2008;102(3):257–65.
20. Menown IB, Allen J, Anderson JM, et al. ST depression only on the initial 12-lead ECG: early diagnosis of acute myocardial infarction. Eur Heart J 2001;22(3): 218–27.
21. Owens CG, McClelland AJ, Walsh SJ, et al. Prehospital 80-LAD mapping: does it add significantly to the diagnosis of acute coronary syndromes? J Electrocardiology 2004;37(Suppl):223–32.
22. Carley SD, Jenkins M, Mackway Jones K. Body surface mapping versus the standard 12 lead ECG in the detection of myocardial infarction amongst emergency department patients: a Bayesian approach. Resuscitation 2005;64(3): 309–14.
23. Abboud S, Zlochiver S. High-frequency QRS electrocardiogram for diagnosing and monitoring ischemic heart disease. J Electrocardiology 2006;39(1):82–6.
24. Tragardh E, Schlegel TT. High-frequency QRS electrocardiogram. Clin Physiol Funct Imaging 2007;27(4):197–204.
25. Thygesen K, Alpert JS, White HD, et al. Universal definition of myocardial infarction. Circulation 2007;116(22):2634–53.
26. Apple FS, Wu AH, Mair J, et al. Future biomarkers for detection of ischemia and risk stratification in acute coronary syndrome. Clin Chem 2005;51(5):810–24.
27. Wood FO, de Lemos JA, Wood FO, et al. Sorting through new biomarkers. Curr Cardiol Rep 2008;10(4):319–26.
28. Steg PG, FitzGerald G, Fox KA, et al. Risk stratification in non-ST-segment elevation acute coronary syndromes: troponin alone is not enough. Am J Med 2009; 122(2):107–8.
29. Reichlin T, Hochholzer W, Stelzig C, et al. Incremental value of copeptin for rapid rule out of acute myocardial infarction. J Am Coll Cardiol 2009;54(1):60–8.
30. Brennan ML, Penn MS, Van Lente F, et al. Prognostic value of myeloperoxidase in patients with chest pain. N Engl J Med 2003;349(17):1595–604.
31. Jaffe AS, Babuin L, Apple FS. Biomarkers in acute cardiac disease: the present and the future. J Am Coll Cardiol 2006;48(1):1–11.
32. Wu AH. Markers for early detection of cardiac diseases. Scand J Clin Lab Invest Suppl 2005;240:112–21.
33. Ilva T, Lund J, Porela P, et al. Early markers of myocardial injury: cTnl is enough. Clinica Chimica Acta 2009;400(1–2):82–5.
34. Rathore S, Knowles P, Mann AP, et al. Is it safe to discharge patients from accident and emergency using a rapid point of care Triple Cardiac Marker test to rule out acute coronary syndrome in low to intermediate risk patients presenting with chest pain? Eur J Intern Med 2008;19(7):537–40.
35. Ng SM, Krishnaswamy P, Morissey R, et al. Ninety-minute accelerated critical pathway for chest pain evaluation. Am J Cardiol 2001;88(6):611–7.
36. Kontos MC, Anderson FP, Hanbury CM, et al. Use of the combination of myoglobin and CK-MB mass for the rapid diagnosis of acute myocardial infarction. Am J Emerg Med 1997;15(1):14–9.

37. McCord J, Nowak RM, McCullough PA, et al. Ninety-minute exclusion of acute myocardial infarction by use of quantitative point-of-care testing of myoglobin and troponin I. Circulation 2001;104(13):1483–8.
38. Dadkhah S, Sharain K, Sharain R, et al. The value of bedside cardiac multibio-marker assay in rapid and accurate diagnosis of acute coronary syndromes. A Journal of Evidence-Based Medicine. Crit Pathw Cardiol 2007;6(2):76–84.
39. Straface AL, Myers JH, Kirchick HJ, et al. A rapid point-of-care cardiac marker testing strategy facilitates the rapid diagnosis and management of chest pain patients in the emergency department. Am J Clin Pathol 2008;129(5):788–95.
40. Newby LK, Storrow AB, Gibler WB, et al. Bedside multimarker testing for risk stratification in chest pain units: The chest pain evaluation by creatine kinase-MB, myoglobin, and troponin I (CHECKMATE) study. Circulation 2001;103(14): 1832–7.
41. Apple FS, Jesse RL, Newby LK, et al. National Academy of Clinical Biochemistry and IFCC Committee for Standardization of Markers of Cardiac Damage Laboratory Medicine Practice Guidelines: analytical issues for biochemical markers of acute coronary syndromes. Circulation 2007;115(13):e352–5.
42. Apple FS, Pearce LA, Smith SW, et al. Role of monitoring changes in sensitive cardiac troponin I assay results for early diagnosis of myocardial infarction and prediction of risk of adverse events. Clin Chem 2009;55(5):930–7.
43. Macrae AR, Kavsak PA, Lustig V, et al. Assessing the requirement for the 6-hour interval between specimens in the American Heart Association Classification of Myocardial Infarction in Epidemiology and Clinical Research Studies. Clin Chem 2006;52(5):812–8.
44. Fesmire FM, Fesmire CE, Fesmire FM, et al. Improved identification of acute coronary syndromes with second generation cardiac troponin I assay: utility of 2-hour delta cTnI > or = +0.02 ng/mL. J Emerg Med 2002;22(2):147–52.
45. Apple FS, Smith SW, Pearce LA, et al. Use of the bioMerieux VIDAS troponin I ultra assay for the diagnosis of myocardial infarction and detection of adverse events in patients presenting with symptoms suggestive of acute coronary syndrome. Clin Chim Acta 2008;390(1–2):72–5.
46. Gupta S, de Lemos JA. Use and misuse of cardiac troponins in clinical practice. Prog Cardiovasc Dis 2007;50(2):151–65.
47. Budoff MJ, Achenbach S, Blumenthal RS, et al. Assessment of coronary artery disease by cardiac computed tomography: a scientific statement from the American Heart Association Committee on Cardiovascular Imaging and Intervention, Council on Cardiovascular Radiology and Intervention, and Committee on Cardiac Imaging, Council on Clinical Cardiology. Circulation 2006;114(16): 1761–91.
48. Raman SV, Shah M, McCarthy B, et al. Multi-detector row cardiac computed tomography accurately quantifies right and left ventricular size and function compared with cardiac magnetic resonance. Am Heart J 2006;151(3):736–44.
49. Rubinshtein R, Halon DA, Gaspar T, et al. Usefulness of 64-slice cardiac computed tomographic angiography for diagnosing acute coronary syndromes and predicting clinical outcome in emergency department patients with chest pain of uncertain origin. Circulation 2007;115(13):1762–8.
50. Rubinshtein R, Halon DA, Gaspar T, et al. Usefulness of 64-slice multidetector computed tomography in diagnostic triage of patients with chest pain and negative or nondiagnostic exercise treadmill test result. Am J Cardiol 2007;99(7): 925–9.

51. Hollander JE, Chang AM, Shofer FS, et al. Coronary computed tomographic angiography for rapid discharge of low-risk patients with potential acute coronary syndromes. Ann Emerg Med 2009;53(3):295–304.

52. Hollander JE, Litt HI, Chase M, et al. Computed tomography coronary angiography for rapid disposition of low-risk emergency department patients with chest pain syndromes. Acad Emerg Med 2007;14(2):112–6.

53. Hoffmann U, Bamberg F, Chae CU, et al. Coronary computed tomography angiography for early triage of patients with acute chest pain: the ROMICAT (Rule Out Myocardial Infarction using Computer Assisted Tomography) trial. J Am Coll Cardiol 2009;53(18):1642–50.

54. Gallagher MJ, Raff GL. Use of multislice CT for the evaluation of emergency room patients with chest pain: the so-called "triple rule-out". Catheter Cardiovasc Interv 2008;71(1):92–9.

55. Gallagher MJ, Ross MA, Raff GL, et al. The diagnostic accuracy of 64-slice computed tomography coronary angiography compared with stress nuclear imaging in emergency department low-risk chest pain patients. Ann Emerg Med 2007;49(2):125–36.

56. Cury RC, Feutchner G, Pena CS, et al. Acute chest pain imaging in the emergency department with cardiac computed tomography angiography. J Nucl Cardiol 2008;15(4):564–75.

57. Hoffmann U, Moselewski F, Nieman K, et al. Noninvasive assessment of plaque morphology and composition in culprit and stable lesions in acute coronary syndrome and stable lesions in stable angina by multidetector computed tomography. J Am Coll Cardiol 2006;47(8):1655–62.

58. Motoyama S, Kondo T, Sarai M, et al. Multislice computed tomographic characteristics of coronary lesions in acute coronary syndromes. J Am Coll Cardiol 2007;50(4):319–26.

59. Ambrose JA. In search of the "vulnerable plaque": can it be localized and will focal regional therapy ever be an option for cardiac prevention? J Am Coll Cardiol 2008;51(16):1539–42.

60. Salah A, Moliterno DJ, Humphries R, et al. Role of cardiac computed tomography and magnetic resonance imaging in the evaluation of acute chest pain in the emergency department. Int J Cardiovasc Imaging 2008;24(3):331–42.

61. Ingkanisorn WP, Kwong RY, Bohme NS, et al. Prognosis of negative adenosine stress magnetic resonance in patients presenting to an emergency department with chest pain. J Am Coll Cardiol 2006;47(7):1427–32.

62. Di Cesare E, Battisti S, Riva A, et al. Parallel imaging and dobutamine stress magnetic resonance imaging in patients with atypical chest pain or equivocal ECG not suitable for stress echocardiography. Radiol Med 2009;114(2):216–28.

63. Lockie T, Nagel E, Redwood S, et al. Use of cardiovascular magnetic resonance imaging in acute coronary syndromes. Circulation 2009;119(12):1671–81.

64. Di Carli MF, Dorbala S. Cardiac PET-CT. J Thorac Imaging 2007;22(1):101–6.

65. Di Carli MF, Dorbala S, Hachamovitch R. Integrated cardiac PET-CT for the diagnosis and management of CAD. J Nucl Cardiol 2006;13(2):139–44.

66. Bassand JP, Hamm CW, Ardissino D, et al. Guidelines for the diagnosis and treatment of non-ST-segment elevation acute coronary syndromes. Eur Heart J 2007;28(13):1598–660.

67. Kline JA, Zeitouni RA, Hernandez-Nino J, et al. Randomized trial of computer-ized quantitative pretest probability in low-risk chest pain patients: effect on safety and resource use. Ann Emerg Med 2009;53(6):727–35 e1.

68. Goldman L, Weinberg M, Weisberg M, et al. A computer-derived protocol to aid in the diagnosis of emergency room patients with acute chest pain. N Engl J Med 1982;307(10):588–96.

69. Selker HP, Beshansky JR, Griffith JL, et al. Use of the acute cardiac ischemia time-insensitive predictive instrument (ACI-TIPI) to assist with triage of patients with chest pain or other symptoms suggestive of acute cardiac ischemia. A multicenter, controlled clinical trial. Ann Intern Med 1998;129(11):845–55.

70. Kennedy RL, Burton AM, Fraser HS, et al. Early diagnosis of acute myocardial infarction using clinical and electrocardiographic data at presentation: deriva-tion and evaluation of logistic regression models. Eur Heart J 1996;17(8): 1181–91.

71. Mitchell AM, Garvey JL, Chandra A, et al. Prospective multicenter study of quan-titative pretest probability assessment to exclude acute coronary syndrome for patients evaluated in emergency department chest pain units. Ann Emerg Med 2006;47(5):447.

72. Kline JA, Johnson CL, Pollack CV Jr, et al. Pretest probability assessment derived from attribute matching. BMC Med Inform Decis Mak 2005;5:26.

73. Harrison RF, Kennedy RL. Artificial neural network models for prediction of acute coronary syndromes using clinical data from the time of presentation. Ann Emerg Med 2005;46(5):431–9.

74. Kline J. Randomized trial of pretest probability in low risk patients with chest pain. Ann Emerg Med 2007;50:S78.

75. Goldman L, Cook EF, Johnson PA, et al. Prediction of the need for intensive care in patients who come to the emergency departments with acute chest pain. N Engl J Med 1996;334(23):1498–504.

76. Antman EM, Cohen M, Bernink PJ, et al. The TIMI risk score for unstable angina/non-ST elevation MI: A method for prognostication and therapeutic decision making. JAMA 2000;284(7):835–42.

77. Hess EP, Thiruganasambandamoorthy V, Wells GA, et al. Diagnostic accuracy of clinical prediction rules to exclude acute coronary syndrome in the emergency department setting: a systematic review. CJEM 2008;10(4):373–82.

78. Cullen L, Than M, Brown AFT, et al. Comprehensive standardised data defini-tions for acute coronary syndrome research in emergency departments in Aus-tralasia. Emerg Med Australas 2010;22:35–55.

79. Gurbel PA, Bliden KP, Hiatt BL, et al. Clopidogrel for coronary stenting: response variability, drug resistance, and the effect of pretreatment platelet reactivity. Circulation 2003;107(23):2908–13.

80. Lau WC, Gurbel PA, Watkins PB, et al. Contribution of hepatic cytochrome P450 3A4 metabolic activity to the phenomenon of clopidogrel resistance. Circulation 2004;109(2):166–71.

81. Morrow DA, Wiviott SD, White HD, et al. Effect of the novel thienopyridine prasu-grel compared with clopidogrel on spontaneous and procedural myocardial infarction in the Trial to Assess Improvement in Therapeutic Outcomes by Opti-mizing Platelet Inhibition with Prasugrel-Thrombolysis in Myocardial Infarction 38: an application of the classification system from the universal definition of myocardial infarction. Circulation 2009;119(21):2758–64.

82. Price MJ. Bedside evaluation of thienopyridine antiplatelet therapy. Circulation 2009;119(19):2625–32.

83. Thomas D, Giugliano RP. Antiplatelet therapy in percutaneous coronary intervention: integration of prasugrel into clinical practice. Crit Pathways Cardiol 2009;8(1):12–9.
84. Wallentin L, Becker RC, Budaj A, et al. Ticagrelor versus clopidogrel in patients with acute coronary syndromes. N Engl J Med 2009;361(11): 1045–57.
85. Gibson CM, Kirtane AJ, Murphy SA, et al. Early initiation of eptifibatide in the emergency department before primary percutaneous coronary intervention for ST-segment elevation myocardial infarction: results of the Time to Integrilin Therapy in Acute Myocardial Infarction (TITAN)-TIMI 34 trial. Am Heart J 2006; 152(4):668–75.
86. Zeymer U, Zahn R, Schiele R, et al. Early eptifibatide improves TIMI 3 patency before primary percutaneous coronary intervention for acute ST elevation myocardial infarction: results of the randomized integrilin in acute myocardial infarction (INTAMI) pilot trial. Eur Heart J 2005;26(19): 1971–7.
87. Montalescot G, Barragan P, Wittenberg O, et al. Platelet glycoprotein IIb/IIIa inhibition with coronary stenting for acute myocardial infarction. N Engl J Med 2001;344(25):1895–903.
88. Pels K, Schroder J, Witzenbichler B, et al. Prehospital versus periprocedural abciximab in ST-elevation myocardial infarction treated by percutaneous coronary intervention. Eur J Emerg Med 2008;15(6):324–9.
89. Giugliano RP, Newby LK, Harrington RA, et al. The early glycoprotein IIb/IIIa inhibition in non-ST-segment elevation acute coronary syndrome (EARLY ACS) trial: a randomized placebo-controlled trial evaluating the clinical benefits of early front-loaded eptifibatide in the treatment of patients with non-ST-segment elevation acute coronary syndrome—study design and rationale. Am Heart J 2005;149(6):994–1002.
90. Kaul S. Sonothrombolysis: a universally applicable and better way to treat acute myocardial infarction and stroke? Who is going to fund the research? Circulation 2009;119(10):1358–60.
91. Siegel RJ, Suchkova VN, Miyamoto T, et al. Ultrasound energy improves myocardial perfusion in the presence of coronary occlusion. J Am Coll Cardiol 2004;44(7):1454–8.
92. Atoui R, Shum-Tim D, Chiu RC, et al. Myocardial regenerative therapy: immunologic basis for the potential "universal donor cells". Ann Thorac Surg 2008;86(1): 327–34.
93. Hirsch A, Nijveldt R, van der Vleuten PA, et al. Intracoronary infusion of autologous mononuclear bone marrow cells in patients with acute myocardial infarction treated with primary PCI: Pilot study of the multicenter HEBE trial. Catheter Cardiovasc Interv 2008;71(3):273–81.
94. Than MP, Helm J, Calder K, et al. Comparison of high specificity with standard versions of a quantitative latex D-dimer test in the assessment of community pulmonary embolism: HaemosIL D-dimer HS and pulmonary embolism. Thromb Res 2009;124(2):230–5.
95. Nordenholz KE, Mitchell AM, Kline JA. Direct comparison of the diagnostic accuracy of fifty protein biological markers of pulmonary embolism for use in the emergency department. Acad Emerg Med 2008;15(9):795–9.
96. Linkins LA, Bates SM, Ginsberg JS, et al. Use of different D-dimer levels to exclude venous thromboembolism depending on clinical pretest probability. J Thromb Haemost 2004;2(8):1256–60.

97. Suleyman T, Tevfik P, Abdulkadir G, et al. Ischemia-modified albumin in the diagnosis of pulmonary embolism: an experimental study. Am J Emerg Med 2009; 27(6):635–40.

98. Sainaghi PP, Alciato F, Carnieletto S, et al. Gas6 evaluation in patients with acute dyspnea due to suspected pulmonary embolism. Respir Med 2009;103(4): 589–94.

99. Mitchell AM, Nordenholz KE, Kline JA. Tandem measurement of D-dimer and myeloperoxidase or C-reactive protein to effectively screen for pulmonary embolism in the emergency department. Acad Emerg Med 2008; 15(9):800–5.

100. Collart JP, Roelants V, Vanpee D, et al. Is a lung perfusion scan obtained by using single photon emission computed tomography able to improve the radionuclide diagnosis of pulmonary embolism? Nucl Med Commun 2002;23(11): 1107–13.

101. Lemb M, Pohlabeln H. Pulmonary thromboembolism: a retrospective study on the examination of 991 patients by ventilation/perfusion SPECT using Technegas. Nuklearmedizin 2001;40(6):179–86.

102. Stein PD, Gottschalk A, Sostman HD, et al. Methods of Prospective Investigation of Pulmonary Embolism Diagnosis III (PIOPED III). Semin Nucl Med 2008;38(6): 462–70.

103. Morris TA, Macfarlane DJ, Eisenberg PR, et al. Clinical diagnostic imaging of pulmonary emboli using radiolabeled anticrosslinked fibrin antibodies Thrombo-View [abstract]. Chest 2006;130:S275.

104. Macfarlane D, Socrates A, Eisenberg P, et al. Imaging of deep venous thrombosis in patients using a radiolabelled anti-D-dimer Fab' fragment (99mTc-DI-DD3B6/22-80B3): results of a phase I trial. Eur J Nucl Med Mol Imaging 2009; 36(2):250–9.

105. Kline JA, Novobilski AJ, Kabrhel C, et al. Derivation and validation of a Bayesian network to predict pretest probability of venous thromboembolism. Ann Emerg Med 2005;45(3):282–90.

106. Runyon MS, Webb WB, Jones AE, et al. Comparison of the unstructured clinician estimate of pretest probability for pulmonary embolism to the Canadian score and the Charlotte rule: a prospective observational study. Acad Emerg Med 2005;12(7):587–93.

107. Baxt WG, Shofer FS, Sites FD, et al. A neural computational aid to the diagnosis of acute myocardial infarction. Ann Emerg Med 2002;39(4):366–73.

108. Kline JA, Mitchell AM, Kabrhel C, et al. Clinical criteria to prevent unnecessary diagnostic testing in emergency department patients with suspected pulmonary embolism. J Thromb Haemost 2004;2(8):1247–55.

109. Kline J, Courtney D, Than M. Accuracy of very low pretest probability estimates for pulmonary embolism using the method of attribute matching compared with the Wells' score. Acad Emerg Med 2010;17:133–41.

110. Pauker SG, Kassirer JP. The threshold approach to clinical decision making. N Engl J Med 1980;302(20):1109–17.

111. Kline JA, Courtney DM, Kabrhel C, et al. Prospective multicenter evaluation of the pulmonary embolism rule-out criteria. J Thromb Haemost 2008;6(5): 772–80.

112. Kline JA, Johns KL, Colucciello SA, et al. New diagnostic tests for pulmonary embolism. Ann Emerg Med 2000;35(2):168–80.

113. Brown MD, Lau J, Nelson RD, et al. Turbidimetric D-dimer test in the diagnosis of pulmonary embolism: a metaanalysis. Clin Chem 2003;49(11):1846–53.

114. Stein PD, Hull RD, Patel KC, et al. D-dimer for the exclusion of acute venous thrombosis and pulmonary embolism: a systematic review. Ann Intern Med 2004;140(8):589–602.
115. Eid-Lidt G, Gaspar J, Sandoval J, et al. Combined clot fragmentation and aspiration in patients with acute pulmonary embolism. Chest. 2008;134(1):54–60.
116. Wan S, Quinlan DJ, Agnelli G, et al. Thrombolysis compared with heparin for the initial treatment of pulmonary embolism: a meta-analysis of the randomized controlled trials. Circulation 2004;110(6):744–9.
117. Stevinson BG, Hernandez-Nino J, Rose G, et al. Echocardiographic and functional cardiopulmonary problems 6 months after first-time pulmonary embolism in previously healthy patients. Eur Heart J 2007;28(20):2517–24.
118. Tran TP, Khoynezhad A. Current management of type B aortic dissection. Vasc Health Risk Manag 2009;5(1):53–63.
119. Suzuki T, Distante A, Zizza A, et al. Diagnosis of acute aortic dissection by D-dimer: the International Registry of Acute Aortic Dissection Substudy on Biomarkers (IRAD-Bio) experience. Circulation 2009;119(20):2702–7.
120. Patel DP, Arora RR. Pathophysiology, diagnosis, and management of aortic dissection. Ther Adv Cardiovasc Dis 2008;2:439–68.
121. Suzuki T, Katoh H, Tsuchio Y, et al. Diagnostic implications of elevated levels of smooth-muscle myosin heavy-chain protein in acute aortic dissection. The smooth muscle myosin heavy chain study. Ann Intern Med 2000;133(7):537–41.
122. Suzuki T, Distante A, Zizza A, et al. Preliminary experience with the smooth muscle troponin-like protein, calponin, as a novel biomarker for diagnosing acute aortic dissection. Eur Heart J 2008;29(11):1439–45.
123. Sodeck G, Domanovits H, Schillinger M, et al. D-dimer in ruling out acute aortic dissection: a systematic review and prospective cohort study. Eur Heart J 2007;28(24):3067–75.
124. Salvagno GL, Targher G, Franchini M, et al. Plasma D-dimer in the diagnosis of acute aortic dissection. Eur Heart J 2008;29(9):1207.
125. Clevert D-A, Weckbach S, Kopp R, et al. Imaging of aortic lesions with color coded duplex sonography and contrast-enhanced ultrasound versus multislice computed tomography (MS-CT) angiography. Clin Hemorheol Microcirc 2008;40(4):267–79.
126. Svensson LG, Kouchoukos NT, Miller DC, et al. Expert consensus document on the treatment of descending thoracic aortic disease using endovascular stent-grafts. Ann Thorac Surg 2008;85(Suppl 1):S1–41.
127. Liu JC, Zhang JZ, Yang J, et al. Combined interventional and surgical treatment for acute aortic type A dissection. Int J Surg 2008;6(2):151–6.
128. Halpern EJ. Triple-rule-out CT angiography for evaluation of acute chest pain and possible acute coronary syndrome. Radiology 2009;252(2):332–45.
129. Takakuwa KM, Halpern EJ, Gingold EL, et al. Radiation dose in a "triple rule-out" coronary CT angiography protocol of emergency department patients using 64-MDCT: the impact of ECG-based tube current modulation on age, sex, and body mass index. Am J Roentgenol 2009;192(4):866–72.
130. Modlin IM, Hunt RH, Malfertheiner P, et al. Diagnosis and management of non-erosive reflux disease—the Vevey NERD Consensus Group. Digestion 2009;80(2):74–88.
131. Schmulson MJ, Valdovinos MA. Current and future treatment of chest pain of presumed esophageal origin. Gastroenterol Clin North Am 2004;33(1):93–105.

132. Christensen HW, Vach W, Gichangi A, et al. Cervicothoracic angina identified by case history and palpation findings in patients with stable angina pectoris. J Manipulative Physiol Ther 2005;28(5):303–11.
133. Stochkendahl MJ, Christensen HW, Vach W, et al. Diagnosis and treatment of musculoskeletal chest pain: design of a multi-purpose trial. BMC Musculoskelet Disord 2008;9:40. Available at: www.biomedcentral.com/1471-2474/9/40. Accessed October, 2009.
134. Harding G, Yelland M. Back, chest and abdominal pain - is it spinal referred pain? Aust Fam Physician 2007;36(6):422–3, 425, 427–9.

BONUS ARTICLE:
Preoperative Evaluation of the Oncology Patient

Sunil K. Sahai, MD, Ali Zalpour, PharmD, Marc A. Rozner, PhD, MD

Edited by Lee A. Fleisher, MD, and Stanley H. Rosenbaum, MD

Preoperative Evaluation of the Oncology Patient

Sunil K. Sahai, MD[a,b], Ali Zalpour, PharmD, BCPS[a],
Marc A. Rozner, MD, PhD[c,d],*

KEYWORDS

• Cancer • Preoperative evaluation • Surgery • Chemotherapy

Although surgery remains the mainstay of cancer care, the advent of multidisciplinary approaches and the use of multiple therapeutic modalities has increased treatment complexity.[1] In patients with solid tumor malignancies, 75% undergo a surgical procedure for a cure. Some 90% will have surgery for other reasons,[2,3] which include diagnostic or palliative procedures, brachytherapy (the implanting of radiation seeds or devices), or surgery unrelated to cancer (eg, vascular surgery or hysterectomy for postmenopausal bleeding). The increasing age of patients with cancer, the increasing number of comorbid conditions, and the complexity of care before surgery often affect their perioperative course. A previous article in this publication addressed these issues from the internist's view point,[4] and reviews have also been written for anesthesiologists.[5,6] This article provides an update for all providers involved in the delivery of perioperative medical care for patients with cancer. Even today, there remains no set of guidelines for these patients. This review focuses primarily on perioperative aspects of chemotherapy, because it is unique to cancer medicine. Because many of the chemotherapeutic agents discussed herein have been used for many decades, some of the references to these agents are old.

A version of this article originally appeared in the 27:4 issue of *Anesthesiology Clinics.*
[a] Department of General Internal Medicine, Ambulatory Treatment, and Emergency Care, The University of Texas M.D. Anderson Cancer Center, 1515 Holcombe Boulevard, Unit 1465, Houston, TX 77030, USA
[b] Internal Medicine Perioperative Assessment Center, Department of General Internal Medicine, Ambulatory Treatment, and Emergency Care, The University of Texas M.D. Anderson Cancer Center, 1515 Holcombe Boulevard, Unit 1465, Houston, TX 77030, USA
[c] The University of Texas M.D. Anderson Cancer Center, Department of Anesthesiology and Perioperative Medicine, 1400 Holcombe Boulevard, Unit 0409, Houston, TX 77030, USA
[d] The University of Texas Health Science Center at Houston, Department of Integrative Biology and Pharmacology, 6431 Fannin Street, Houston, TX 77030, USA
* Corresponding author. The University of Texas M.D. Anderson Cancer Center, 1400 Holcombe Boulevard, Unit 0409, Houston, TX 77030.
E-mail address: mrozner@mdanderson.org

Med Clin N Am 94 (2010) 403–419
doi:10.1016/j.mcna.2010.01.012
0025-7125/10/$ – see front matter © 2010 Elsevier Inc. All rights reserved.
medical.theclinics.com

GOALS OF PREOPERATIVE ASSESSMENT

Ideally, the preoperative assessment serves as a roadmap to guide the patient safely through surgery and the perioperative period. For the medically complex patient whose cancer is complicated by comorbid conditions, this guidance often requires close cooperation between internal medicine consultants, anesthesiologists, critical care physicians, and the surgeons. Sometimes, other medical needs of these patients are ignored because of their cancer treatment. For example, in a study of 161 patients with cancer and a pacemaker presenting for cancer surgery, 32% had not undergone interrogation of their devices for more than 1 year.[7]

In many settings, preoperative patients are routed to an internal medicine consultant before surgery. In general, nonsurgical medical comorbidities should be identified at this visit, and targeted preoperative testing and other consultations should be ordered with attention to appropriate optimization and perioperative risk assessment. Many patients are then evaluated at a preoperative anesthesiology clinic that provides anesthetic risk assessment for a variety of surgical and nonsurgical procedures requiring anesthesia.[6]

Probably the most difficult issue surrounding cancer surgery is its timing, because cancer surgery often is neither truly elective nor truly emergent. Delaying cancer surgery to embark on an extended diagnostic evaluation of a new finding, or to achieve ideal medical optimization of a comorbid condition can render surgical intervention impossible because of tumor growth or extension.[8] As a result, customary perioperative guidelines might not be applicable to patients with cancer who are undergoing surgery.

CANCER, CANCER TREATMENT, AND PERIOPERATIVE IMPLICATIONS

In its most fundamental form, cancer represents a disruption of the body's homeostasis, and chemotherapy and/or radiation therapy can further disrupt this homeostasis from the subcellular level to the functional level. Many patients who were functionally vigorous before their cancer diagnosis become unable to achieve an adequate exercise tolerance as a result of the effects of treatment. Therefore, preoperative evaluation must take into account all previous treatments and their effects on the patient. An updated list of the most commonly used chemotherapy agents, their mechanisms of action, and perioperative implications of their side effects is given in **Table 1**. Common combinations of chemotherapeutic and adjunctive agents are listed in **Table 2** because many patients with cancer will be able to identify their protocols but not the specific agents. Many chemotherapy combinations involve administration of steroids (see **Table 2**), which can produce immunosuppression and glucose intolerance. Throughout this document, common brand/index names are shown in the text.

CARDIOVASCULAR EFFECTS AND EVALUATION

A variety of chemotherapeutic agents directly affect the heart and the cardiovascular system, and these effects often outlast the acute treatment stage. Although most practitioners are aware of the link between doxorubicin (Adriamycin) and the development of heart failure, many are unaware that the anthracycline class includes daunorubicin, epirubicin, idarubicin, mitoxantrone, and valrubicin. All of these drugs are similar to doxorubicin except for their potency.[9] The risk of developing cardiomyopathy increases greatly if the total dose is more than 550 mg/m^2 for daunorubicin and doxorubicin, and 900 mg/m^2 for epirubicin.[10–12] The likelihood of developing cardiomyopathy further depends on the presence of preexisting cardiac disease, concomitant administration of other chemotherapeutic agents (particularly cyclophos-phamide [Cytoxan], paclitaxel [Taxol], and trastuzumab [Herceptin]), chest irradiation, and extremes of age. In addition, any preexisting cardiomyopathy can exacerbate the cardiotoxicity of other agents in these patients.[13,14]

Other chemotherapeutic agents have been associated with cardiomyopathy, including taxanes such as paclitaxel and docetaxel (Taxotere). In addition, newer agents such as the tyrosine kinase inhibitors (see **Table 1**) have been associated with cardiomyopathy.[15]

Cardiac effects are not limited to cardiomyopathy; some agents can produce myocardial ischemia from coronary artery spasm or bradyarrhythmias.[16] The pyrimi-dine analogue 5-fluorouracil (5-FU) is used to treat several cancers, and it has the potential to induce myocardial ischemia, with or without progression to myocardial infarction. Co-administration of 5-FU with cisplatin seems to increase the incidence of ischemic events.[11] Capecitabine (Xeloda) is an oral, prodrug formulation of 5-FU. Because activation of the drug takes place mainly in cancer cells, the toxicity profile of capecitabine is believed to be lower than that of 5-FU.[17] Nevertheless, capecitabine use has produced myocardial ischemia and infarction, presumably by mechanisms similar to that of 5-FU.[10]

Electrocardiographic changes as well as chest pain have been found in patients during the administration of 5-FU. Any patient experiencing chest pain during 5-FU administration should be referred to a cardiologist to identify any underlying coronary artery disease,[18] although some might have normal coronary anatomy.[19]

Some other agents deserve mention: thalidomide can cause severe bradycardia necessitating pacemaker implantation.[20] In addition, co-administration of doxorubicin and vincristine has been reported to change pacing threshold.[21]

Radiation therapy to the thorax or mediastinum might damage the heart and its associated vascular structures. The potential adverse effects of mediastinal or mantle irradiation include coronary artery disease, pericarditis, cardiomyopathy, valvular disease, and conduction abnormalities.[22] A significantly higher risk of death as a result of ischemic heart disease has been reported for patients treated with radiation therapy to the chest for Hodgkin disease and breast cancer,[23] although not all investigators agree that breast irradiation leads to increased heart disease.[24] Coronary artery endo-thelial cell damage from radiation has been proposed as one mechanism for heart disease after chest irradiation. Factors affecting development of coronary artery disease include the percentage of the left ventricle irradiated, concurrent hormonal treatment, and a history of hypercholesterolemia.[25] As noted earlier, the risk of cardio-myopathy increases when radiation therapy is combined with doxorubicin (or any of the anthracyclines), because there seems to be a synergistic toxic effect on the myocardium.[23]

For the perioperative cardiac evaluation of the patient with cancer undergoing noncardiac surgery, many practitioners rely on the latest *Guidelines for Perioperative Evaluation* from the American College of Cardiology/American Heart Association (ACC/AHA).[26] However, the multiple toxicities associated with previous cancer treat-ment, along with decreases in a patient's functional status, increase the importance of a complete history of the patient's symptoms. The patient who presents with fatigue and dyspnea on exertion may have symptoms consistent with a particularly vigorous course of chemotherapy or cardiomyopathy secondary to prior chemotherapy or radi-ation therapy. As a result, application of the ACC/AHA guidelines may lead to unnec-essary testing based on the use of functional status. In these patients, their functional status before the onset of treatment becomes an important factor in their planned preoperative course. The patient with cancer with cardiomyopathy probably benefits

Table 1
Common chemotherapeutic agents

Class	Agents	Mechanism	Perioperative Implications
Alkylating Agents			
Nitrosoureas	Carmustine (BiCNU) Lomustine (CeeNU)	Inhibits DNA and RNA synthesis	Pulmonary fibrosis
Methylating agents	Procarbazine (Matulane)	Methylation of nucleic acid that leads to DNA and RNA synthesis inhibition	Hemorrhage Seizure Hemolysis Ototoxicity Edema Tachycardia
	Dacarbazine (DTIC-Dome)		Hepatic necrosis and occlusion Hepatic vein thrombosis
	Temozolamide (Temodar)		Seizure and gait abnormality Peripheral edema
Platinums	Cisplatin (Platinol; Platinol-AQ) Carboplatin (Paraplatin) Oxaliplatin (Eloxatin)	Inhibition of DNA replication	Acute renal tubular necrosis Magnesium wasting Peripheral sensory neuropathy Paresthesias Ototoxicity
Nitrogen mustards	Cyclophoshamide (Cytoxan; Neosar) Ifosfamide (Ifex)	Cross-linking DNA strands	Pericarditis Pericardial effusions Pulmonary fibrosis Hemorrhagic cystitis Water retention Anemia SIADH SIDAH Seizures
	Melphalan (Alkeran) Chlorambucil (Leukeran)		
Antimetabolites			

Anthracyclines/anthraquinolones	Doxorubicin (Adriamycin PFS; Adriamycin RDF) Daunorubicin (Cerubidine) Epirubicin (Ellence) Idarubicin (Idamycin) Mitoxantrone (Novantrone) Valrubicin (Valstar)	Interruption of DNA synthesis Inhibition of topisomerase type II	Cardiomyopathy ECG changes
Antitumor antibiotics: natural product	Bleomycin (Blenoxane) Mitomycin C (Mutamycin)	Inhibition of DNA and RNA synthesis	Pulmonary fibrosis Pneumonitis Pulmonary hypertension
Pyrimidine analogue	Capecitabine (Xeloda) Cytarabine (Ara-C) Fluorouracil (5-FU) Adrucil; Efudex) Gemcitabine (Gemzar)	Pyrimidine antimetabolite that interferes with DNA synthesis	Myocardial ischemia/infarction Coronary vasospasm Edema Proteinuria
Purine analog	Thioguanine (6-TG; 6-thioguanine; TG; tioguanine) Pentostatin (Nipent; 2'-deoxycoformycin; DCF) Cladribine (Leustatin, 2-CdA) Fludarabine (Fludara) Mercaptopurine (Purinethol; 6-mercaptopurine; 6-MP)	Purine antimetabolite that interferes with DNA synthesis	Hepatotoxicity Pulmonary toxicity Deep vein thrombophlebitis Chest pain Edema AV block Arrhythmia Hypo and hypertension Thrombosis tachycardia Acute renal failure Tumor lysis syndrome CVA/TIA Angina Thrombosis Arrhythmia CHF Acute renal failure Tumor lysis syndrome Intrahepatic cholestasis and focal centralobular necrosis

(continued on next page)

Table 1
(continued)

Class	Agents	Mechanism	Perioperative Implications
Folate antagonist	Methotrexate (Mexate; Rheumatrex)	Methotrexate is a folate antimetabolite that inhibits DNA synthesis	Elevated liver enzymes Pulmonary edema Pleural effusions Encephalopathy Meningismus Myelosuppression Seizure Edema
Substituted urea	Hydroxyurea (Hydrea)		
Microtubule Assembly Inhibitors			
Taxanes	Paclitaxel (Taxol) docetaxel (Taxotere)	Microtubule assembly Inhibitor	Peripheral neuropathy Bradycardia Autonomic dysfunction Hypertension Angina
Alkaloids	Vinblastine (Vincaleukoblastine; VLB)		Cerebrovascular accident Coronary ischemia ECG abnormalities, Raynaud phenomenon SIADH
	Vincristine (Vincasar)		GI bleed Paresthesias Recurrent laryngeal nerve palsy Autonomic dysfunction Orthostasis Hypo and hypertension SIADH
Biologic Agents			

Monoclonal antibodies	Alemtuzumab (Campath)	Binding to immune cells to accelerate antibody dependent lysis of tumor cells	Dysrhythmia/tachycardia/SVT Hypotension and hypertension
	Bevacizumab (Avastin)		Pulmonary bleeding Hypertension Thromboembolic events Cardiopulmonary arrest
	Cetuximab (Erbitux) Rituximab (Rituxan)		Tumor lysis syndrome Electrolyte abnormality
	Trastuzumab (Herceptin)		Cardiomyopathy Thrombus formation Pulmonary toxicity Tachycardia Hypertension Chest pain
	Daclizumab (Zenapax)		Hyper and hypotension Thrombosis Peripheral edema
	Ibritumomab (Zevalin) Palivizumab (Synagis) Muromonab-CD3 (Orthoclone OKT3)		Arrhythmia Tachycardia Hyper and hypotension
Biologic Response Modulators			
Interleukins	Aldesleukin (IL-2; Proleukin) Denileukin diftitox (Ontak)	Promotes proliferation and differentiation of T and B cells	Capillary leak syndrome Peripheral edema Hypotension ECG changes
Interferon	Interferon alfa-2b (Intron A) Interferon alfacon-1 (Infergen)	Alteration in cellular differentiation	Arrhythmia Chest pain Pulmonary pneumonitis Ischemic disorders Hyperthyroidism Hypothyroidism
	Peginterferon alfa-2a (Pegasys) Peginterferon alfa-2b (PEG-Intron)		Pulmonary infiltrates Ischemic disorders Hyperthyroidism Hypothyroidism

(continued on next page)

Table 1
(continued)

Class	Agents	Mechanism	Perioperative Implications
Vascular Endothelial Growth Factor (VEGF) Inhibitor			
Tyrosine kinase inhibitors	Imatinib (Gleevec)	Inhibition of angiogenesis through VEGF receptor blockade	Edema
	Sorafenib (Nexavar)		Left ventricular dysfunction Cardiac ischemia and infarction Hypertension Thromboembolism
	Sunitinib (Sutent)		Cardiac ischemia and infarction Thromboembolism Adrenal insufficiency Pulmonary hemorrhage Hypertension Hypothyroidism Cardiomyopathy QT prolongation Torsade de pointes
	Dasatinib (Sprycel)	BCR-ABL tyrosine kinase inhibitor	Fluid retention Cardiomyopathy QT prolongation Pulmonary hemorrhage Platelet dysfunction
	Nilotinib (Tasigna)		QT prolongation Hypertension Peripheral edema
Epidermal Growth Factor Receptor (EGFR) Inhibitor			
	Erlotinib (Tarceva)	Epidermal growth factor receptor (HER1/EGFR)–tyrosine kinase	Deep venous thrombosis Arrhythmia Pulmonary toxicity Cerebrovascular accidents Myocardial ischemia, Syncope Edema
	Lapatinib (Tykerb)		Cardiomyopathy Pulmonary toxicity QT prolongation Pulmonary fibrosis
	Panitumumab (Vectibix)		Peripheral edema

Angiogenesis Inhibitors

Immunomodulators	Thalidomide (Thalomid) Lenalidomide (Revlimid)	Blocks tissue necrosis factor (TNF), suppression of angiogenesis, prevention of free-radical–mediated DNA damage, and increased cell-mediated cytotoxic effects	Thromboembolism Edema Bradycardia
Enzymes	Asparginase (Elspar; Kidrolase)	Inhibits protein synthesis by hydrolyzing asparagine to aspartic acid and ammonia	Thrombosis Glucose intolerance Coagulopathy
Miscellaneous			
Topoisomerase I inhibitor	Irinotecan (Camptosar, CPT-11) Topotecan (Hycamtin) Rubitecan (Orathecin)	Inhibits topoisomerase I and causes DNA breakdown	Neutropenia Diarrhea Cholinergic syndrome
Epipodophyllotoxin topoisomerase II inhibitor	Etoposide (Vepesid, VP-16)	Inhibits topoisomerase II and causes DNA breakdown	Neutropenia Stevens-Johnson syndrome Toxic epidermal necrolysis Myocardial infarction Congestive heart failure

Generic and brand names are used in this table. Some chemotherapy agents have Index names that are used as well.
Data from Refs. [51–54]

Table 2
Common chemotherapeutic combinations

Combination Abbreviation	Chemotherapy Components	Steroids
A-CMF	Doxorubicin, cyclophosphamide, methotrexate, 5-fluorouracil	
ABVD	Bleomycin, doxorubicin, vinblastine, dacarbazine	
BEP	Bleomycin, etoposide, cisplatin	
BEACOPP	Bleomycin, etoposide, vincristine, cyclophosphamide, vincristine, procarbazine	Prednisone
CAPP	Cyclophosphamide, doxorubicin, cisplatin	Prednisone
CAPOX	Capecitabine, oxaliplatin;	
CHOP ± rituximab[a]	Cyclosphosphamide, doxorubicin, vincristine	Prednisone
CHOEP ± rituximab[a]	Cyclosphosphamide, doxorubicin, etoposide, vincristine	Prednisone
CHOP-Bleo	Cyclosphosphamide, doxorubicin, vincristine, bleomycin	Prednisone
DHAP	Cisplatin, cytarabine	Dexamethasone
ESHAP	Cisplatin, cytarabine, etoposide	Methylprednisolone
FAC	5-Fluorouracil, cyclophosphamide, doxorubicin	
FEC	5-Fluorouracil, cyclophosphamide, epirubicin	
FOLFIRI	5-Fluorouracil, irinotecan, leucovorin	
FOLFOX	5-Fluorouracil, leucovorin, oxaliplatin	
hyper-CVAD	Course A: cyclophosphamide, doxorubicin, methotrexate, vincristine (± MESNA) Course B: cytarabine, leucovorin, methotrexate	Dexamethasone (course A only)
M-VAC	Methotrexate, vinblastine, doxorubicin, cisplatin	
R-CHOP	Rituximab + CHOP	
TAC	Cyclophosphamide, docetaxel, doxorubicin	
TCG	Paclitaxel, cisplatin, gemcitabine	
VAD	Doxorubicin, vincristine	Dexamethasone
VIM	Etoposide, ifosfamide, methotrexate	
VIP	Etoposide, ifosfamide, cisplatin, MESNA	

Only generic names are used in this table. Commonly, the brand name Adriamycin is used for the drug doxorubicin. Another generic name is hydroxydaunorubicin, and this name is the source of the "H" in many abbreviations that include this drug.
[a] CHOP or CHOEP plus rituximab are often abbreviated R-CHOP or R-CHOEP.
Data from LEXI-Comp ONLINE. Available at: http://www.crlonline.com. Accessed February 15, 2010.

from beta blocker therapy.[27] In the absence of significant contraindications, these patients should be treated according to the ACC/AHA guidelines for heart failure.[16,28] These patients can be followed with serial echocardiography or repeated evaluations of serum B-type natriuretic peptide.[16]

As previously mentioned, complications from cancer and cancer care can include cardiomyopathy, ischemic heart disease, congestive heart failure, hypertension, hypotension, pericarditis, and bradyarrhythmias. In high-risk patients, noninvasive testing might be useful to predict postoperative cardiac complications.[29] Any decision to delay surgery in high-risk patients should be made in consultation with the patient's other physicians, because preoperative angiography and coronary artery stent placement can lead to significant surgical delay,[30] which might render a previously resectable cancer unresectable.

PULMONARY AND AIRWAY EFFECTS AND EVALUATION

As in the cardiovascular system, previous chemotherapy and radiation treatment can adversely affect the lungs. Bleomycin (BLM), an antitumor antibiotic used in treatment of germ cell tumors and certain hematological malignancies, causes interstitial pneumonitis followed by pulmonary fibrosis. BLM-induced pneumonitis occurs in 3% to 5% of patients receiving cumulative doses of less than 300 mg. At doses greater than 500 mg, 20% of patients experience pneumonitis. Lung fibrosis can develop even 10 years after cessation of therapy.[31] Advanced age, preexisting lung disease, or previous radiation therapy to the chest seems to predispose patients to pulmonary fibrosis.[32] In addition to BLM, other chemotherapeutic agents can cause interstitial pneumonia or pulmonary fibrosis in up to 25% of patients, including busulfan; chlorambucil; cyclophosphamide; melphalan; methotrexate; the nitrosoureas (carmustine [BCNU], lomustine [CCNU], or semustine-methyl [CCNU]), and vinca alkaloids with mitomycin. Many of these agents have also been associated with other pulmonary toxic effects including bronchiolitis obliterans with organizing pneumonia, pulmonary infiltrates with eosinophilia, noncardiac pulmonary edema, and pleural effusion. Vinca alkaloids with mitomycin have been reported to induce or exacerbate asthma.[33]

During the preoperative evaluation of patients with agents known to cause pulmonary toxicities, signs and symptoms of pulmonary compromise (dyspnea, nonproductive cough, pleurisy, crackles on examination) must be thoroughly vetted, because postoperative pulmonary complications are common. Although routine pulmonary testing is not usually warranted, chest radiograph, spirometry, arterial blood gases, and assessment of diffusing capacity should be considered if the patient will benefit from medical optimization before surgery.[34] Patients found to have restrictive lung disease, an increased alveolar-arterial oxygen gradient, and/or a decreased diffusing capacity may require special pulmonary care in the perioperative period.[35]

Pulmonary function testing may be indicated in those patients with known pulmonary fibrosis who have a poor functional status and have received radiation to the chest and/or BLM therapy if the treatment plan will be modified based on untoward results. A preoperative therapeutic thoracentesis for a pleural effusion may increase a patient's pulmonary reserve during surgery. In addition, patients with chronic obstructive pulmonary disease may benefit from pulmonary rehabilitation before surgery.[36] For appropriate patients with pulmonary compromise who will undergo neoadjuvant therapy before their surgical intervention, referral to a pulmonary rehabilitation program can make good use of this interval.

Radiation therapy to the head and neck area can compromise the airway. Many patients who undergo head and neck radiation develop trismus, limited mouth opening, limited neck extension, and limited mobility of pharyngeal structures, all of which can complicate the anesthesiologist's access to the airway for intubation. Even though many patients continue to demonstrate a normal external airway on physical examination, they might be difficult to ventilate or intubate after induction of general anesthesia or during a medical emergency. Thus, alternatives to direct laryngoscopy must be readily available for use in these patients.

GASTROINTESTINAL AND HEPATOBILIARY CONCERNS

Although all patients with cancer are at risk for malnutrition, patients with gastrointestinal (GI) tract malignancies are especially vulnerable. Radiation therapy to the abdomen can cause radiation-induced enteritis, leading to malabsorption and diarrhea. Low serum albumin levels are a marker for malnutrition, and an albumin level less than 3.0 g/dL has been shown to increase the risk of postoperative pneumonia according to a recent meta-analysis.[37] However, there seems to be no effective short-term treatment of this problem at this time.

Cancer that involves the liver, either as a primary site or through metastatic disease, as well as chemotherapy, may complicate the perioperative course through coagulopathy, biliary dysfunction, and malnutrition. Agents known to cause liver dysfunction are methotrexate, L-asparaginase, cytosine arabinoside, plicamycin, streptozocin, and 6-mercaptopurine.

GENITOURINARY AND RENAL

Several chemotherapeutic agents can cause renal insufficiency. In addition, tumor location can affect renal function, either through direct tumor invasion (eg, a primary urologic malignancy) or through mechanical issues leading to obstructive hydronephrosis. Cisplatin, used in a variety of head and neck, GI, genitourinary, and gynecologic malignancies can produce a dose-related nephrotoxicity, which represents its major dose-limiting toxicity. Toxicity occurs in 28% to 36% of patients after a single 50 mg/m^2 dose, manifested by increases in blood urea nitrogen, serum creatinine, and serum uric acid levels. A significant number of patients receiving cisplatin (and other platinum-based agents) develop magnesium wasting and hypomagnesemia,[38,39] and magnesium supplementation might ameliorate the sensory peripheral neuropathy that can develop with cisplatin[40] or oxaliplatin.[41]

Cyclophosamide, used to treat breast cancer and hematogenous malignancies, can cause hemorrhagic cystitis, producing obstructive uropathy from blood clot accumulation in the bladder. Treatment can require emergent cystoscopy or placement of percutaneous nephrostomy tubes. Hematuria from bladder cancer can influence perioperative anticoagulation strategies, especially in the patient with a cardiac stent; concern about bleeding from the antiplatelet therapy must be balanced with the protection conferred against stent stenosis. Tumor lysis syndrome can cause renal insufficiency.[42]

HEMATOLOGY

Cancer produces a hypercoagulable state caused by higher levels of cytokines, clotting factors, and cancer procoagulant.[43,44] Some chemotherapy agents, especially thalidomide, can exacerbate this issue.[10] As a result, venous thromboembolism (VTE) prophylaxis in the perioperative period should be used in all patients with cancer unless a specific contraindication is present.[45]

Patients who are undergoing chemotherapy and multiple laboratory draws often have wide variability in blood counts. Anemia has been treated with erythropoietin agents, but their use has been associated with shorter survival,[46] and controversy exists about the role of erythropoietin receptors on tumor cells.[47] Pancytopenia, thrombocytosis, and polycythemia are common, either as a result of treatment, or the disease itself. Phlebotomy and/or transfusions may be needed depending on the specific situation. Some patients may be taking hydroxyurea and/or anagrelide (Agrylin) to assist in the management of the thrombocytosis. In general, hydroxyurea inhibits platelet formation and may be safely continued throughout the perioperative period. Anagrelide inhibits platelet formation and aggregation and may need to be stopped in the perioperative period to avoid bleeding complications.[48]

NEUROLOGY

Tumors or metastatic disease of the brain or spinal cord may complicate postoperative VTE prophylaxis. In addition, many of these patients take steroids to limit or reduce cerebral swelling and pressure, and their blood sugar levels can be increased, leading to steroid-induced diabetes. Myasthenia gravis occurs as a paraneoplastic syndrome in about 30% of those with thymomas.[49] Eaton-Lambert syndrome, another paraneoplastic event, is associated with small cell lung cancer, and appropriate perioperative precautions need to be considered in both conditions.[50] The presence of a neurologic malignancy can complicate anticoagulation therapy (ie, coumadin for atrial fibrillation, clopidogrel for coronary athersclerosis) and VTE prophylaxis in these patients.

ENDOCRINOLOGY

Cushing syndrome resulting from ectopic production of adrenocorticotropic hormone has been associated with small cell lung cancer, pancreatic cancer, carcinoid, and thymic tumors. The syndrome of inappropriate secretion of antidiuretic hormone (SIADH) can accompany several types of lung cancer, including small cell, large cell, and adenocarcinoma. SIADH can be found in patients with pancreatic and duodenal cancers. Many of these patients will have mild, asymptomatic hyponatremia, which is generally not a contraindication to surgery.

Several conditions can lead to hypercalcemia, including ectopic production of parathyroid hormone, prostaglandins, and metastatic bone disease. Patients with elevated calcium levels should be investigated for occult hyperparathyroidism. Tumors associated with hypercalcemia include breast cancer, non–small cell lung cancer, and multiple myeloma.

Hypoglycemia can accompany mesenchymal tumors, adrenocortical tumors, pancreatic non–islet cell tumors, and hepatocellular cancer. Treatment is symptomatic, and some of these patients will need glucose supplementation on the day of their surgery in view of their nil-per-os status.

Hyperglycemia often accompanies chemotherapy, especially when steroids are co-administered. Many of these patients also have multiple risk factors for diabetes, and a glycosylated hemoglobin determination can be used to help determine the extent of the disease. Standard recommendations for diabetes management in the perioperative period also apply to patients with cancer, although special attention is required for the patient who requires a multiple day preoperative diet/caloric restriction regimen.

Adrenal insufficiency is common in patients who have received steroids in the course of their cancer care, and, as noted earlier, hypothyroidism can develop in those patients who have received radiation for head and neck cancers.

SPECIAL CONSIDERATIONS

Patients with complex head and neck cancers need careful evaluation by an anesthesiologist for any potential airway issues. Those patients undergoing head and neck surgery with obstructive sleep apnea and who have already obtained a positive pressure mask might benefit from evaluation by a pulmonologist, because their mask might not fit correctly after surgery, or its position might jeopardize any skin or tissue grafts placed for reconstructive procedures.

With regard to traditional laboratory testing, most practitioners realize that perioperative medicine has moved away from the comprehensive metabolic screening panel before surgery. However, selective laboratory testing (eg, electrolyte, renal function, and magnesium determination for the patient exposed to recent steroid therapy or nephrotoxic chemotherapy) may uncover secondary metabolic or hematologic issues that need to be addressed in the perioperative period. Chest radiograph and electro-cardiographic evaluation might be indicated for those with a history of thoracic cancer, previous thoracic surgery, or radiotherapy to the chest wall. Thyroid function screening before surgery in a patient with a history of irradiation to the neck and the chest seems warranted, as these patients can develop occult thyroid insufficiency. In this cost conscious era, many of these studies may have been obtained during the work-up of a patient with cancer and need not be repeated for the planned surgical procedure if the test values have been obtained recently and there seems no change in a patient's status.

SUMMARY

Although the perioperative care of the patient with cancer is, in many ways, unchanged from the usual patient without a history of cancer, the broad systemic effects of cancer and cancer therapy pose challenges that need to be addressed. The role of physicians familiar with cancer, cancer treatment, and cancer-related comorbidities can play an integral part in the management of the patient who has cancer in the perioperative period.

REFERENCES

1. Geraci JM, Escalante CP, Freeman JL, et al. Comorbid disease and cancer: the need for more relevant conceptual models in health services research. J Clin Oncol 2005;23(30):7399–404.
2. Daly JM, Decosse JJ. Principles of surgical oncology. In: Calabrese P, Schein PS, Rosenberg SA, editors. Medical oncology. Toronto: Macmillan; 1995. p. 261.
3. Fox KR. Surgery in the patient with cancer. In: Goldmann DR, Brown FH, Guarnieri DM, editors. Perioperative medicine: medical care of the surgical patient. 2nd edition. New York: McGraw-Hill; 1994. p. 283–93.
4. Manzullo EF, Weed HG. Perioperative issues in patients with cancer. Med Clin North Am 2003;87(1):243–56.
5. Davis MM, Rozner MA. Effects of cancer treatment on perioperative anesthetic care. In: Lake CL, Johnson JO, McLoughlin TM, editors. Advances in anesthesia. New York: Mosby; 2004. p. 121–42.
6. Andrabi TR, Rozner MA. Preoperative anesthesia evaluation. In: Shaw AD, Riedel BJ, Burton AW, et al, editors. Acute care of the cancer patient. Boca Raton (FL): Taylor and Francis; 2005. p. 243–58.
7. Rozner MA, Nguyen AD, Roberson JC. Inadequate pacemaker follow-up detected at the preanesthetic visit. Anesthesiology 2002;96:A1071.
8. Ewer MS. Specialists must communicate in complex cases. Int Med World Rep 2001;16(5):17.
9. Gharib MI, Burnett AK. Chemotherapy-induced cardiotoxicity: current practice and prospects of prophylaxis. Eur J Heart Fail 2002;4(3):235–42.
10. Micromedix(R) Healthcare Series. Thompson Healthcare: Greenwood Village (CO); 2008. Available at: http://www.micromedex.com/about_us/legal/cite/. Accessed February 15, 2010.
11. Ewer MS, Benjamin RS. Cardiac complications. In: Bast RC, Kufe DW, Pollock RE, et al, editors. Cancer medicine. 5th edition. London: B.C. Decker, Incorporated; 2000. p. 2324–39.

12. Zambetti M, Moliterni A, Materazzo C, et al. Long-term cardiac sequelae in operable breast cancer patients given adjuvant chemotherapy with or without doxorubicin and breast irradiation. J Clin Oncol 2001;19(1):37–43.

13. Philips JA, Marty FM, Stone RM, et al. Torsades de pointes associated with voriconazole use. Transpl Infect Dis 2007;9(1):33–6.

14. Bdair FM, Graham SP, Smith PF, et al. Gemcitabine and acute myocardial infarction–a case report [review]. Angiology 2006;57(3):367–71.

15. Chu TF, Rupnick MA, Kerkela R, et al. Cardiotoxicity associated with tyrosine kinase inhibitor sunitinib. Lancet 2007;370(9604):2011–9.

16. Youssef G, Links M. The prevention and management of cardiovascular complications of chemotherapy in patients with cancer [review]. Am J Cardiovasc Drugs 2005;5(4):233–43.

17. Kaklamani VG, Gradishar WJ. Role of capecitabine (Xeloda) in breast cancer. Expert Rev Anticancer Ther 2003;3(2):137–44.

18. Anand AJ. Fluorouracil cardiotoxicity. Ann Pharmacother 1994;28(3):374–8.

19. Akpek G, Hartshorn KL. Failure of oral nitrate and calcium channel blocker therapy to prevent 5-fluorouracil-related myocardial ischemia: a case report. Cancer Chemother Pharmacol 1999;43(2):157–61.

20. Kaur A, Yu SS, Lee AJ, et al. Thalidomide-induced sinus bradycardia. Ann Pharmacother 2003;37(7–8):1040–3.

21. Wilke A, Hesse H, Gorg C, et al. Elevation of the pacing threshold: a side effect in a patient with pacemaker undergoing therapy with doxorubicin and vincristine. Oncology 1999;56(2):110–1.

22. Adams MJ, Hardenbergh PH, Constine LS, et al. Radiation-associated cardiovascular disease. Crit Rev Oncol Hematol 2003;45(1):55–75.

23. Basavaraju SR, Easterly CE. Pathophysiological effects of radiation on atherosclerosis development and progression, and the incidence of cardiovascular complications. Med Phys 2002;29(10):2391–403.

24. Vallis KA, Pintilie M, Chong N, et al. Assessment of coronary heart disease morbidity and mortality after radiation therapy for early breast cancer. J Clin Oncol 2002;20(4):1036–42.

25. Lind PA, Pagnanelli R, Marks LB, et al. Myocardial perfusion changes in patients irradiated for left-sided breast cancer and correlation with coronary artery distribution. Int J Radiat Oncol Biol Phys 2003;55(4):914–20.

26. Fleisher LA, Beckman JA, Brown KA, et al. ACC/AHA 2007 guidelines on perioperative cardiovascular evaluation and care for noncardiac surgery: a report of the American College of Cardiology/American Heart Association Task Force on practice guidelines (Writing Committee to revise the 2002 guidelines on perioperative cardiovascular evaluation for noncardiac surgery). Published 9-27-2007. Available at: http://circ.ahajournals.org/cgi/content/short/116/17/e418. Accessed November 18, 2008.

27. Mukai Y, Yoshida T, Nakaike R, et al. Five cases of anthracycline-induced cardiomyopathy effectively treated with carvedilol. Intern Med 2004;43(11):1087–8.

28. Hunt SA. ACC/AHA 2005 guideline update for the diagnosis and management of chronic heart failure in the adult: a report of the American College of Cardiology/American Heart Association Task Force on practice guidelines (Writing Committee to update the 2001 guidelines for the evaluation and management of heart failure). J Am Coll Cardiol 2005;46(1):1116–43.

29. Chang K, Sarkiss M, Won KS, et al. Preoperative risk stratification using gated myocardial perfusion studies in patients with cancer. J Nucl Med 2007;48(3):344–8.

30. Grines CL, Bonow RO, Casey DE Jr, et al. Prevention of premature discontinuation of dual antiplatelet therapy in patients with coronary artery stents: a science advisory from the American Heart Association, American College of Cardiology, Society for Cardiovascular Angiography and Interventions, American College of Surgeons, and American Dental Association, with representation from the American College of Physicians. Circulation 2007;115(6):813–8.

31. Tashiro M, Izumikawa K, Yoshioka D, et al. Lung fibrosis 10 years after cessation of bleomycin therapy. Tohoku J Exp Med 2008;216(1):77–80.

32. Einhorn L, Krause M, Hornback N, et al. Enhanced pulmonary toxicity with bleomycin and radiotherapy in oat cell lung cancer. Cancer 1976;37(5):2414–6.

33. Copper JA Jr. Drug-induced lung disease. Adv Intern Med 1997;42:231–68.

34. Smetana GW. Preoperative pulmonary evaluation: identifying and reducing risks for pulmonary complications. Cleve Clin J Med 2006;73(Suppl 1):S36–41.

35. Klein DS, Wilds PR. Pulmonary toxicity of antineoplastic agents: anaesthetic and postoperative implications. Can Anaesth Soc J 1983;30(4):399–405.

36. Sekine Y, Chiyo M, Iwata T, et al. Perioperative rehabilitation and physiotherapy for lung cancer patients with chronic obstructive pulmonary disease. Jpn J Thorac Cardiovasc Surg 2005;53(5):237–43.

37. Smetana GW, Lawrence VA, Cornell JE. Preoperative pulmonary risk stratification for noncardiothoracic surgery: systematic review for the American College of Physicians. Ann Intern Med 2006;144(8):581–95.

38. Stohr W, Paulides M, Bielack S, et al. Nephrotoxicity of cisplatin and carboplatin in sarcoma patients: a report from the late effects surveillance system. Pediatr Blood Cancer 2007;48(2):140–7.

39. Kintzel PE. Anticancer drug-induced kidney disorders. Drug Saf 2001;24(1): 19–38.

40. Lajer H, Daugaard G. Cisplatin and hypomagnesemia. Cancer Treat Rev 1999; 25(1):47–58.

41. Grothey A. Oxaliplatin-safety profile: neurotoxicity [review]. Semin Oncol 2003; 30(4:Suppl 15):5–13.

42. Coiffier B, Altman A, Pui CH, et al. Guidelines for the management of pediatric and adult tumor lysis syndrome: an evidence-based review. J Clin Oncol 2008; 26(16):2767–78.

43. Adcock DM, Fink LM, Marlar RA, et al. The hemostatic system and malignancy. Clin Lymphoma Myeloma 2008;8(4):230–6.

44. Gouin-Thibault I, Achkar A, Samama MM. The thrombophilic state in cancer patients. Acta Haematol 2001;106(1–2):33–42.

45. Lyman GH, Khorana AA, Falanga A, et al. American Society of Clinical Oncology guideline: recommendations for venous thromboembolism prophylaxis and treatment in patients with cancer. J Clin Oncol 2007;25(34):5490–505.

46. Tovari J, Pirker R, Timar J, et al. Erythropoietin in cancer: an update [review]. Curr Mol Med 2008;8(6):481–91.

47. Fandrey J. Erythropoietin receptors on tumor cells: what do they mean? [review]. Oncologist 2008;13(Suppl 3):16–20.

48. Harrison CN. Essential thrombocythaemia: challenges and evidence-based management. Br J Haematol 2005;130(2):153–65.

49. Maggi L, Andreetta F, Antozzi C, et al. Thymoma-associated myasthenia gravis: outcome, clinical and pathological correlations in 197 patients on a 20-year experience. J Neuroimmunol 2008;201–202:237–44.

50. O'Neill GN. Acquired disorders of the neuromuscular junction. Int Anesthesiol Clin 2006;44(2):107–21.

51. MICROMEDEX Healthcare Series. Available at: http://www.thomsonhc.com/home/dispatch. Accessed February 15, 2010.

52. LEXI-Comp ONLINE. Available at: http://www.crlonline.com. Accessed February 15, 2010.

53. Skeel RT. Biologic and pharmacologic basis of cancer chemotherapy. In: Lippincott's handbook of cancer chemotherapy. 6th edition. Philadelphia (PA): Lippincott Williams and Wilkins; 2003.

54. Balmer CM, Valley AW, Lannucci A. Cancer treatment and chemotherapy. In: DiPiro JT, Talbert RL, Yee GC, et al, editors. Pharmacotherapy: a pathophysiologic approach. 6th edition. New York: McGraw-Hill Book Co; 2005. p. 2279–328.

Index

Note: Page numbers of article titles are in **boldface** type.

A

Achalasia, dysphagia in, 251
Acid reflux. *See* Gastroesophageal reflux disease.
Acute coronary syndrome, 354–356, 364, 368
    future developments in, 376–382
        body surface mapping, 377
        earlier diagnosis, 376
        high-frequency QRS analysis, 377
        new imaging modalities, 380–381
        novel biomarkers, 377–380
        risk stratification tools, 381–382
        treatment advances, 382
Acyclovir, for herpes zoster, 321
Adenosine, for stress testing, 207
Adrenal gland, preoperative cancer surgery evaluation of, 413
Albumin, ischemia modified
    for acute coronary syndrome, 379
    for pulmonary embolism, 383
Aldesleukin, perioperative implications of, 407
Alememtuzumab, perioperative implications of, 407
Allodynia, in fibromyalgia, 279
Amlodipine, for angina, 210
Amyotrophic lateral sclerosis, dysphagia in, 251
Anemia, preoperative cancer surgery evaluation of, 412
Aneurysms
    aortic, 339
    coronary artery, 337
Angina, 354–356. *See also* Nonacute coronary syndrome anginal chest pain.
    cervical, 266
    Prinzmetal, 202–203
Angiography
    computed tomography
        for acute coronary syndrome, 380
        for aortic dissection, 390
    coronary, 209
    magnetic resonance imaging, for pulmonary embolism, 384
Angioleiomyomas, 322–323
Angiolipomas, 323
Angiotensin-converting enzyme inhibitors, for angina, 209
Anticoagulants, for pulmonary embolism, 386–387

Med Clin N Am 94 (2010) 421–434
doi:10.1016/S0025-7125(10)00031-3
0025-7125/10/$ – see front matter © 2010 Elsevier Inc. All rights reserved.

Moving?

Make sure your subscription moves with you!

To notify us of your new address, find your **Clinics Account Number** (located on your mailing label above your name), and contact customer service at:

Email: journalscustomerservice-usa@elsevier.com

800-654-2452 (subscribers in the U.S. & Canada)
314-447-8871 (subscribers outside of the U.S. & Canada)

Fax number: 314-447-8029

Elsevier Health Sciences Division
Subscription Customer Service
3251 Riverport Lane
Maryland Heights, MO 63043

*To ensure uninterrupted delivery of your subscription, please notify us at least 4 weeks in advance of move.

ELSEVIER